CHILDREN'S ISSUES, LAWS AND PROGRAMS

YOUTH

PRACTICES, PERSPECTIVES AND CHALLENGES

CHILDREN'S ISSUES, LAWS AND PROGRAMS

Additional books in this series can be found on Nova's website
under the Series tab.

Additional e-books in this series can be found on Nova's website
under the e-book tab.

SOCIAL ISSUES, JUSTICE AND STATUS

Additional books in this series can be found on Nova's website
under the Series tab.

Additional e-books in this series can be found on Nova's website
under the e-book tab.

CHILDREN'S ISSUES, LAWS AND PROGRAMS

YOUTH

PRACTICES, PERSPECTIVES AND CHALLENGES

ELIZABETH TREJOS-CASTILLO
EDITOR

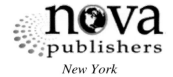

New York

Copyright © 2013 by Nova Science Publishers, Inc.

All rights reserved. No part of this book may be reproduced, stored in a retrieval system or transmitted in any form or by any means: electronic, electrostatic, magnetic, tape, mechanical photocopying, recording or otherwise without the written permission of the Publisher.

For permission to use material from this book please contact us:
Telephone 631-231-7269; Fax 631-231-8175
Web Site: http://www.novapublishers.com

NOTICE TO THE READER

The Publisher has taken reasonable care in the preparation of this book, but makes no expressed or implied warranty of any kind and assumes no responsibility for any errors or omissions. No liability is assumed for incidental or consequential damages in connection with or arising out of information contained in this book. The Publisher shall not be liable for any special, consequential, or exemplary damages resulting, in whole or in part, from the readers' use of, or reliance upon, this material. Any parts of this book based on government reports are so indicated and copyright is claimed for those parts to the extent applicable to compilations of such works.

Independent verification should be sought for any data, advice or recommendations contained in this book. In addition, no responsibility is assumed by the publisher for any injury and/or damage to persons or property arising from any methods, products, instructions, ideas or otherwise contained in this publication.

This publication is designed to provide accurate and authoritative information with regard to the subject matter covered herein. It is sold with the clear understanding that the Publisher is not engaged in rendering legal or any other professional services. If legal or any other expert assistance is required, the services of a competent person should be sought. FROM A DECLARATION OF PARTICIPANTS JOINTLY ADOPTED BY A COMMITTEE OF THE AMERICAN BAR ASSOCIATION AND A COMMITTEE OF PUBLISHERS.

Additional color graphics may be available in the e-book version of this book.

Library of Congress Cataloging-in-Publication Data

ISBN: 978-1-62618-067-3

Published by Nova Science Publishers, Inc. † New York

To my sons, Pablo Jr. and Isaac,

*who remind me every day of the miracle of life
and how precious youth are!*

Contents

Preface ix

Section 1. Youth Health 1

Chapter 1 Evaluation of Nutrition Outcomes in Youth: Challenges and Opportunities
Lucia Kaiser, Constance Schneider, Marisa Neelon, Chutima Ganthavorn, Brenda Roche, Concepcion Mendoza and Timothy Matthiessen 3

Chapter 2 The Risk of Cardiovascular Disease and its Associations between Obesity and Physical Activity in Adolescents: International Perspective**s**
Duncan S. Buchan, Non. E. Thomas, Lon Kilgore, Juliette M. Mason and Julien S. Baker 17

Chapter 3 TDM as a Tool for the Personalization of Psychiatric Treatment in Children and Adolescents
Ioanna Vardakou, Constantinos Pistos, Chara Spiliopoulou and Giorgos Alevizopoulos 37

Chapter 4 The Assessment of Schizotypal Experiences in Adolescent Population
Eduardo Fonseca-Pedrero, Mercedes Paino, Serafín Lemos-Giráldez and José Muñiz 67

Section 2. Contextual Effects and Socialization Processes 87

Chapter 5 Youth Violence: Risks, Causes, Management Strategies and Directions for Future Inquiry
Suman Sarkar 89

Chapter 6 Determining Adolescents' Risk for Involvement in Bullying or Cyberbullying: A Review of Two Studies
Elizabeth L. W. McKenney, Amanda M. Cole, Lisa M. Young, Emily J. Krohn, Stephen D. A. Hupp and Jeremy D. Jewell 111

Chapter 7	Cannabis Use Disorders Predispose to the Development of Sexually Transmitted Diseases among Youth *Jack R. Cornelius and Levent Kirisci*	131
Chapter 8	Beyond School and Family: The Basis and the Structure of the Tertiary Socialisation Field and the "Youth-affairs" as an Autonomous Area *Adam Nagy and Levente Székely*	137
Chapter 9	Hispanic Adolescent Challenges in the School Environment *Fernando Valle and Francisco B. Debaran*	159

Section 3. Treatment and Intervention Issues — 179

Chapter 10	Aggression Replacement Training for Disruptive Adolescents: Efficacy, Effectiveness, and New Directions Involving Families *Robert Weis and Ellen R. Pucke*	181
Chapter 11	When Words Fail – A Role Specific Perspective on the Treatment of Youths *Nikolas Anastasiadis*	207
Chapter 12	Earning Grades with Excellent Intelligence Assessed by Raven's Matrices *Chau-kiu Cheung and Elisabeth Rudowicz*	223
Chapter 13	Family Dysfunction in Pediatric Bipolar Disorder and Associated Family-Based Interventions *Brendan A. Rich and Heather R. Rosen*	245
Chapter 14	Achieving Academic Resilience for Mexican American Students: Issues and Challenges *Alfredo H. Benavides and Eva Midobuche*	263

Section 4. Social Policy and Institutional Support — 287

Chapter 15	Youth Participation and Protection: From Theory to Practice *Maria Manuela Calheiros, Joana Patrício and Sónia Bernardes*	289
Chapter 16	Reforming Juvenile Justice: Case Studies in Reinvestment and Realignment *Douglas N. Evans and Lisa Marie Vasquez*	311
Chapter 17	System Maturation: Leveraging Change and Reducing Disproportionate Contact through Risk Assessment *Eyitayo Onifade*	331
Chapter 18	Human Capital Development among Immigrant Youth *Elizabeth Trejos-Castillo, Sherley Bedore and Nancy Treviño Schafer*	349

Index — 365

PREFACE

Youth is the trustee of prosperity.
Benjamin Disraeli (1804-1881)

If help and salvation are to come, they can only come from the children, for the children are the makers of men.
Maria Montessori (1870-1952)

Youth development represents a complex set of individual transitions embedded in a particular socio-political environment, cultural context, and historical timing. Though turning points are experienced across the life span, changes may possibly be even more salient in youth given the fundamental biological, cognitive, psychological, and social transformations occurring at this developmental stage. From a global perspective, industrialization and progress continue to differentially impact youth across countries exposing some but not others to limited access to resources, educational attainment, rapid demographic growth, and declining economies. Differential rates in education opportunities, health and social services, technological advances, and financial stability among adolescents within and across nations are creating a greater gap among social groups and populations. Nevertheless, adolescents are able to transition into adulthood supported by their families, traditional and non-traditional educational opportunities, supportive community agencies and faith-based organizations, and local governments committed to providing a future for adolescents. At this point in time, we are able to signal the continuing growth of the youth development field as we welcome the development of new methodologies and scientific tools to further our knowledge on the unique events shaping our children into adolescents and supporting them in their journey to adulthood.

"Youth Practices, Perspectives, and Challenges" is a joint effort by American, European, and Asian scholars who provide a multi and inter-disciplinary view of the current state of youth development and discuss a world-wide range of timely issues. The chapters are organized in four main sections: Health, Contextual Effects–Socialization Processes, Treatment-Intervention, and Social Policy-Institutional Support. A brief description of the book sections and the chapters included in each section is provided below.

YOUTH HEALTH

The first section of the book focuses on health issues affecting the physical and mental health of youth. In "*Evaluation of Nutrition Outcomes in Youth: Challenges and Opportunities*" in which Kaiser, Schneider, Neelon, Ganthavorn, Roche, Mendoza, and Matthiessen (USA) describe innovative practices related to evaluation of nutrition programs in children and youth and compare nutrition outcomes in real-world settings using multiple methods such as Teacher Observation Tool (TOT), a Food Taste Test Tool (TTT), and Digital Image Food Records (DIFR). Buchan, Thomas, Kilgore, Mason, and Baker (Scotland-Wales, UK) provide an in-depth overview about the prevalence of cardiovascular disease (CVD) risk in youth while examining the evidence concerning its associations between obesity and physical activity and raise awareness about public health strategies that aim to reduce the prevalence of obesity and being overweight among youth to protect them against poor cardiometabolic profiles in "*The Risk of Cardiovascular Disease and Its Associations Between Obesity and Physical Activity in Adolescents: International Perspectives.*" Vardakou, Pistos, Spiliopoulou, and Alevizopoulos (Greece) discuss in "*TDM as a Tool for the Personalization of Psychiatric Treatment in Children and Adolescents*" safety and effectiveness of the use of psychotropic drugs use in children and youth given the risk of under or overdosing young patients, the risk of long-term side effects, and an evaluation of the Therapeutic Drug Monitoring (TDM) tool to optimize pharmacotherapy by maximizing therapeutic efficacy and minimizing adverse events in this particular population. In "*The assessment of schizotypal experiences in adolescent population*", Fonseca-Pedrero, Paino, Lemos-Giraldez, and Muñiz (Spain) discuss the importance of having a measuring instrument with adequate psychometric properties (reliability-validity) to screen youth at-risk for later development of psychotic disorders and to examine the rates of schizotypal experiences in nonclinical adolescents.

CONTEXTUAL EFFECTS AND SOCIALIZATION PROCESSES

The second section includes five chapters on contextual effects and socialization processes effecting youth developmental outcomes. Sarkar (India) examines the trend of increasing youth violence in India, both victimization and criminal behaviors, discusses strategies for combating the problem of youth violence, and provides some recommendations on the basis of various social, psychological and scientific evidences available today in "*Youth Violence: Risks, Causes, Management Strategies and Directions for Future Inquiry*". In "*Determining Adolescents' Risk for Involvement in Bullying or Cyberbullying: A Review for Two Studies*", McKenney, Cole, Young, Krohn, Hupp, and Jewell (USA) examine the role of gender, time spent online, time spent sending and receiving text messages ("texting"), parenting styles, and relationship dynamics within families in predicting involvement in bullying either as a bully or as a victim and discuss implications for future research into school- and community-based interventions targeting family interaction patterns to preventing or reducing bullying. Cornelius and Kirisci (USA) in "*Assessing TLI as a Predictor of Treatment Seeking for SUD among Youth Transitioning to Young Adulthood*" discuss a longitudinal etiology study assessing whether the behavioral undercontrol Transmissible

Liability Index (TLI) serve as a predictor of the development of substance use disorders (SUD) and of treatment utilization during young adulthood. Based on existing theories of socialization environments, Nagy and Székely (Hungary) propose a new conceptual model of youth activities related to extra familiar and curricular environment—a tertiary socialization environment—as an alternative way to explain the potential existence of a homogeneous socialization field beyond the school and the family in *"Beyond School and Family: The Basis and the Structure of the Tertiary Socialization Field and the "Youth-Affairs" as an Autonomous Area"*. Using person environment fit theory as a framework, Valle and Debaran (USA) examine existing structures in the pipeline of Hispanic adolescent education, discuss a re-examination of obstacles faced by Hispanic students during adolescent development to fit into U.S. school environments, and provide conclusions and recommendations for policy makers and educational leaders to scrutinize Hispanic adolescent realities and create inclusive spaces for educational opportunities in *"Fitting In: Hispanic Adolescent Challenges in the School Environment."*

TREATMENT AND INTERVENTION ISSUES

The third section of the book centers on issues pertaining to the treatment and intervention efforts for children and youth. In "Aggression *Replacement Training for Disruptive Adolescents: Efficacy, Effectiveness, and New Directions involving Families*", Weis and Pucke (USA) review the existing research on Aggression Replacement Training (ART)—multimodal treatment for disruptive, aggressive, and antisocial adolescents—and provide empirical evidence supporting the effectiveness of a new development in (ART) research, namely the practice of including parents and other caregivers in ART sessions, as well as examining social skills, anger management, and moral reasoning training for disruptive adolescents and their families. Based on Verhofstadt-Deneve's Phenomenological-Dialectical personality model as well as Schacht's developmental theory, Anastasiadis (Austria) introduce Psychodrama techniques as a well-established method in the treatment of psychologically malaffected youths and discuss the relevance of Psychodrama techniques where traditional conversational methods are difficult, or where the developmental age of the young person does not match their expected maturity in *"When Words Fail – A Role-specific Perspective on the Treatment of Youths."* In "Earning Grades with Excellent Intelligence Assessed by Raven's Matrices" Cheung and Rudowicz (China) based on the theoretical premise that intelligence promotes learning effort and contributes to good grades, examine excellence in intelligence and learning effort using Raven's Standard Progressive Matrices, school grades, and learning effort among Hong Kong Chinese students and report that excellent intelligence based on the most difficult items contributed to grades, partly through mediation by learning effort. In *"Family Dysfunction in Pediatric Bipolar Disorder and Associated Family-Based Intervention",* Rich and Rosen (USA) review emerging empirical efforts to understand the causes, longitudinal outcomes, and optimal treatments for Pediatric bipolar disorder (PBD) focusing on family functioning and discuss family-based approaches to treating PBD as well as identifying shared psychotherapeutic approaches for ameliorating core PBD symptomatology and family dysfunction. In *"Achieving Academic Resilience for Mexican American Students: Issues and Challenges",* Benavides & Midobuche (USA) review the existing literature on the issue of resiliency among Mexican American students and examine the classification of resilient and non-resilient students including criteria such as achievement test results, grades, percentile rank, and teacher identification and nominating procedures and criteria, including teacher expectations and attitudes towards the students.

SOCIAL POLICY AND INSTITUTIONAL SUPPORT

The final section of the book addresses social policy and institutional support endeavors targeting youth. Calheiros, Patricio, and Bernardes (Portugal) in *"Youth Participation and Protection: From Theory to Practice"* review different perspectives, models and practices to promote youth participation and discuss two studies undertaken within the health-care and youth protection systems to further illustrate how the right of youth to participation can be promoted through participatory research, namely through needs assessment and youth involvement in social and health services design. Evans and Vasquez (USA) discuss in *"Reforming Juvenile Justice: Case Studies in Reinvestment and Realignment"* two different strategies for juvenile justice reform, namely reinvestment strategies to promote the creation of financial incentives that encourage county governments to limit the number of juvenile offenders sent to secure state facilities, and second, realignment which is the shifting of management and responsibility, typically from the state to the county level. In *"System Maturation: Leveraging Change and Reducing Disproportionate Contact through Risk Assessment"*, Onifade (USA) provides a brief background on the underlying conceptual framework of reducing Disproportionate Minority Contact (DMC) through risk assessment, describes the experiences of the county juvenile justice system attempting to implement the strategy over a nearly decade long period, and discusses the challenges and successes of a juvenile justice system in the mid-west that attempted to reduce disproportionate minority contact using the risk assessment approach. Finally, Trejos-Castillo, Bedore, & Trevino Schafer (USA) in *"Human Capital Development among Immigrant Youth"* review the main theoretical views on human capital, development and transmission, and provide a critical discussion of extant empirical research and existing socio-political policies on the development of human capital in immigrant families and youth, particularly the most underserved minority groups such as refugees and illegal immigrants.

As a final note, I would like to express my sincere gratitude to all authors for their contributions to this edited volume. Your committed leadership and your enthusiastic support to advance the field of youth development are deeply inspiring!

Section 1. Youth Health

In: Youth: Practices, Perspectives and Challenges
Editor: Elizabeth Trejos-Castillo

ISBN: 978-1-62618-067-3
© 2013 Nova Science Publishers, Inc.

Chapter 1

EVALUATION OF NUTRITION OUTCOMES IN YOUTH: CHALLENGES AND OPPORTUNITIES

Lucia Kaiser[1,]*, Constance Schneider[1], Marisa Neelon[2], Chutima Ganthavorn[3], Brenda Roche[4], Concepcion Mendoza[1] and Timothy Matthiessen[5]

[1]Dept. of Nutrition, UC Davis, US
[2]University of California Cooperative Extension, Contra Costa County, US
[3]University of California Cooperative Extension. Riverside County, US
[4]University of California Cooperative Extension, Los Angeles County, US
[5]University of Virginia Health System, US

ABSTRACT

To determine the effectiveness of programs and policies for the prevention of obesity in youth, more robust and varied evaluation methods are needed. Traditional nutrition assessment methods are often problematic to implement in youth and can yield evaluation data that are neither valid nor reliable. The purpose of this chapter is to describe innovative practices related to the evaluation of nutrition programs in children and youth. Faced with the challenge of obtaining data from youth among whom cognitive ability and cultural factors may vary widely, capturing the perspective of teachers and parents, as well as the youth themselves, can enhance the evaluation of nutrition programs. The University of California Cooperative Extension has developed and tested the validity of different approaches to evaluate and compare nutrition outcomes in real-world settings. Some promising methods include a Teacher Observation Tool (TOT), a Food Taste Test Tool (TTT), and Digital Image Food Records (DIFR). Use of new technology and different perspectives can strengthen program evaluations and improve the delivery of nutritional interventions.

---

* E-mail: llkaiser@ucdavis.edu.

INTRODUCTION

During the past thirty years, the prevalence of childhood obesity, defined as a body mass index for age $\geq 95^{th}$ percentile, has become a serious health issue, particularly among some racial/ethnic groups.[1] Among 12-19 year olds in 2005-2008, Mexican American boys and African American girls had the highest rate of obesity, at 26.2% and 29.4% respectively. These health disparities emerge early in life and are associated with chronic disease risk factors in adolescence.[2] Children who are overweight or obese at eight years are six times more likely to have elevated blood pressure, glucose, triglycerides, and insulin by 15 years of age. A systematic review of 13 high-quality studies found consistent evidence that overweight and obese youth become overweight adults.[3]

Experts recommend that childhood obesity prevention include efforts at family and community levels, as well as at school, industry, and government levels.[4] Stronger evaluation methods are needed on all fronts to assess the progress of prevention efforts and refine or improve intervention strategies. However, measuring nutrition outcomes in youth, particularly those related to diet, poses several problems. Cognitive ability, age, and body weight are key factors that affect the accuracy and validity of assessments.[5] In evaluating dietary intake of children and adolescents, researchers are encouraged to exercise caution because dietary data is prone to reporting error. The cognitive ability of youth under the age of 12 may be limited to accurately report intake, especially among those from low-income households [6], and their parents do not always know what kids eat outside of home. Overweight children and adolescents are also likely to under-report intake. [7, 8] Whether it is conscious or unconscious, under-reporting among obese individuals increases with age.[7] Both under- and over-reporting of foods are common with traditional dietary assessment methods, including food frequency questionnaires, 24-hour dietary recalls, written food records, and diet histories, mainly due to the subject's inability to correctly quantify the foods (or ingredients) consumed. The most accurate methods, including the weighed food record and direct observation, can be overly burdensome and costly to implement, prompting changes in the behavior of people in general. [9]

For a program evaluation in real world settings, there may be other challenges. If the findings are intended to be shared, informed parental consent is often required to collect data directly from the youth. Selection bias can limit the usefulness of or ability to generalize the results if some youth are excluded from the evaluation due to lack of parental consent and differ from the rest of the sample (for example, lower parental education or non-English speaking parents). Generalizability may also be limited if lower-performing classrooms and schools choose not to participate in the evaluation. Getting matched sets of pre-post data can also be difficult, especially if youth have unstable home environments and/or are frequently absent from the program. Finally, instruments or methods that work in one audience may not be valid or reliable in another. Thus, the cultural adaptation and validation of instruments may be necessary prior to implementing a program evaluation.

Cultural adaptation or development of new evaluation instruments to measure nutrition outcomes involves mixed methods of qualitative and quantitative data collection. Many validation studies have employed quantitative testing to assess validity and reliability of food behavior assessment tools; however, very few have used qualitative testing procedures. Careful cognitive testing during in-depth individual interviews or focus groups explores the interpretation of each question, identifies wording that may be confusing or ambiguous, and alternative ways to ask questions that are clearer to the target audience, especially where differences may exist in cultural foods, meal and snacking patterns, literacy, and language. [10] For example, in adapting a pictorial food behavior checklist to a Latino audience, items related to beverage intake were modified to show both Mexican and American brands of soft drinks. Even where the same food is consumed, the form of that food may differ among cultural groups (i.e., fish sticks compared to whole fish). Cognitive testing is a *critical phase* of instrument development and adaptation of dietary assessment tools, and is essential even where funding may not support further validation and reliability testing. [11]

However, wherever possible, all new instruments should be validated by comparing data to other traditional or standard methods (convergent validity) or, preferably, to the most accurate method that is considered to be a "gold standard" (criterion validity). [12,13] Establishing instrument reliability is equally important, considering both test-retest or repeat reliability and internal consistency. Test-retest reliability determines whether the subject responses are the same when the instrument is administered on two separate occasions in the absence of an intervention. Internal consistency can be determined using the Cronbach's alpha coefficient to measure the level of agreement among several items that are designed to capture the same construct. [14]

It is a challenge to obtain data from youth whose cognitive ability and cultural factors may vary widely. Therefore, capturing the perspective of teachers and parents, as well as the youth themselves, can result in a more robust and thorough evaluation of nutrition outcomes. With this in mind, the University of California Cooperative Extension (UCCE) has developed and tested the validity of different approaches to evaluate and compare nutrition outcomes in real-world settings. The purpose of this chapter is to describe innovative practices related to the evaluation of nutrition programs in children and youth. A discussion will focus on the development, validation, and application of three evaluation methods that have been used in extension programs in California, including the Teacher Observation Tool, the Taste Test Tool, and Digital Image Food Records.

USING A TEACHER OBSERVATION TOOL (TOT) FOR ELEMENTARY SCHOOL STUDENTS

Development of the TOT

In 2009, an evaluation taskforce of UCCE nutrition advisors and one specialist began developing an evaluation tool to capture changes in student food-related attitudes and behaviors that are due to participation in the University of California Food Stamp Nutrition Education Program (now known as UC CalFresh Nutrition Education). All research procedures were reviewed and approved by the University of California at the Davis Institutional Review Board (IRB).

Since the researchers did not plan to observe the students directly and the procedures posed minimal risk, the IRB waived the requirement of obtaining informed consent from parents. Using open-ended questions, the nutrition advisors conducted individual in-depth interviews with six elementary school teachers to determine key student outcomes that could be linked to the UC CalFresh program and cognitively test the wording of the questions. The questions focused on whether the teachers had observed any changes in their students related to: 1) being aware of the importance of good nutrition; 2) making healthier meal and snack choices; 3) eating breakfast more often; 4) being willing to try new foods; 5) washing hands and using other food safety practices; and 6) increasing physical activity. Teachers were asked to provide specific examples of behaviors in their students that they had observed in the school setting.

During the interviews, the teachers also mentioned several changes that they had implemented in their classrooms as a result of their participation in the nutrition education program. Emerging themes from the interviews, along with the teachers' suggestions on the wording of questions, were used to draft the questions that are shown in Figure 1.

The ten TOT questions (Figure 1) were added to an online survey, enabling UC CalFresh staff to send the web link to the classroom teachers at the end of the school year.

Although the online survey takes less than 10 minutes to complete, many counties used paper versions of the survey to make sure they obtained evaluation data from their teachers. After a small feasibility test in 2009, TOT has been distributed statewide in California to elementary school classroom teachers to complete at the end of the school year. In 2010-11, n= 976 teachers (reporting for 23,990 students, preschool through 6th grade) completed the TOT survey (Figures 2 and 3).

The findings consistently indicate that the strongest student outcomes are identifying healthy foods, washing hands more often, and being willing to try new foods, whereas teachers are less able to report changes in bringing fruit as a snack and choosing fruit and vegetables in the school environment.

Validity and Reliability

In examining validity, an important question to ask is how the retrospective version of TOT compares to the traditional method of the pre-post survey administration. In other words, would a pre-post version of TOT actually show significant changes?

In ten California counties, UCCE staff recruited first- to fifth-grade teachers who planned to deliver nutrition education during most of the school year instead of teaching nutrition as a short-term unit. The teachers completed the pre-TOT before delivering nutrition lessons and post-TOT after teaching all the lessons.

They also completed the retrospective TOT a minimum of 2 weeks after the post TOT and before the start of the new school year.

TOT student scores were calculated by summing up the responses for the five student knowledge, attitude, and behavior items. A greater TOT score (regardless of pre-, post-, or retrospective TOT) indicates more desirable outcomes. Matching sets of pre-post TOT and retrospective TOT were obtained for 52 classrooms.

In this sample of classrooms, a significant difference in TOT scores was observed in the pre-post administration of the TOT. For 5 student items, mean TOT scores were as follows: pre-TOT: 16.3 (ranges 6-23); post-TOT; 19.7 (ranges 13-25); and retrospective TOT: 20.7 (14-25).

Using a paired t-test, significant differences were observed in the post vs. pre TOT (p <0.0001) and in the retro vs. pre TOT (p < 0.0001). However, post-TOT and retro-TOT are strongly correlated (Spearman correlation coefficient: r=0.47, p< 0.0002).

Figure 1. Teacher Observation Tool (TOT) Questions

Identifier	Question	Scale
Snack	Compared to the beginning of the school year, *more* students *now* bring fruit as a snack.	5=Strongly agree; 4=Agree; 3=Not sure/unable to observe; 2=Disagree; 1=Strongly disagree
Wash	Compared to the beginning of the school year, *more* students *now* wash hands more often.	5=Strongly agree; 4=Agree; 3=Not sure/unable to observe; 2=Disagree; 1=Strongly disagree
Identify	Compared to the beginning of the school year, *more* students *now* can identify healthy food choices.	5=Strongly agree; 4=Agree; 3=Not sure/unable to observe; 2=Disagree; 1=Strongly disagree
Willing	Compared to the beginning of the school year, *more* students *now* are willing to try new foods offered at school.	5=Strongly agree; 4=Agree; 3=Not sure/unable to observe; 2=Disagree; 1=Strongly disagree
Choose	Compared to the beginning of the school year, *more* students *now* choose fruits and/or vegetables in the cafeteria or during classroom parties.	5=Strongly agree; 4=Agree; 3=Not sure/unable to observe; 2=Disagree; 1=Strongly disagree
Offer	Compared to the beginning of the school year, I (the teacher) *now* offer healthy food choices to the students (at parties, snacks, rewards).	3= A lot more often; 2=Somewhat more often; 1=About the same as before
Breakfast	Compared to the beginning of the school year, I (the teacher) *now* encourage students to eat breakfast.	3= A lot more often; 2=Somewhat more often; 1=About the same as before
Parties	Compared to the beginning of the school year, I (the teacher) *now* remind families to bring healthy snacks for school parties.	3= A lot more often; 2=Somewhat more often; 1=About the same as before
Active	Compared to the beginning of the school year, I (the teacher) *now* encourage the students to be physically active. 3= A lot more often; 2=Somewhat more often; 1=About the same as before.	3= A lot more often; 2=Somewhat more often; 1=About the same as before
Role Model	Compared to the beginning of the school year, I (the teacher) *now* make healthier personal food choices.	3= A lot more often; 2=Somewhat more often; 1=About the same as before

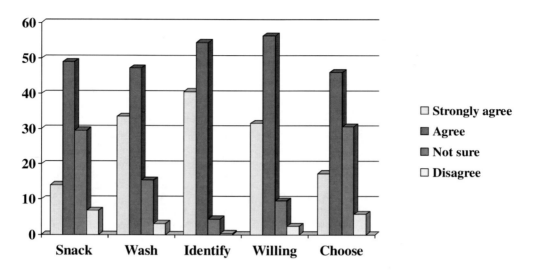

Figure 2. TOT Responses Related to Student Outcomes.

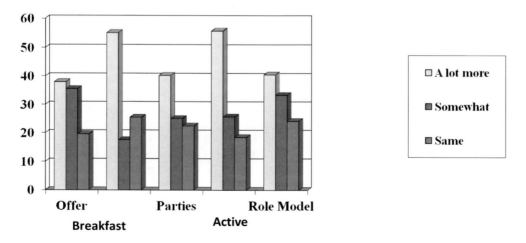

Figure 3. TOT Responses Related to Teacher Outcomes.

These findings show that the teachers' perceptions of the students' nutrition knowledge, attitudes, and behaviors change during the course of the school year. Nonetheless, their final perception at the end of the lessons remains consistent at two separate time points.

Based on statewide data from 2010-11 (n=976 teachers), the internal reliability or consistency of TOT was examined using the Cronbach's coefficient alpha. The Cronbach's alpha for the 10 TOT items is $\alpha=0.81$, well above the cut-off of 0.70 generally used as an indication of acceptable consistency or internal reliability for a scale.

Application of TOT

Teachers who are recruited into the UC CalFresh program decide which curricula and how many lessons they want to deliver during the school year, resulting in considerable variability in delivery.

Since teachers perceive stronger outcomes in some areas than others, the application of TOT will permit an exploration of factors that contribute to better outcomes. Areas not showing strong outcomes can be targeted for additional intervention using TOT as the evaluation tool. For example, the "students bringing fruit as a snack" was not a strong outcome in the teachers' perception. An educational program for parents can be designed to promote students bringing fruit as a snack to school.

Thus, TOT can be used to examine outcomes that differ depending on the dose and content of the nutrition education.

EVALUATING FOOD EXPERIENCES WITH THE TASTE TEST TOOL (TTT)

Development of the TTT

Since limited resources may discourage parents from offering new fruits and vegetables that their children might reject, a goal of UC CalFresh is to increase willingness to try new foods, especially fruits and vegetables, and encourage children to ask for them at home, which has been associated with greater household purchases of fruits and vegetables [15], and fruit and vegetable consumption in school-aged children. [16] Having a tool to evaluate youth acceptance of new foods was deemed to be useful in examining program outcomes. Thus, along with TOT in 2009, the UCCE Evaluation Taskforce developed a tool that could be used to evaluate food tasting activities that are coupled with nutrition education in the UC CalFresh youth program. The protocols for the development of the TTT were approved by the University of California at the Davis Institutional Review Board. A pilot study, conducted to validate TTT, involved parental informed consent forms. The other activities, during which teachers administered the TTT at a classroom level without identifying individual students, were covered under a separate protocol as exempt from full review and did not require a parent's informed consent.

Like TOT, a prototype of TTT was cognitively tested among nine elementary school teachers. [17] The modified and final wording of the questions is shown below in Figure 4.

Based on the initial cognitive testing, the UCCE Evaluation Taskforce also developed a teacher guide for conducting a food tasting, adhering to food safety guidelines, and recording the student responses (available upon request from the authors). According to the guide, each food tasting is expected to focus on one food item, although in many cases the target food is paired with another food (for example, fat-free yogurt—the target food—with strawberries). After presenting a food for tasting, the teacher asks the students and counts (by show of hands) how many: 1) have ever seen or tried the food before; 2) are willing to try it again (both at school and at home); and 3) are willing to ask for the food at home.

1. Before today's class, how many students have ever seen this food before?
2. Before today's class, how many students have ever tasted this food before?
3. How many students ate (or tasted) the food today?
4. How many students were willing to eat the food at school again?
5. How many students were willing to eat this food at home?
6. How many students were willing to ask for this food at home?

Figure 4. Taste Test Tool Questions.

Validation and Reliability

The procedures and results of the pilot study to examine the validity and reliability of TTT have been reported elsewhere. [17] Briefly, the study involved 114 youth, ages 9-17 years, who were participating in UC CalFresh nutrition education program in summer day camps in three California counties. On the first day of camp, the parents provided informed consent. The camp counselors conducted food tastings among 29 small groups of campers (with 7-12 youth per group), and then administered the TTT. At the same time, the campers privately recorded their degree of liking the food they tasted in a log (3=It's great. I would ask for it at home; 2=It is okay. I might eat it again; and 1= I really did not like it.).

A strong degree of liking a food, based on the logs, was positively correlated with a willingness to try the food again at school ($r=+0.52$, $p=0.004$); to try the food again at home ($r=+0.37$, $p =0.05$); and to ask for the food at home ($r=+0.36$, $p =0.06$).

At the next camp meeting, youth were asked to record in their logs if they had made a request for a specific fruit or vegetable sampled at day camp. To determine the validity of the student reports, the researchers surveyed the parents at the end of the six-week day camp session to see if they had received requests from their children during the previous month for any of the four foods presented during the tastings (tomato, cabbage, nectarine, cantaloupe). Matched parent and youth were available for 40 dyads. Among the 27 youth who reported requesting cantaloupe, 23 (85%) of their parents confirmed receiving such a request (Fisher's exact test: $p = 0.003$). Among the 29 youth who reported requesting nectarines, 23 (79%) of their parents confirmed the request (Fisher's exact test: $p = 0.02$). Fewer requests were made for tomatoes or cabbage and these could not be confirmed by their parents (data not shown).

Consistency (or reliability) of youth responses to the TTT questions was also very good. The overall Cronbach's $\alpha= 0.86$ (cutoff for acceptability is above 0.70).

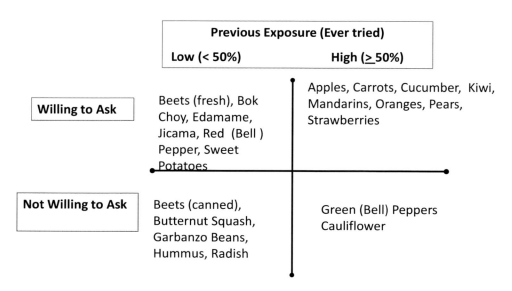

Figure 5. Use of TTT data to categorize foods by previous exposure and willingness to ask for the food.

In 2010-11, the TTT was administered statewide in n=514 classrooms, capturing the response of 16,664 students (preschool through eighth grade, ages 4 to 14) to food tastings. [17] The proportion of the classrooms who had ever tried the foods before was 0.65, and 0.82 were willing to try the foods again at school.

As shown in Figure 5, TTT data can be used to categorize foods by level of previous exposure (high or low) and willingness of the students to ask for the food (yes or no). This can help teachers identify which fruits and vegetables are well-known and well-liked and thus would be good candidates for pairing with unfamiliar and/or less popular fruits and vegetables. For example, carrots and cucumbers (both familiar and well-liked) might be selected for pairing with hummus at another food tasting. Sharing the results with food service administration, school wellness committees, and teachers may encourage them to offer certain foods, particularly those with low previous exposure and good response, again at school.

More research is needed on administration of the TTT among middle-school and high-school aged youth. Use of hand-held clickers appears promising to record student responses discreetly and thus, limits the influence of peer pressure.

Although no differences in responses were observed among preschool and elementary school students, this finding should be replicated in other studies.

CAPTURING DIETARY PATTERNS THROUGH DIGITAL IMAGES

Especially among youth who find traditional dietary methods "boring", use of digital image food records (DIFR) holds great promise in collecting data on dietary patterns.

Boushey and colleagues have developed a method using a camera-equipped, mobile, computing device that works in conjunction with a remote server to automatically identify and quantify foods. [18,19] Use of the image-based food record has also been validated in free-living adolescents (10-16 years) by comparing dietitians' analyses of food images recorded by adolescent participants to records of the pre-weighed foods, prepared in a research laboratory. [20]

Validation and Reliability

Recently, UCCE has validated the use of DIFR to describe food patterns among youth ages 9-12 years in a home setting. [21] After obtaining parental consent and youth assent, a graduate student instructed the youth (n=28) on using small digital cameras (Canon PowerShot A470) to take images of foods and beverages before and after meals and snacks consumed from 5PM until bedtime. The youth also filled out a brief log to help the analysts identify the foods. During the same week, the graduate student conducted three 24-hour dietary recalls to be able to examine the convergent validity of the DIFR method. Two analysts, including the graduate student and a nutrition undergraduate student, independently viewed the images taken by each youth to determine his or her intake of each food group.

MyPyramid food group[1] intakes, determined by the DIFR method, were significantly correlated with food group intakes, assessed by the dietary recall method for the two analysts and for all food groups (p< 0.001, n=26). Inter-analyst reliability of food group intakes was also very good, with Spearman correlations ranging from 0.635 for grains to 0.926 for fruit (p < 0.001).

Application of DIFR

While DIFR has been successfully used in school settings to examine food choices of youth [22], our work has shown that the method can also be used at home.

To apply DIFR, some tips are listed below as a guide for the researchers in using DIFR. From this list, researchers should develop their own simplified subject instructions.

1) Use a placement, 11 X 17 inches, with one-inch marks along one side and instructions as an easy reference (see Figure 6 below).
2) Capture the whole plate, bowl, cup or dish in the image. To do this, put all food and drinks on the placemat, including condiments and water, and frame the borders of the placemat with the camera.
3) Make sure the photo is clear and readable. To do this, ensure that the inch-marks on the placemat are not covered, and the flash is on.
4) Uncover all food items to make them visible in the image. For example, sandwiches and burritos need to be opened up or unrolled before the photo is taken. Where opening the food is not possible (such as in a piece of lasagna), write details about the food in the log. If food is eaten from a large multi-serving bag, like chips or pretzels, a handful of the food should be taken out of the bag. An image of the food should be taken before and after it is eaten. Repeat for every handful. In the food log, record how many handfuls are eaten.

---

[1] MyPyramid food groups include grains, vegetables, fruit, dairy, and meat and beans.

5) Hold the camera directly above the food, framing the placemat in the viewfinder. Push the button and review the screen to be sure the image is captured. Take a second snap-shot of the food from a 45° angle and a third shot from a 0° angle. This will give depth to the images and allow the height of foods to be evaluated. Repeat after the completion of the meal. If no food is left, only a 90° shot needs to be taken.
6) Take multiple images. If an image does not turn out well, just take another. Make sure additional helpings are recorded. To do this, take a picture of the plate before adding the additional food; another picture after adding the additional food; and a final picture before clearing the dishes. When the meal is done, take an image of the plate, whether or not there is still food on it. If a subject forgets to capture the meal, he/she can try to re-create it with leftover foods.

CONCLUSION

Evaluations of nutrition education programs that target youth face many challenges. For routine program evaluations, methods commonly employed in research studies may not be practical or cost-effective. The TTT and TOT are relatively easy to administer and capable of being used to set realistic objectives and measure outcomes in a large statewide sample. For example, a program objective, based on TOT data, might include the following: at least 50% of the teachers strongly agree that their students are now more able to identify healthy food choices, compared to the beginning of the school year. With additional information related to the program delivery, including the number and content of the lessons delivered, program managers can then identify the best practices to achieve better outcomes. The TTT can likewise be used to set targets, by encouraging educators to offer fruits and vegetables that most children have not seen before and to evaluate a variety of strategies, like the use of dips [23], attractive visual presentation [24], or garden-based learning [25] to determine which are most successful in gaining student acceptance and willingness to try the foods again.

The DIFR is not intended for use in large samples but it does provide a method that is both appealing to youth [18] and accurate in assessing dietary intake. This method has been used with youth in non-laboratory settings, including a school cafeteria [22]. The findings presented here indicate that youth, 9-12 years, are capable of using the method at home to describe their usual food intake in the evening. Since family meals appear to foster healthier diets and body weight among youth [26], having a method to capture food intake during meals at home is useful.

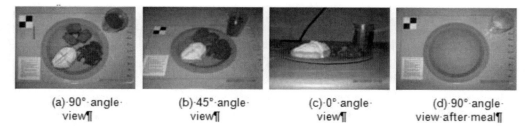

(a) 90° angle view (b) 45° angle view (c) 0° angle view (d) 90° angle view after meal

Figure 6. Capturing food images at different angle views before and after a meal.

The development and validation of evaluation methods that can be applied in real-world settings is critical not only to identify effective intervention strategies, but also to advocate for continued support of programs. UCCE used the findings generated through these evaluations to describe program outcomes to local partners and stakeholders, by generating one-page reports that incorporate the TOT or TTT outcomes, as well a testimonial statements from clientele. These reports are used to educate legislators and other policy-makers about the outcomes and impact of UCCE nutrition programs (http://ucanr.org/delivers/?topicnumber=13).

Strengths of the evaluation research described above include the use of mixed qualitative and quantitative methods for instrument development and the availability of large statewide samples to examine outcomes. A limitation is the use of small, nonrandomly selected subsamples for validation studies, which may limit generalizing results to other groups. More research is needed to refine methods of evaluation, appropriate for real-world settings, particularly in older youth, as well as preschool students.

A teacher's perspective on student improvement in nutrition-related behaviors is most useful among classroom teachers who spend the entire day with the students. Therefore, planning evaluation strategies that capture multiple perspectives of youth, parents, and teachers may be the best approach. Capitalizing on new technology and different perspectives can strengthen program evaluation and improve the delivery of nutrition interventions designed for youth.

REFERENCES

[1] Centers for Disease Control Health, United States 2010. Available at http://www.cdc.gov/nchs/data/hus10.pdf. Accessed March 23, 2010. 2011.

[2] Garnett SP, Baur LA, Srinivasan S, Lee JW, Cowell CT. Body mass index and waist circumference in midchildhood and adverse cardiovascular disease risk clustering in adolescence. *Am. J. Clin. Nutr.* 2007;86(3):549-55.

[3] Singh AS, Mulder C, Twisk JW, van Mechelen W, Chinapaw MJ. Tracking of childhood overweight into adulthood: a systematic review of the literature. *Obes. Rev.* 2008;9(5):474-488.

[4] Institute of M. Progress in preventing childhood obesity : how do we measure up? Washington DC: National Academies Press; 2007.

[5] Livingstone MB, Robson PJ, Wallace J. Issues in dietary intake assessment of children and adolescents. *Br. J. Nutr.* 2004;92:S213-222.

[6] Moore GF, Tapper K, Moore L, Murphy S. Cognitive, behavioral, and social factors are associated with bias in dietary questionnaire self-reports by schoolchildren aged 9 to 11 years. *J. Am. Diet. Assoc.* 2008;108(11):1865-73.

[7] Lanctot JQ, Klesges RC, Stockton MB, Klesges LM. Prevalence and characteristics of energy underreporting in African-American girls. *Obesity. (Silver Spring)* 2008;16(6):1407-12.

[8] Sichert-Hellert W, Kersting M, Schoch G. Underreporting of energy intake in 1 to 18 year old German children and adolescents. *Z Ernahrungswiss.* 1998;37(3):242-51.

[9] Livingstone MB, Prentice AM, Strain JJ, et al. Accuracy of weighed dietary records in studies of diet and health. *BMJ* 1990;300:708-712.

[10] Banna JC, Vera Becerra LE, Kaiser L, Townsend MS. Using qualitative methods to improve questionnaires for Spanish speakers: assessing face validity of a food behavior checklist. *J. Am. Diet. Assoc.* 2010;110:80-90.

[11] Carbone E, Campbell M, Honess-Morreale L. Use of cognitive interview techniques in the development of nutrition surveys and interactive nutrition messages for low-income populations. *JADA*. 2002;102:690-695.

[12] Townsend MS. Evaluating food stamp nutrition education: Process for development and validation of evaluation measures. *J. Nutr. Educ. Behav.* 2006;38:18-34.

[13] Townsend MS, Kaiser LL, Allen LH, Joy AB, Murphy SP. Selecting items for a food behavior checklist for a limited resource audience. *J. Nutr. Educ. Behav.* 2003;35: 69-82.

[14] Santos JR. Cronbach's alpha: a tool for assessing reliability of scales. Available at: http://www.joe.org/joe/1999april/tt3.php. Accessed 9/1/2011. 1999.

[15] Busick DB, Brooks J, Pernecky S, Dawson R, Petzoldt J. Parent food purchases as a measure of exposure and preschool-aged children's willingness to identify and taste fruit and vegetables. *Appetite*. 2008;51(3):468-73.

[16] Sandeno C, Wolf G, Drake T, Reicks M. Behavioral strategies to increase fruit and vegetable intake by fourth- through sixth-grade students. *J. Am. Diet. Assoc.* 2000;100(7):828-30.

[17] Kaiser L, Schneider C, Mendoza C, et al. Development and use of an evaluation tool for taste testing activities in children. *J. Academy of Nutrition and Dietetics.* In Press.

[18] Boushey CJ, Kerr DA, Wright J, Lutes KD, Ebert DS, Delp EJ. Use of technology in children's dietary assessment. *Eur. J. Clin. Nutr.* 2009;63(Supple 1):S50-57.

[19] Six BL, Schap TE, Zhu FM, et al. Evidence-based development of a mobile telephone food record. *J. Am. Diet. Assoc.* 2010;110:74-79.

[20] Higgins JA, LaSalle AL, Zhaoxing P, et al. Validation of photographic food records in children: are pictures really worth a thousand words? . *Eur. J. Clin. Nutr.* 2009;63:1025-1033.

[21] Matthiessen T, Steinberg F, Kaiser L. Convergent validity of a digital image-based food record to assess food group intake in youth. *J. Am. Diet. Assoc.* 2011; 111; 756-761.

[22] Swanson M. Digital photography as a tool to measure school cafeteria consumption. *J. Sch. Health.* 2008;78:432-437.

[23] Fisher JO, Mennella JA, Hughes SO, Liu Y, Mendoza PM, Patrick H. Offering "dip" promotes intake of a moderately-liked raw vegetable among preschoolers with genetic sensitivity. *J. Acad. Nutr. Diet.* 2012;112(2):235-245.

[24] Jansen E, Mulkens S, Jansen A. How to promote fruit consumption in children. Visual appeal versus restriction. *Appetite*. 2010;54(3):599-602.

[25] Morris JL, Zidenberg-Cherr S. Garden-enhanced nutrition curriculum improves fourth-grade school children's knowledge of nutrition and preferences for some vegetables. *J. Am. Diet. Assoc.* 2002;102(1):91-3.

[26] Berge JM. A review of familial correlates of child and adolescent obesity: what has the 21st century taught us so far? *Int. J. Adolesc. Med. Health.* 2009;21(4):457-83.

In: Youth: Practices, Perspectives and Challenges
Editor: Elizabeth Trejos-Castillo

ISBN: 978-1-62618-067-3
© 2013 Nova Science Publishers, Inc.

Chapter 2

THE RISK OF CARDIOVASCULAR DISEASE AND ITS ASSOCIATIONS BETWEEN OBESITY AND PHYSICAL ACTIVITY IN ADOLESCENTS: INTERNATIONAL PERSPECTIVES

Duncan S. Buchan[1]*, Non. E. Thomas[2], Lon Kilgore[1], Juliette M. Mason[1] and Julien S. Baker[1]

[1]Health and Exercise Sciences, School of Science,
University of the West of Scotland, Hamilton, Scotland, UK
[2]Centre for Children and Young People's Health and Well-Being,
School of Human and Health Sciences, Swansea University,
Swansea, Wales, UK

ABSTRACT

The prevalence of cardiovascular disease (CVD) is increasing and has become the leading cause of death around the world. Though once thought of as an adult problem, it is now recognised that the early manifestations of disease may occur during childhood. Numerous risk factors have been linked to CVD with much of the research focusing on understanding the prevalence and relationship of traditional risk factors such as dyslipidemia, smoking, diabetes mellitus, hypertension, obesity, psychosocial stress, poor diet, physical inactivity and alcohol consumption to the early etiology of disease. Needless to say, the majority of our understanding is from adult studies though evidence from youth populations is beginning to accumulate. It is well established that obesity is linked to nearly all CVD risk factors though untangling the precise reasons whereby individuals become overweight are challenging and complex. The need to untangle this complex web is nonetheless vital. Estimates suggest that at least 20 million children under 5 years of age were overweight while by 2015 it is predicted that approximately 2.3 billion adults will be overweight and more than 700 million will be obese [1]. Public health strategies that aim to reduce the prevalence of obesity and overweight encourage

---
* Email: duncan.buchan@uws.ac.uk. Telephone: 01698 283100.

youth to increase their physical activity levels as a means of protecting against poor cardiometabolic profiles. This is in part due to several epidemiological studies involving adults which have demonstrated that high physical activity levels are associated with favorable risk profiles. Whether the same relationships are seen in youth populations though are unclear. Studies have shown that interventions that increase physical activity can lead to a reduction in certain CVD risk factors but the lack of agreement between findings makes it impossible to give precise recommendations. Yet it is important that research continues and examines the associations between lifestyle behaviors, physical activity behavior and CVD risk factors in order to identify individuals who may be at most need of intervention. Thus, this chapter will provide an in-depth overview of what is currently known about the prevalence of CVD risk in youth while examining the evidence concerning its associations between obesity and physical activity.

INTRODUCTION

Cardiovascular Disease (CVD) has been the leading cause of death in developed countries since the early 1900's [2]. CVD relates to any disease that affects the cardiovascular system which comprises the heart, blood and blood vessels. In 2005, the World Health Organization (WHO) estimated that 30% of the annual 58 million deaths in this year was attributed to CVD [3]. Though there has been a significant reduction in cardiovascular mortality during the preceding four decades [2, 4], improvements in mortality rates have now begun to slow if not already at a plateau. Understandably the prevalence of CVD is presenting a growing financial and social challenge for many developed and developing countries and is rightly deemed a global concern. Thus, in order to prevent and reverse current CVD mortality rates it is vital that a clear understanding of its development, risk factors and preventable measures are understood. While the risk of cardiovascular mortality was once relatively low in youth, accumulating evidence through several large scale epidemiological studies suggests that CVD has its origins in childhood [5-8]. Findings from large prospective population studies such as the Muscatine Study [9], the Bogalusa Heart Study [7], the Cardiovascular Risk in Young Finns Study [10] and the European Youth Heart Study [5, 11] have all shown that a number of CVD risk factors are prevalent in both children and adolescents and tend to track into adulthood. Indeed, the clustering of risk factors are prevalent in youth with estimates ranging from 0 – 60% depending on the definitions used and the population under surveillance, though the higher prevalence figures are almost always observed in obese youth populations [12].

Numerous risk factors have been linked to the development of CVD and include; poor dietary habits, overweight/obesity, hypertension, insulin resistance or diabetes mellitus, alcohol consumption, smoking, poor physical activity levels and dyslipidemia (disorder of fats within the blood) [13, 14]. These major risk factors often occur in combination and are seen as primary modifiable factors that can reduce the risk of current and future CVD. Unlike the prevalence of other CVD risk factors such as smoking, obesity rates during both childhood and adolescence is on the rise and is now considered a pandemic [14]. Furthermore, evidence has shown that children who are obese in their preschool years are more likely to be obese in adolescence and adulthood [1]. Given that childhood obesity increases the risk of becoming obese in adulthood, and that obesity at any age is associated with numerous co-morbidities such as, type 2 diabetes, CVD risk, hypertension, asthma, depression, certain cancers, and sleep apnoea [1, 7, 15, 16], reversing current trends in obesity prevalence is of vital concern.

Understanding the underlying factors and mechanisms whereby individuals become overweight or obese is challenging. There are a wide range of behavioural, genetic, cultural, environmental and biological variables that act both independently and amongst one another which contribute to its development in youth [17]. Nonetheless, it is generally accepted that the resultant energy imbalance produced from excessive energy intake and low physical activity are widely considered to be the most important contributors to the current overweight and obese rates within youth populations. In adults, being obese is known to double an individual's risk of all-cause mortality [18]. Numerous studies have also reported that unfavourable CVD risk profiles are associated with adiposity (accumulation of excess fat) in youth [7, 10]. Nonetheless, low physical activity levels are also independently associated with CVD risk factors [19]. Though the relative importance of fatness and physical activity in youth remains unclear [20, 21], low physical activity levels and excess adiposity often occur concurrently [22]. Increasing physical activity levels can have a direct effect upon measures of adiposity providing that the stimulus is appropriate. It seems that in order to protect against poor cardiometabolic (diseases of the heartand metabolic disorders) profiles, reducing weight status while increasing physical activity seems to be the best approach to recommend to improve the health status of those most vulnerable of risk.

In order to prevent future CVD there is a need to implement established health strategies early in life. Before any physical activity intervention is undertaken it is vital that an assessment of risk is carried out. Though the clinical symptoms of CVD may be absent in youth populations, understanding the prevalence of CVD risk factors and how they are manifested may provide the best means of implementing health enhancing strategies which have a chance of preventing the occurrence of CVD or other co-morbidities once adulthood is reached. Thus, this chapter will provide an in-depth overview of what is currently known about the prevalence of CVD in youth and will examine the evidence concerning the associations between obesity and physical activity while suggesting the need for authors to consider the use of alternative physical activity intervention strategies as a means of improving the health and well-being of youth populations

CARDIOVASCULAR DISEASE

The incidence of CVD results from a complex interaction of many risk factors all of which predispose individuals to its incidence over their lifetime. Several landmark epidemiological studies [7, 9, 10] have greatly enhanced our knowledge and understanding of the key risk factors implicated in the prevalence of CVD. These studies have led to the acceptance that nine modifiable risk factors – dyslipidemia, smoking, diabetes mellitus, hypertension, obesity, psychosocial stress, poor diet, physical inactivity, and alcohol consumption – are fundamental to the prevalence and reversal of CVD risk. Though some believe that these nine risk factors account for approximately 90% of the CVD risk evident in populations [23] others believe this estimate to be more like 50% [24]. The WHO meanwhile estimate that 80% of premature mortality can be prevented through a comprehensive assessment and management of these potent risk factors [1]. Nonetheless, while these risk factors account for a large proportion of CVD events, they do not fully explain cardiovascular risk and mortality.

More than a hundred emerging risk factors have been suggested as potential markers for improving CVD risk classification [25]. Several of these novel biomarkers have generated significant interest within the scientific community since they may provide additional means of improving risk assessment. Some of the more widely investigated biomarkers include C-reactive protein (CRP), adiponectin, plasminogen activator inhibitor-1 (PAI-1), interleukin-6 (IL-6) and fibrinogen (Fg). Much of the evidence linking these markers to CVD though has been derived from adult populations. Though cardiovascular events tend to typically occur during mid adulthood, it is now accepted that CVD risk factors have their origins in childhood and tend to track into adulthood [10, 26]. Despite the extremely low risk of early mortality in youth, early and continued exposure to an unhealthy risk profile may accentuate early mortality. In the study by Raitakari et al. (2003) the authors were able to track CVD risk factors from youth into adulthood and predict the extent of CVD disease, independently of current risk status. This emphasizes the importance of early identification to ensure that preventable measures are put in place early to prevent unfavourable risk profiles tracking into adulthood.

Evidence from the Bogalusa study in the United States (US) found that approximately 60% of overweight children aged between 5 – 10 years of age had one CVD risk factor such as hypertension, hyperlipidemia or elevated insulin levels [7]. Of the same cohort, approximately 25% of those who were overweight had two or more CVD risk factors. Comparable findings have also been seen from an earlier investigation in Muscatine, US where the prevalence of risk factors was documented in 4,829 school children aged between 6 and 18 years [9]. From the data the authors found that a considerable number of individuals had risk profiles which in adults are predictive of early mortality. Evidence from the longitudinal Bogalusa Heart Study [27] in the US found that 60% of 10 year old children who were overweight had at least one risk factor with a further 25% presenting with three or more. It is clear from these studies that poor weight status in youth is continually associated with poor risk profiles.

Though one could argue that this problem may just be prevalent in North America, similar findings have also been reported in Europe through the European Heart study [11]. Here the authors conducted a cross-sectional analysis of 1020 randomly selected Danish boys and girls aged between 9 and 15 years for the presence of multiple CVD risk factors. From their analysis the authors found that 8–9 times as many individuals from a random distribution had five risk factors with three times as many having four risk factors. Though these findings are limited to a Danish population, the author also carried out a similar investigation with N=1732 randomly selected 9-year-old and 15-year-old school children from Denmark, Estonia and Portugal [5]. Once again the authors found comparable results with their previous investigation with 11% of the sample presenting with a number of CVD risk factors.

It is clear that the identification of individuals presenting with an abnormal CVD risk profile, or a profile just below accepted levels of risk, is central to the development and implementation of appropriate health strategies in youth. Poor weight status and low physical activity levels are continually linked to the prevalence of unfavourable health profiles, thus, it is important that at risk individuals are identified early in youth. Thus, the subsequent section will provide an overview of the current literature concerning the measurement and prevalence of obesity in youth populations.

OBESITY

Overweight and obesity can be defined as an excessive or abnormal fat accumulation that may impair health [28]. Obesity is the leading public health crisis of our time with some suggesting that current prevalence levels are of pandemic proportions [14]. Understanding the underlying factors and mechanisms whereby individuals become overweight or obese is challenging. There are a wide range of behavioural, genetic, cultural, environmental and biological variables that act both independently and synergistically with one another which contribute to the development of overweight and obesity in youth [17]. Adult body mass index (BMI) cut-off values of 25 kg/m^2 for overweight and 30 kg/m^2 for obesity are internationally recognized and widely used as criterion measures to define the weight status of adult populations [28]. Similar age and sex specific BMI cut-off values have also been developed for use in children and adolescents and are based on pooled international data that provide cut-offs to define thinness, overweight and obesity [29, 30].

With the estimated cost to the UK economy of treating obesity related disorders at a staggering £3.5 billion ($5.5 billion) per annum [31], the seriousness of the current situation is evident. Each year the WHO estimate that 2.6 million people die as a result of being overweight or obese [1]. With reference to youth, current global estimates suggest that at least 10% are overweight or obese with the Americas leading at 32%, Europe at 20% and the Middle East at 16% [32]. Similar estimates have also been reported in the Oceania region [33] with 10% of youth classed as being obese and 20% overweight in Australia. Though some contend that obesity prevalence may be beginning to level off [34], others predict a continued increase over the next few years. Indeed some believe that not only is the prevalence of overweight and obesity increasing but the rate of new cases each year is rising too, particularly in countries that have had low prevalence rates in the past [32]. Needless to say the prevalence of overweight and obesity in youth is widespread around the globe and has led the WHO to refer to the current situation as "one of the greatest public health challenges of the 21st century" [28].

The US, for instance, has seen the prevalence of obesity among youths rise by 14.6% in just 40 years [35]. The authors further exacerbate this plight by reporting that one in three US adolescents are either overweight or obese with the prevalence more than tripling between 1970 and 2004 [35]. Similar findings have also been observed in Canada, China, Germany, Brazil, North Africa, Australia, Saudi Arabia, France and Finland [36]. Within the UK, recent investigations denote worrying figures also. Recent estimates from England purport that around three in ten boys and girls aged 2 to 15 can be classed as either overweight or obese (31% and 28% respectively) [37]. Within Scotland estimates suggest that for 2-15 year olds, 29% of boys and 27% of girls are either overweight or obese while in adults, this figure increases to 66% for men and 58% for women, respectively [38]. Other reports predict that if current trends continue 40% of all adults within Scotland will be obese by 2030 with the total cost to Scottish society of treating obesity related conditions, including both direct and indirect costs, ranging from £0.9 billion - £3 billion ($1.4 billion– $4.7 billion)[39]. When you consider that recent reports estimate that 10% of all youth globally will become overweight [14] and that 80% of obese adolescents will become obese adults [40] action is urgently required to abate and reverse these current trends.

A troubling consequence of this expected trend in weight status from youth to adulthood is exemplified in the excellent longitudinal Harvard growth study conducted by Must and colleagues [41]. Here the authors examined the relationship between weight status and morbidity and mortality in adolescent participants samples during the 1920's and 1930's. Follow up data on participants were then captured in the late 80's on those who were still alive where information was obtained about their medical history, weight, functional capacity, and other risk factors. Cause of death in those that were deceased was obtained from death certificates. Interestingly the authors found that individuals who were overweight a adolescents had increased age-specific morbidity and mortality relating to CVD and other chronic diseases 55 years later [41]. It was also documented that obese adolescents who had subsequently lost the excess weight in adulthood were still at an increased risk, independent of adult weight status. Collectively these findings seem to suggest that in the presence of adolescent obesity a series of mechanisms are set in motion that is associated with adverse risk which may be difficult to reverse through weight loss alone in adulthood.

Further evidence is also provided through the Bogalusa Heart study which showed that childhood overweight is related to the development of adverse risk profiles in adulthood. he authors examined the CVD risk profiles of 2617 participants who were examined initially at ages 2 to 17 years and then re-examined at ages 18 – 37 years [8]. Of particular importance was the finding that adverse risk factors such as BMI, dyslipidemia, diabetes mellitus and blood pressure in adulthood was directly associated to the poor weight status of individuals from childhood to adulthood. Furthermore, the authors noted that of the children identified as overweight at the initial examination, 77% of those remained obese into adulthood. Given that childhood obesity frequently tracks into adulthood it is clear that if current prevalence rates continue to rise then childhood overweight and obesity will become major contributors to the adult obesity epidemic in the forthcoming years. The importance of implementing preventative measures early in one's life before adverse weight status is reached is thus vital to promote health and well-being not only in youth, but in future adulthood also.

Though contentious, BMI can be used as a standard for identifying those at risk of obesity [29]. Some have questioned the utility of BMI measurements as it does not distinguish between weight associated with muscle and weight associated with fat and thus provides only a crude measure of body fatness. Although less sensitive than other measures of adiposity such as percentage body fat (%BF), waist circumference (WC) and waist to hip ratio (WHR) [28], measures of BMI are inexpensive and simple to administer. They are routinely used in adult populations and now more so within youth populations [29, 30] which can provide a means of direct comparisons between the prevalence of overweight and obesity rates throughout the world. Though it has been firmly established that a greater BMI is associated with increased risk of early mortality from CVD in both adults [42] and youth [8], some question its diagnostic value [23]. Moreover despite the strong associations between BMI and body fat estimates in youth, this association is somewhat attenuated for boys when compared to girls and in pre-pubertal adolescents when compared to pubertal adolescents [43]. At present there is no universal agreement over the most appropriate measure of body composition in youth populations. BMI is the most common measure used to define weight status in youth populations though other measures are also being used more readily [44].

WC is becoming increasingly recognized as an important measure within the overall assessment of CVD risk. Measuring WC is a relatively simple procedure and is increasingly used as a surrogate measure of abdominal or central obesity. Its measurement is also now included as a pre-requisite for the diagnosis of the metabolic syndrome in both adult and youth populations [45]. To date there is no universal cut-off value for WC or WHR that can be applied worldwide so researchers are advised to use country specific values when considering their aims and available resources [46]. At present there are no recommended centile thresholds for WC to grade British Caucasian youth (<16 years) as being at risk. Recent recommendations proposed by the International Diabetes Foundation (IDF) suggest that in European individuals of 16 years of age or older, central obesity can be classified if individuals present with a WC ≥ 94 cm for men and ≥ 80 cm for women [45]. These are similar to previous thresholds proposed for Scottish Caucasians [47] and provide a means to identify individuals at increased risk. For those of South and South-East Asian, Japanese, and ethnic South and Central American origin, the cut-offs should be ≥ 90 cm for men, and ≥ 80 cm for women [45]. Though this is a simple measurement, it is useful for health practitioners in indentifying those at most risk of unfavourable lifestyles.

Evidence has shown that measuring central adiposity rather than overall adiposity may provide a more accurate indication of CVD risk in adults [23]. Findings from the INTERHEART study which involved N=27,000 participants from 52 countries found that measures of WC was more strongly associated with the risk of CVD than BMI. This finding has also been confirmed within youth populations [7, 48]. In the study by Savva et al. (2006) proxy measures of central adiposity were used as independent predictors to determine the prevalence of CVD risk factors within pre-pubescent European youth. From their findings the authors noted that WC was seen to be the most significant predictor of all CVD risk factors measured in both boys and girls whereas BMI was seen as the poorest. More recent investigations involving European children and adolescents have also demonstrated a negative association between time spent in vigorous physical activity and WC [49, 50]. Interestingly, these authors also found that the strength of these associations differed in terms of the participant's cardiorespiratory fitness levels and amount of vigorous physical activity undertaken which suggests that fitness and physical activity levels may impact independently upon the WC of youth participants. Finally, in a recent review there was strong evidence that WC is a good measure to estimate central adiposity in youth populations and its measurement to estimate the presence of central adiposity seems worthwhile to improve risk identification [44].

There has been increasing attention given to the measurement of the WHR for detecting central obesity and those at increased risk of CVD. Like the measurement of WC, the WHR is another proxy measure of central obesity that includes the measurement of hip circumference, which measures fat accumulation on the hips, to provide an overall score. WHR is calculated by dividing the circumference of the waist by the distance around the hips and buttocks [51]. As highlighted previously, there is no agreed cut-off values proposed for WHR for youth populations. For British adults aged ≥ 16 years a threshold of 1.0 for men and 0.85 for women has been proposed with values above this indicating an increased risk of early mortality [52]. As the authors contend nonetheless this threshold should be viewed with caution given the lack of age and gender specific growth charts currently available within the UK. Cut-off points vary considerably between nations and should be considered when measuring the risk status of individuals. Within the US for instance, the widely used recommendations from the

National Cholesterol Education Program (NCEP) suggest a single set of sex-specific cut-offs, of above 102 cm for men and above 88 cm for women [53].

Though it may be difficult to use WHR as a measure of central obesity within a clinical and diagnostic setting, like WC it is a simple measure that has shown to be more predictive of CVD risk than BMI alone [23]. Findings from the INTERHEART study showed that for adults, WHR demonstrated highly significant associations with myocardial infarction risk with those at most risk having a WHR above approximately 0.95 for men and 0.80 for women [23]. These findings have also been confirmed somewhat in other studies involving European adult populations [54]. In this study, the authors examined the association of BMI, WC, and WHR with the risk of death among N = 359,387 participants over a period of just less than 10 years. When controlling for BMI, central adiposity was positively associated with the risk of death though surprisingly these associations seemed to be stronger among individuals with a lower BMI than those with a higher BMI. Of particular importance was the recommendation that when predicting the risk of death, measures of both central and total adiposity are required to improve the prediction. While the evidence pertaining to the utility of WHR as a measure of CVD risk in youth populations is questionable [44, 55], measuring either WC or WHR in addition to BMI may improve the assessment and identification of individuals at risk of early mortality. Particularly when it is known that poor weight status and unfavourable behaviours tend to track from childhood into adulthood [10]. Another method that is used to estimate total adiposity within youth populations is the skinfold measurement. Although there are gold standard measures available that will accurately estimate body composition, including underwater weighing, air displacement plethysmography, labelled water techniques and dual-energy X-ray absorptiometry (DXA) [43], these measures are expensive and impractical within a field setting. Evidence suggests that the commonly used equations proposed by Slaughter et al, (1988) that use the triceps and calf skinfolds to provide an estimate of %BF show the best agreement with the gold standard DXA method for male and female adolescents [43, 56]. This is not surprising since estimates based on BMI have shown measurement errors of between 5 – 6% when compared to gold standard measures whereas %BF estimates derived from the slaughter equations, involving calf and tricep measures, have shown only an 2-3% measurement error [57, 58]. The simplicity, speed and accuracy of the skinfold measurement make the assessment a popular method for estimating total adiposity in youth populations, particularly within the field setting where a large number of individuals have to be measured. Gender specific cut off values for % BF have been established and allow for participants to be classified into 2 groups (normal fat and overfat) which are based on the cut-points for % body fat used in the FITNESSGRAM test assessment programme [58]. These cut-points correspond to body fat ≥25% in boys and ≥30% in girls as overfat, and <25% and <30% in boys and girls, respectively, as normal fat and are derived from the Bogalusa Heart Study which involved over 2000 boys and girls aged between 6 – 18 years that were tracked from childhood into adulthood [59]. From their findings the authors noted that individuals were at an increased risk of elevated atherogenic blood lipids and blood pressure at higher levels of body fat (25% in boys and 30-35% in girls). Nevertheless, conclusions from a recent review highlight the need for caution when considering the best method for assessing total adiposity in youth populations [44]. Within this review the authors scrutinized a total of 40 investigations involving children and adolescents that examined the validity of BMI and skinfold measure as estimates of total adiposity. The authors concede that while both skinfold measures and BMI are good predictors of total adiposity, BMI seems to be the best indicator within obese youth while for non-obese youth, skinfold measures seems the best predictor. They continue by stating that the accuracy of BMI varies with the degree of total adiposity, improving significantly at higher levels of total adiposity [44]. Overall, the evidence reviewed by the authors supports the notion that no one measure may accurately predict the body composition in youth populations. Thus it seems that when possible, researchers should undertake a series of body composition measures in order to best identify those individuals at most risk of obesity related disorders.

PHYSICAL ACTIVITY

Though the terms physical fitness, exercise and physical activity are often used interchangeably within the exercise science literature it is important to realise that these concepts are not one and the same. Physical activity is a behaviour and can be defined as any bodily movement produced by the skeletal muscles which results in a substantial increase in energy expenditure over resting levels [60]. Exercise can be defined as "a subset of physical activity that is planned, structured, and repetitive bodily movements done to improve or maintain one or more components of physical fitness" [61]. Physical fitness on the other hand is a physiological trait which refers to the capacity to perform physical activity. This section will focus on the importance of physical activity and its effects upon the health and wellbeing of individuals.

PHYSICAL ACTIVITY AND HEALTH

Physical inactivity in known to be a leading risk factor for global mortality and is estimated to account for 6% of all deaths throughout the world, behind only high blood pressure (13%) and tobacco use (9%) [62]. This has predictably led to a leading Exercise Scientist claiming that "physical inactivity is one of the most important public health problems of the 21st century"[63]. The importance and promotion of regular physical activity to human health has been recognised for some time and is now deemed a major component of public health policies. Within youth, physical activity is required to ensure optimal growth patterns and for the development of physical fitness (cardiorespiratory fitness, muscular power, agility and speed) [62]. Physical activity is also an important means of treatment and prevention of overweight and obesity prevalence in youth, notably through its positive effects on body composition through increased energy expenditure.

In adults, the pioneering work led by British scientist Jerry Morris in the 1950's was the first to provide empirical evidence that regular physical activity was associated with positive health outcomes [64, 65]. Frequently termed the London bus study, Morris and colleagues demonstrated that individuals who were physically active (bus conductors) were less likely to develop coronary heart disease in comparison to those who were almost sedentary in the work place (i.e. bus drivers). Further work undertaken by Ralph Paffenbarger in the US continued to build upon this evidence with the commencement of the seminal Harvard Alumni Health study in 1960 [66, 67]. Here the authors focused on the effects on the relationship between physical activity and CVD in Harvard male alumni who had graduated between 1916 and

1950. Through the use of periodic self-report questionnaires over three decades evidence on the health status and lifestyle of the cohort was collected. From their data the authors were able to confirm that those who were physically active had a lower risk of mortality attributable to CVD. An interesting assertion made by the authors was that of those alumni in their 4th decade, vigorous exercise and increased energy expenditure predicted a lower risk of CVD and early mortality in comparison to those who were sedentary or moderately active. It is no surprise then that the first formal guidelines produced by the American College of Sports Medicine recommended aerobic fitness training through vigorous exercise as a means to promote health, fitness and well-being [68].

Table 1. Comparison of the key physical activity recommendations for school aged youth from the UK, USA and the WHO

	Age Group	
World Health Organization	5 – 17 years of age	1. Children and young people aged 5–17 years old should accumulate at least 60 minutes of moderate to vigorous-intensity physical activity daily. 2. Physical activity of amounts greater than 60 minutes daily will provide additional health benefits. 3. Most of daily physical activity should be aerobic. Vigorous-intensity activities should be incorporated, including those that strengthen muscle and bone, at least 3 times per week.
	Age Group	
UK Department of Health	5 – 18 years of age	1. All children and young people should engage in moderate to vigorous intensity physical activity for at least 60 minutes and up to several hours every day. 2. Vigorous intensity activities, including those that strengthen muscle and bone, should be incorporated at least three days a week. 3. All children and young people should minimise the amount of time spent being sedentary (sitting) for extended periods.
U.S. Department of Health and Human Services.	6 – 17 years of age	Children and adolescents should do 60 minutes (1 hour) or more of physical activity daily. Aerobic: Most of the 60 or more minutes a day should be either moderate- or vigorous-intensity aerobic physical activity, and should include vigorous-intensity physical activity at least 3 days a week. Muscle-strengthening: As part of their 60 or more minutes of daily physical activity, children and adolescents should include muscle-strengthening physical activity on at least 3 days of the week. Bone-strengthening: As part of their 60 or more minutes of daily physical activity, children and adolescents should include bone-strengthening physical activity on at least 3 days of the week. It is important to encourage young people to participate in physical activities that are appropriate for their age, that are enjoyable, and that offer variety.

Source: Adapted from [96, 103, 104].

The work undertaken by Paffenbarger and colleagues was the first study to quantify the relationship between adverse health status and physical activity and is the foundation from which future epidemiological studies have been built upon. Since then position statements and reports from leading organizations have consistently reported the benefits of regular physical activity upon the health and well-being of adults [61, 62, 69, 70]. Strong evidence from the U.S. Department of Health and Human Services found that when compared to inactive adults, active adults are less likely to suffer from hypertension, stroke, type 2 diabetes, breast cancer and coronary heart disease [70]. It has also been stated that increased levels of physical activity are also associated with increased longevity by limiting the development and progression of chronic disease and debilitating conditions [61].

Though the evidence base is rather less for youths in comparison to adults, recent reviews have demonstrated similar protective effects of physical activity on health related measures [62, 70-74]. Collectively, the scientific evidence currently available on youth demonstrates that physical activity provides fundamental health benefits for children and adolescents that include; increased physical fitness (both cardiorespiratory fitness and muscular strength), reduced body fatness, favourable cardiovascular and metabolic disease risk profiles, enhanced bone health and reduced symptoms of depression [62, 70, 72, 73]. Based on this substantial body of evidence the Department of Health within the UK agreed that for the first time a review of current physical activity recommendations would be undertaken as a national collaboration between the four UK home countries; Wales, Scotland, England and Northern Ireland. The new UK physical activity guidelines have since been published [69] in part to reflect the new scientific evidence but also to ensure consistency between all of the four home countries. These updated guidelines relative to youth populations can be found in table 1 in addition to the recommendations proposed by the US Government and the World Health Organization.

BENEFICIAL EFFECTS OF PHYSICAL ACTIVITY UPON CVD RISK FACTORS

In recent years, cross sectional studies have begun to examine the relationship between physical activity and traditional risk factors of CVD [49, 75-77]. Much of this new research has also been able to objectively assess physical activity levels through the use of accelerometers which have improved our understanding of the relationship between physical activity and CVD risk. Two recent studies involving participants from the European Youth Heart Study have both demonstrated a negative relationship between physical activity levels and measures of total adiposity [75, 76]. In the study by Ekelund et al, (2004) a large cohort of children aged between 9 and 10 years from four European countries (Norway, Estonia, Denmark and Portugal) participated with the aim to examine the associations between objective measures of physical activity and two indicators of total adiposity (BMI and 5 skinfold thickness measures). In one of the first large scale studies of its kind, the authors found a small association between physical activity and total adiposity though the effect on total adiposity was only significant for the amount of time spent at moderate and vigorous physical activity.

Similar findings were also seen by Ruiz et al, (2006) involving a cohort from Estonia and Sweden of the same age though in this study the authors found that total adiposity measured from 5 skinfolds was significantly associated with higher levels of vigorous physical activity, but not with moderate or total physical activity. These findings have also been confirmed in older cohorts too from the US, 4-19 year olds [78] and 16 year olds [79]. In these studies dual-energy X-ray absorptiometry was used to estimate total adiposity with the authors reporting strong negative associations between vigorous physical activity and total adiposity. Comparable findings have also been reported when waist circumference is used as a measure of adiposity in children and adolescents [49].

Contradictory evidence exists regarding the effects of physical activity on measures of BP. A previous meta-analysis study conducted in 2003 and a more recent systematic review from 2009 reported no clear association between physical activity and BP in normotensive children [80] or indeed a positive effect on BP of increasing physical activity levels in both children and adolescents [74]. Nevertheless, cross sectional studies have repeatedly shown that total levels of physical activity [81] and moderate to vigorous physical activity [77] are negatively associated with lower BP values in both children and adolescents. One explanation for the contradictory findings may relate to the intensity of the activity performed. In the meta-analysis conducted in 2003, the authors reported that no statistically significant changes were observed for body weight, BMI or %BF in any of the studies that met their inclusion criteria [80]. Concomitantly, Dobbins et al, (2009) in their review only examined the effects of increasing physical activity levels upon measures of BP but were unable to compare this association with measures of adiposity and/or improvements in cardiorespiratory fitness. It may be that if exercise interventions are to be employed to examine its effects upon measures of BP, increases in cardiorespiratory fitness and/or reduction in measures of adiposity may be required rather than just an increase in total physical activity levels.

Though these recent investigations during the last decade seem to support the benefits of vigorous physical activity upon CVD risk, this is not new and has been known for well over 30 years [66] and has been advised previously [68]. It seems that the inability for most adults of the Western World to comply with the "3 x 20" recommendation resulted in a change of focus from policy makers to adopt the "moderate physical activity" message [82]. Now it seems that the policy makers have come full circle though time will tell whether individuals are able to comply with these new recommendations. Recent evidence though suggests otherwise.

Despite the well established benefits of regular physical activity on health and well-being, current levels within school aged youth are widely regarded as insufficient to meet current recommendations [83, 84]. Recent findings from the US purport that only 8% of adolescents (12 - 19 years of age) are sufficiently active to meet these recommendations [84] whereas in Europe, less than one third of youth (11 – 15 yrs) currently engage in 60 minutes of moderate – vigorous physical activity most days [85, 86]. Based on previous physical activity recommendations from Scotland, approximately 71% of Scottish youth aged between 2-15 years meet current recommendations which is significantly greater than other studies involving European youth [38]. Nonetheless, given that self reported physical activity questionnaires were used within this survey caution is warranted. Within adults, only 37% were seen to meet the physical activity recommendations of at least 30 minutes of moderate activity on at least five days a week. In contrast, the number of adults aged between 16-24 years meeting the recommendations for health declined drastically to 50%. It is not clear whether this percentage would increase if the report had included school aged youth from 16-18 years; nevertheless, the trend among late adolescence and young adults raises concerns.

SUMMARY

CVD continues to be the leading cause of death in the Western world. As the prevalence of traditional CVD risk factors seem to becoming more evident in childhood, it is vital that pre-emptive interventions are implemented early in one's life before the associated cardiovascular complications are established. Childhood is seen as an ideal phase for intervention. This is the stage in one's life where behaviors are established which if left unabated may continue into adulthood. Yet, this is also a stage where behaviors can be influenced. The school environment, and in particular physical education, is often cited as an ideal setting to implement health enhancing interventions that can capture a wide range of youth from assorted social and economical backgrounds. Much of the work carried out for identifying individuals at risk of CVD has primarily focused on the detection of nine well established risk factors such as: dyslipidemia, smoking, diabetes mellitus, hypertension, obesity, psychosocial stress, poor diet, physical inactivity and alcohol consumption. These risk factors tend to cluster and its measurement is especially useful for identifying those most vulnerable to unhealthy lifestyle choices and future cardiovascular complications. Nevertheless, these risk factors do not fully explain cardiovascular risk and mortality.

What is clear nonetheless is that being overweight and obese has consistently been identified as a key contributor to CVD risk with nearly all risk factors in one way or another linked to the presence of unhealthy weight status. The burgeoning prevalence rates of obesity throughout the globe, and in particular within youth populations, may mean that the favourable reversal in cardiovascular morbidity and mortality rates seen in recent decades may soon begin to diminish.

Findings from epidemiological and cross-sectional studies have identified the importance of physical activity for the prevention and reversal of unfavourable cardiovascular risk profiles. As physical activity can influence obesity directly, and given the associations between obesity and CVD risk factors, it is important that we endeavor to disentangle this causal relationship. Nevertheless, it is clear from the literature discussed that our understanding of the significance and associations between CVD risk and obesity and physical activity in youth is poorly understood. Findings are often contradictory which makes it difficult to assert conclusively the best means of reversing potentially unfavourable behaviours and cardiovascular and metabolic profiles.

While the contradictions in findings are disappointing, this reflects the limited investigations carried out within youth populations in comparison to adults. Thus, improved understanding of the effects of different physical activity interventions upon CVD risk factors may provide new avenues for intervention that can provide the best means of protection against current and future cardiovascular complications. For instance, low physical activity levels are often identified as a behaviour which can be modified and provide protection against the deleterious effects of being overweight and obese in youth. School based physical activity interventions implemented within the physical education curriculum may be the best hope for practitioners and researchers to investigate the effects of such interventions on CVD risk factors linked to cardiovascular morbidity and mortality. The school environment affords an ideal setting to practice health-promoting behaviors among youth that will reach a large number of individuals from assorted socio-economic surroundings. Since the role of Physical Education is, to some extent, continually marginalized with the curriculum it is important that policy makers realise the importance of this setting and its role in the health of school age youth.

REFERENCES

[1] World Health Organization. Preventing chronic disease: a vital investment Geneva, Switzerland:World Health Organization http://www.who.int/chp/chronic_disease_report/full_report.pdf. Accessed 17th May 2011; 2005

[2] Lloyd-Jones D, Adams RJ, Brown TM, Carnethon M, Dai S, De Simone G, et al. Heart disease and stroke statistics--2010 update: a report from the American Heart Association. Circulation. 2009 Feb 23;121(7):e46-e215.

[3] World Health Organization. A healthy city is an active city: a physical activity planning guide. Available from http://www.euro.who.int/__data/assets/pdf_file/0012/99975/E91883.pdf. Accessed 8th August 2011. Geneva: World Health Organization; 2008.

[4] Unal B, Critchley JA, Capewell S. Explaining the decline in coronary heart disease mortality in England and Wales between 1981 and 2000. Circulation. 2004 Mar 9;109(9):1101-7.

[5] Andersen LB, Harro M, Sardinha LB, Froberg K, Ekelund U, Brage S, et al. Physical activity and clustered cardiovascular risk in children: a cross-sectional study (The European Youth Heart Study). *Lancet.* 2006 07/22/2006 Jul 22-28;368(9532):299-304.

[6] Eisenmann JC, Welk GJ, Wickel EE, Blair SN. Stability of variables associated with the metabolic syndrome from adolescence to adulthood: the Aerobics Center Longitudinal Study. *American Journal of Human Biology.* 2004 Nov-Dec;16(6):690-6.

[7] Freedman DS, Dietz WH, Srinivasan SR, Berenson GS. The relation of overweight to cardiovascular risk factors among children and adolescents: the Bogalusa Heart Study. *Pediatrics.* 1999 Jun;103(6 Pt 1):1175-82.

[8] Freedman DS, Khan LK, Dietz WH, Srinivasan SR, Berenson GS. Relationship of childhood obesity to coronary heart disease risk factors in adulthood: the Bogalusa Heart Study. *Pediatrics.* 2001 Sep;108(3):712-8.

[9] Lauer RM, Connor WE, Leaverton PE, Reiter MA, Clarke WR. Coronary heart disease risk factors in school children: the Muscatine study. *Journal of Pediatrics.* 1975 May;86(5):697-706.

[10] Raitakari OT, Juonala M, Kahonen M, Taittonen L, Laitinen T, Maki-Torkko N, et al. Cardiovascular risk factors in childhood and carotid artery intima-media thickness in adulthood: the Cardiovascular Risk in Young Finns Study. *Journal of the American Medical Association.* 2003 Nov 5;290(17):2277-83.

[11] Andersen LB, Wedderkopp N, Hansen HS, Cooper AR, Froberg K. Biological cardiovascular risk factors cluster in Danish children and adolescents: the European Youth Heart Study. *Preventive Medicine.* 2003 Oct;37(4):363-7.

[12] Steele RM, Brage S, Corder K, Wareham NJ, Ekelund U. Physical activity, cardiorespiratory fitness, and the metabolic syndrome in youth. *Journal of Applied Physiology*. 2008 Jul;105(1):342-51
[13] Ortega FB, Artero EG, Ruiz JR, Espana-Romero V, Jimenez-Pavon D, Vicente-Rodriguez G, et al. Physical fitness levels among European adolescents: the HELENA study. *British Journal of Sports Medicine*. 2011 Jan;45(1):20-9.
[14] Lobstein T. Obesity in children. *BMJ*. 2008;337:a669.
[15] Steinberger J, Daniels SR, Eckel RH, Hayman L, Lustig RH, McCrindle B, et al. Progress and challenges in metabolic syndrome in children and adolescents: a scientific statement from the American Heart Association Atherosclerosis, Hypertension, and Obesity in the Young Committee of the Council on Cardiovascular Disease in the Young; Council on Cardiovascular Nursing; and Council on Nutrition, Physical Activity, and Metabolism. *Circulation*. 2009 Feb 3;119(4):628-47.
[16] Daniels SR, Arnett DK, Eckel RH, Gidding SS, Hayman LL, Kumanyika S, et al. Overweight in children and adolescents: pathophysiology, consequences, prevention, and treatment. *Circulation*. 2005 Apr 19;111(15):1999-2012.
[17] Story M, Sallis JF, Orleans CT. Adolescent obesity: towards evidence-based policy and environmental solutions. *Journal of Adolescent Health*. 2009 Sep;45(3 Suppl):S1-5.
[18] Department of Health. At least 5 a week: Evidence of the impact of physical activity and its relationship to health. A report from the Chief Medical Officer. London: *Department of Health*; 2004
[19] Andersen LB, Sardinha LB, Froberg K, Riddoch CJ, Page AS, Anderssen SA. Fitness, fatness and clustering of cardiovascular risk factors in children from Denmark, Estonia and Portugal: the European Youth Heart Study. *International Journal of Pediatric Obesity*. 2008;3 Suppl 1:58-66.
[20] Martins CL, Andersen LB, Aires LM, Ribeiro JC, Mota JA. Association between Fitness, Different Indicators of Fatness, and Clustered Cardiovascular Diseases Risk Factors in Portuguese Children and Adolescents. *Open Sport Sciences Journal*. 2010;3:149-54.
[21] Jago R, Drews KL, McMurray RG, Thompson D, Volpe SL, Moe EL, et al. Fatness, fitness, and cardiometabolic risk factors among sixth-grade youth. *Medicine and Science in Sports and Exercise*. 2010 Aug;42(8):1502-10.
[22] Eisenmann JC. Aerobic fitness, fatness and the metabolic syndrome in children and adolescents. *Acta Paediatrica*. 2007 Dec;96(12):1723-9.
[23] Yusuf S, Hawken S, Ounpuu S, Dans T, Avezum A, Lanas F, et al. Effect of potentially modifiable risk factors associated with myocardial infarction in 52 countries (the INTERHEART study): case-control study. *Lancet*. 2004 Sep 11-17;364(9438):937-52.
[24] Wei M, Mitchell BD, Haffner SM, Stern MP. Effects of cigarette smoking, diabetes, high cholesterol, and hypertension on all-cause mortality and cardiovascular disease mortality in Mexican Americans. The San Antonio Heart Study. *American Journal of Epidemiology*. 1996 Dec 1;144(11):1058-65.
[25] Brotman DJ, Walker E, Lauer MS, O'Brien RG. In search of fewer independent risk factors. *Archives of Internal Medicine*. 2005 Jan 24;165(2):138-45.
[26] Andersen LB, Hasselstrom H, Gronfeldt V, Hansen SE, Karsten F. The relationship between physical fitness and clustered risk, and tracking of clustered risk from adolescence to young adulthood: eight years follow-up in the Danish Youth and Sport

Study. *International Journal of Behavioral Nutrition and Physical Activity.* 2004 Mar 8;1(1):6.

[27] Berenson GS, Srinivasan SR, Bao W, Newman WP, 3rd, Tracy RE, Wattigney WA. Association between multiple cardiovascular risk factors and atherosclerosis in children and young adults. The Bogalusa Heart Study. *New England Journal of Medicine.* 1998 Jun 4;338(23):1650-6.

[28] World Health Organization. The challenge of obesity in the WHO European Region and the strategies for response World Health Organisation Copenhagen, Denmark Available from http://www.euro.who.int/data/assets/pdf_file/0010/74746/E90711.pdf Accessed 21st July 2011; 2007

[29] Cole TJ, Bellizzi MC, Flegal KM, Dietz WH. Establishing a standard definition for child overweight and obesity worldwide: international survey. *BMJ.* 2000 May 6;320(7244):1240-3.

[30] Cole TJ, Flegal KM, Nicholls D, Jackson AA. Body mass index cut offs to define thinness in children and adolescents: international survey. *BMJ.* 2007 Jul 28;335(7612):194.

[31] Haslam D, Sattar N, Lean M. ABC of obesity. Obesity--time to wake up. *BMJ.* 2006 Sep 23;333(7569):640-2.

[32] Jackson-Leach R, Lobstein T. Estimated burden of paediatric obesity and co-morbidities in Europe. Part 1. The increase in the prevalence of child obesity in Europe is itself increasing. *International Journal of Pediatric Obesity.* 2006;1(1):26-32.

[33] Barnett AH. How well do rapid-acting insulins work in obese individuals? *Diabetes, Obesity and Metabolism.* 2006 Jul;8(4):388-95.

[34] British Heart Foundation. Couch Kids: The Nation's Future... London: British Heart Foundation; 2009.

[35] Ogden CL, Carroll MD, Flegal KM. High body mass index for age among US children and adolescents, 2003-2006. *The Journal of the American Medical Association.* 2008 May 28;299(20):2401-5.

[36] Lobstein T, Baur L, Uauy R. Obesity in children and young people: a crisis in public health. *Obesity Reviews.* 2004 May;5 Suppl 1:4-104.

[37] The Health and Social Care Information Centre. Statistics on obesity, physical activity and diet: England, 2011: The Health and Social Care Information Centre; 2011.

[38] The Scottish Government. The Scottish Health Survey Volume 1: Main Report. Edinburgh, Scotland: The Scottish Government http://www.scotland.gov.uk/Resource/Doc/325403/0104975.pdf. Accessed 18th July 2011; 2010.

[39] The Scottish Government. Preventing Overweight and Obesity in Scotland: A Route Map Towards Healthy Weight. Available from http://www.scotland.gov.uk/Resource/Doc/302783/0094795.pdf. Accessed 2nd August 2011. Edinburgh: The Scottish Government; 2010.

[40] Schonfeld-Warden N, Warden CH. Pediatric obesity. An overview of etiology and treatment. *Pediatric Clinics of North America.* 1997 Apr;44(2):339-61.

[41] Must A, Jacques PF, Dallal GE, Bajema CJ, Dietz WH. Long-term morbidity and mortality of overweight adolescents. A follow-up of the Harvard Growth Study of 1922 to 1935. *New England Journal of Medicine.* 1992 Nov 5;327(19):1350-5.

[42] Stevens J, Cai J, Pamuk ER, Williamson DF, Thun MJ, Wood JL. The effect of age on the association between body-mass index and mortality. *New England Journal of Medicine*. 1998 Jan 1;338(1):1-7.

[43] Rodriguez G, Moreno LA, Blay MG, Blay VA, Fleta J, Sarria A, et al. Body fat measurement in adolescents: comparison of skinfold thickness equations with dual-energy X-ray absorptiometry. *European Journal of Clinical Nutrition*. 2005 Oct;59(10):1158-66.

[44] Castro-Pinero J, Artero EG, Espana-Romero V, Ortega FB, Sjostrom M, Suni J, et al. Criterion-related validity of field-based fitness tests in youth: a systematic review. *British Journal of Sports Medicine*. 2009 Oct;44(13):934-43.

[45] Zimmet P, Alberti KG, Kaufman F, Tajima N, Silink M, Arslanian S, et al. The metabolic syndrome in children and adolescents - an IDF consensus report. *Pediatric Diabetes*. 2007 Oct;8(5):299-306.

[46] Qiao Q, Nyamdorj R. The optimal cutoff values and their performance of waist circumference and waist-to-hip ratio for diagnosing type II diabetes. *European Journal of Clinical Nutrition*. 2010 Jan;64(1):23-9.

[47] Lean ME, Han TS, Morrison CE. Waist circumference as a measure for indicating need for weight management. *BMJ*. 1995 Jul 15;311(6998):158-61.

[48] Savva SC, Tornaritis M, Savva ME, Kourides Y, Panagi A, Silikiotou N, et al. Waist circumference and waist-to-height ratio are better predictors of cardiovascular disease risk factors in children than body mass index. *International Journal of Obesity and Related Metabolic Disorders*. 2000 Nov;24(11):1453-8.

[49] Ortega FB, Ruiz JR, Sjostrom M. Physical activity, overweight and central adiposity in Swedish children and adolescents: the European Youth Heart Study. *The International Journal of Behavioral Nutrition and Physical Activity*. 2007;4:61.

[50] Ortega FB, Ruiz JR, Hurtig-Wennlof A, Vicente-Rodriguez G, Rizzo NS, Castillo MJ, et al. Cardiovascular fitness modifies the associations between physical activity and abdominal adiposity in children and adolescents: the European Youth Heart Study. *British Journal of Sports Medicine*. 2010 Mar;44(4):256-62.

[51] Ledoux M, Lambert J, Reeder BA, Despres JP. A comparative analysis of weight to height and waist to hip circumference indices as indicators of the presence of cardiovascular disease risk factors. Canadian Heart Health Surveys Research Group. *Canadian Medical Association Journal*. 1997 Jul 1;157 Suppl 1:S32-8.

[52] National Institute of Health and Clinical Excellence. Obesity: the prevention, identification, assessment and management of overweight and obesity in adults and children.[Online].December 2006. Available from: www.nice.org.uk/guidance/CG43. [Accessed 25th July 2011]; 2006

[53] APT III. Third report of the expert panel on detection, evaluation, and treatment of high blood cholesterol in adults, Adult Treatment Panel (APT) III: National Heart, Lung and Blood Institute; 2001. Report No.: 02-5215.

[54] Pischon T, Boeing H, Hoffmann K, Bergmann M, Schulze MB, Overvad K, et al. General and abdominal adiposity and risk of death in Europe. *New England Journal of Medicine*. 2008 Nov 13;359(20):2105-20.

[55] Goran MI, Gower BA, Treuth M, Nagy TR. Prediction of intra-abdominal and subcutaneous abdominal adipose tissue in healthy pre-pubertal children. *International Journal of Obesity and Related Metabolic Disorders*. 1998 Jun;22(6):549-58.

[56] Steinberger J, Jacobs DR, Raatz S, Moran A, Hong CP, Sinaiko AR. Comparison of body fatness measurements by BMI and skinfolds vs dual energy X-ray absorptiometry and their relation to cardiovascular risk factors in adolescents. *International Journal of Obesity* (Lond). 2005 Nov;29(11):1346-52.

[57] Slaughter MH, Lohman TG, Boileau RA, Horswill CA, Stillman RJ, Van Loan MD, et al. Skinfold equations for estimation of body fatness in children and youth. *Human. Biology.* 1988 Oct;60(5):709-23.

[58] Going SB, Lohman TG, Falls HB. Body Composition Assessment. In: Welk GJ, Meredith MD, editors. Fitnessgram / Activitygram Reference Guide (pp Internet Resource). Dallas, TX: *Human Kinetics*; 2008. p. 37-44.

[59] Williams DP, Going SB, Lohman TG, Harsha DW, Srinivasan SR, Webber LS, et al. Body fatness and risk for elevated blood pressure, total cholesterol, and serum lipoprotein ratios in children and adolescents. *American Journal of Public Health.* 1992 Mar;82(3):358-63.

[60] Bouchard C, Blair SN, Haskell WL. Why study physical activity and health? In: Bouchard C, Blair SN, Haskell WL, editors. *In* Physical Activity and Health. Leeds: Human Kinetics; 2007. p. 3-19.

[61] Haskell WL, Lee IM, Pate RR, Powell KE, Blair SN, Franklin BA, et al. Physical activity and public health: updated recommendation for adults from the American College of Sports Medicine and the American Heart Association. *Circulation.* 2007 Aug 28;116(9):1081-93.

[62] World Health Organization. Global Recommendations on Physical Activity for Health. Available from http://whqlibdoc.who.int/publications/2010/9789241599979_eng.pdf. Accessed 8th August 2011. Geneva: World Health Organization; 2010.

[63] Blair SN. Physical inactivity: the biggest public health problem of the 21st century. *British Journal of Sports Medicine.* 2009 Jan;43(1):1-2.

[64] Morris JN, Heady JA. Mortality in relation to the physical activity of work: a preliminary note on experience in middle age. *British Journal of Industrial Medicine.* 1953 Oct;10(4):245-54.

[65] Morris JN, Heady JA, Raffle PA, Roberts CG, Parks JW. Coronary heart-disease and physical activity of work. *Lancet.* 1953 Nov 28;265(6796):1111-20.

[66] Paffenbarger RS, Jr., Wing AL, Hyde RT. Physical activity as an index of heart attack risk in college alumni. *American Journal of Epidemiology.* 1978 Sep;108(3):161-75.

[67] Paffenbarger RS, Jr., Hyde RT, Wing AL, Hsieh CC. Physical activity, all-cause mortality, and longevity of college alumni. *New England Journal of Medicine.* 1986 Mar 6;314(10):605-13.

[68] American College of Sports Medicine. Position statement on the recommended quantity and quality of exercise for developing and maintaining fitness in healthy adults. Medicine & Science in Sports & Exercise. 1978;10:vii-x.

[69] Department of Health. Stay Active: a report on physical activity for health from the four home countries' Chief Medical Officers. London; 2011.

[70] US Department of Health and Human Services. Physical Activity Guidlines for Americans. Advisory Committee report 2008. Available from http://www.health.gov/paguidelines/Report/Default.aspx. Accessed 8th August 2011. Washington DC; 2008.

[71] Andersen LB, Riddoch C, Kriemler S, Hills A. Physical activity and cardiovascular risk factors in children. *British Journal of Sports Medicine*. In Press. Sep;45(11):871-6.

[72] Strong WB, Malina RM, Blimkie CJ, Daniels SR, Dishman RK, Gutin B, et al. Evidence based physical activity for school-age youth. *Journal of Pediatrics*. 2005 Jun;146(6):732-7.

[73] Janssen I, LeBlanc AG. Systematic review of the health benefits of physical activity and fitness in school-aged children and youth. *The International Journal of Behavioral Nutrition and Physical Activity*. 2010;7:40.

[74] Dobbins M, De Corby K, Robeson P, Husson H, Tirilis D. School-based physical activity programs for promoting physical activity and fitness in children and adolescents aged 6-18. Cochrane Database Syst Rev. 2009(1):CD007651.

[75] Ruiz JR, Rizzo NS, Hurtig-Wennlof A, Ortega FB, Warnberg J, Sjostrom M. Relations of total physical activity and intensity to fitness and fatness in children: the European Youth Heart Study. *American Journal of Clinical Nutrition*. 2006 Aug;84(2):299-303.

[76] Ekelund U, Sardinha LB, Anderssen S, Harro M, Franks PW, Brage S, et al. Associations between objectively assessed physical activity and indicators of body fatness in 9- to 10-y-old European children: a population-based study from 4 distinct regions in Europe (the European Youth Heart Study). *American Journal of Clinical Nutrition*. 2004 Sep;80(3):584-90.

[77] Hurtig-Wennlof A, Ruiz JR, Harro M, Sjostrom M. Cardiorespiratory fitness relates more strongly than physical activity to cardiovascular disease risk factors in healthy children and adolescents: the European Youth Heart Study. *European Journal of Cardiovascular Prevention & Rehabilitation*. 2007 Aug;14(4):575-81.

[78] Butte NF, Puyau MR, Adolph AL, Vohra FA, Zakeri I. Physical activity in nonoverweight and overweight Hispanic children and adolescents. *Medicine and Science in Sports and Exercise*. 2007 Aug;39(8):1257-66.

[79] Gutin B, Yin Z, Humphries MC, Barbeau P. Relations of moderate and vigorous physical activity to fitness and fatness in adolescents. *American Journal of Clinical Nutrition*. 2005 Apr;81(4):746-50.

[80] Kelley GA, Kelley KS, Tran ZV. The effects of exercise on resting blood pressure in children and adolescents: a meta-analysis of randomized controlled trials. *Preventive Cardiology*. 2003 Winter;6(1):8-16.

[81] Mark AE, Janssen I. Dose-response relation between physical activity and blood pressure in youth. *Medicine and Science in Sports and Exercise*. 2008 Jun;40(6):1007-12.

[82] Bauman A. Trends in exercise prevalence in Australia. *Community Health Studies*. 1987;11(3):190-6.

[83] McLure SA, Summerbell CD, Reilly JJ. Objectively measured habitual physical activity in a highly obesogenic environment. *Child: Care, Health and Development*. 2009 May;35(3):369-75.

[84] Troiano RP, Berrigan D, Dodd KW, Masse LC, Tilert T, McDowell M. Physical activity in the United States measured by accelerometer. *Medicine and Science in Sports and Exercise*. 2008 Jan;40(1):181-8.

[85] Armstrong N, Welsman JR. The physical activity patterns of European youth with reference to methods of assessment. *Sports Medicine*. 2006;36(12):1067-86.

[86] Riddoch CJ, Bo Andersen L, Wedderkopp N, Harro M, Klasson-Heggebo L, Sardinha LB, et al. Physical activity levels and patterns of 9- and 15-yr-old European children. *Medicine and Science in Sports and Exercise*. 2004 Jan;36(1):86-92.

Reviewed by: Dr Michael Graham, Principal Lecturer, Academic Lead and Head of Sport and Exercise Science, Glyndŵr University, Wrexham, LL11 2AW.

In: Youth: Practices, Perspectives and Challenges
Editor: Elizabeth Trejos-Castillo

ISBN: 978-1-62618-067-3
© 2013 Nova Science Publishers, Inc.

Chapter 3

TDM AS A TOOL FOR THE PERSONALIZATION OF PSYCHIATRIC TREATMENT IN CHILDREN AND ADOLESCENTS

Ioanna Vardakou[1], Constantinos Pistos[1]*, Chara Spiliopoulou[1] and Giorgos Alevizopoulos[2]

[1]Laboratory of Forensic Medicine and Toxicology, Medical School,
University of Athens, Greece
[2]Department of Psychiatry and Behavioral Sciences, Faculty of Nursing,
University of Athens, Greece

ABSTRACT

The safety and effectiveness of psychotropic drugs use in children and youth is widely debated, since both populations are being treated more and more with antipsychotic drugs and the risk of under- or overdosing and a delayed risk of long-term side effects, remains unclear. Recent research supports also the existence of Pharmacogenetic and age-associated differences that do not allow the direct application of pharmacokinetic data from adults to younger ages with simple extrapolation techniques. Since studies in children and adolescents are lacking for most of the psychotropic drugs, and the data are limited concerning genetic or age variabilities and long term effects, Therapeutic Drug Monitoring (TDM) appears to be a significant tool that optimizes pharmacotherapy by maximizing therapeutic efficacy, while minimizing adverse events.

Such TDM studies in these particular age groups, enable the identification of genetic and age dependent therapeutic ranges of blood concentrations and facilitate a more accurate documentation in the children and adolescents antipsychotic treatment, providing data for future research, as a baseline for example for clinically relevant interactions with various co-medications. Phycisians who are involved in the psychiatric

---

* Address Correspondence to: Dr. Constantinos Pistos, Assistant Professor of Toxicology, School of Medicine, University of Athens, Email: cpistos@med.uoa.gr.

treatment of youth must be aware of the therapeutic failure and/or the risk for side effects, if factors that might influence the pharmacokinetic of the prescribed medications would not be considered.

INTRODUCTION

Worldwide, the most prescribed antipsychotic agents are clozapine, quetiapine, amisulpride, olanzapine, aripiprazole, and risperidone (Tale 1). These agents reduce negative symptoms of schizophrenia, are effective in treatment refractory cases, and have a markedly lower incidence of extrapyramidal symptoms (EPS) and tardive dyskinesia (TD). However, there is considerable patient-to-patient variability in therapeutic dose requirements of atypical antipsychotics and the propensity for side effects is frequently observed. This risk of edverse events is increased in specific age groups such as youth, where metabolic enzymes and developmental factors avtivity is different versus other ages like adults or elderly people. The majority of side-effects associated with antipsychotic treatment are dose-related. These include EPS, sedation, postural hypotension, anticholinergic effects, QTc prolongation and sudden cardiac death [1].

In addition, there are significant risks associated with first and second-generation antipsychotics: weight gain, diabetes, hyperlipidemia particularly with the second-generation drugs [2, 3, 4], movement disorders [5, 6], hyperprolactinemia and cardiovascular adverse effects. The pharmacokinetic genes contribute to the differences in plasma level or tissue distribution of drugs and examples of pharmacokinetic genes are those coding for cytochrome P450 (CYP450), a set of enzymes involved in the first phase of metabolism of many antipsychotics. Some of CYP450 genes are highly polymorphic and it is thought that their variations can contribute to side effects of antipsychotics. The function of these genes is known, and the phenotypes resulted from their polymorphisms can be characterized by measuring drug metabolic ratios [7]. It is obvious that CYP450 enzyme sybstrate in children and adolescents possesses particular characteristics due to differential activity comparing to adults.

Developmental changes in physiology produce in addition, many of the age-associated changes in the absorption, distribution, metabolism, and excretion of psychotropic drugs following oral administration (most drugs are administered orally to children and adolescents) that result in altered pharmacokinetics and thus serve as the determinants of age-specific dose requirements. More than 100 years ago Dr. Abraham Jacobi, the father of American paediatrics, recognised the importance of and need for age-appropriate pharmacotherapy when he wrote, "Pediatrics does not deal with miniature men and women, with reduced doses and the same class of disease in smaller bodies, but ... has its own independent range and horizon [8]. The recognition that developmental changes profoundly affect the responses to medications (both efficacy and side effects) produced a need for age-dependent adjustment in doses. However, the selection of doses in paediatric patients requires a consideration of pharmacokinetic parameters, and warrants specific studies in children and adolescents. The term therapeutic drug monitoring (TDM) defines the laboratory measurement of a chemical parameter that, with appropriate clinical interpretation, will directly influence drug prescribing procedures [9].

Otherwise, TDM refers to the individualization of drug dosage by maintaining plasma or blood drug concentrations within a targeted therapeutic range [10]. By combining knowledge of pharmaceutics, pharmacokinetics, and pharmacodynamics, TDM enables the assessment of the efficacy and safety of a particular medication in a variety of clinical settings. The goal of this process is to individualize therapeutic regimens for optimal patient benefit [11].

AIM OF THE REVIEW

The present study gives a general perspective of the antipsychotic treatment in children and adolescents, and focuses on their variability response comparing to adults data due to genetic and age differences. Finally, the utilization of TDM practice is underlined and it is proposed as an appropriate tool for the improvement of dosing and drug safety of antipsychotic treatment of these age groups.

ATYPICAL ANTIPSYCHOTIC AGENTS

Most perscribed antipsychotic agents are clozapine, quetiapine, amisulpride, olanzapine, aripiprazole, and risperidone (Tale 1). These agents reduce negative symptoms of schizophrenia, are effective in treatment refractory cases, and have a markedly lower incidence of extrapyramidal symptoms (EPS) and tardive dyskinesia (TD). However, there is considerable patient-to-patient variability in therapeutic dose requirements of atypical antipsychotics and the propensity for side effects. Phases in dosage recommendations of APs, ensued over the coming decades with trials of very high doses [12] and trials of very low doses [13], with as usual, mixed results. In general, however, once blood levels of psychotropic drugs became widely available, it became apparent that very high doses provided no added value for the average patient and that measuring blood levels might help to some degree in explaining the heterogeneity of response [14].

The identification of dopamine as a key neurotransmitter in the mechanism of action of antipsychotic drugs and the discovery of various dopamine receptors in specific brain regions led to renewed enthusiasm about finding more "rational" pharmacologic agents and again setting the stage for further progress in understanding dosage requirements and heterogeneity of response. Concerns regarding dose-response (and dose-tolerability) relationships were also an important focus in evaluating comparative data between first- and second-generation antipsychotics.

Although some reviews and meta-analyses had suggested that some of the apparent superiority of second- versus first-generation antipsychotics was due to unnecessarily high dosages of first-generation medications [15], other reviews did not support this conclusion [16, 17]. The initial excitement since the introduction of atypical antipsychotics is now shifting towards a focus on individualization of pharmacotherapy and elucidation of the mechanistic basis of interindividual variability in drug response with use of pharmacokinetic and pharmacodynamic biomarkers.

Clozapine

Clozapine, a tricyclic dibenzodiazepine derivative, is classified as an atypical antipsychotic drug, due to its complex pharmacologic properties and different effects that produce comparing to those exhibited by more typical antipsychotic drugs. Clozapine is efficacious for the treatment of patients with schizophrenia who fail to show an acceptable response to standard antipsychotic drugs [18]. Clozapine plasma levels are broadly related to daily dose, but there is sufficient variation to make impossible any precise prediction of plasma level. Plasma levels are generally lower in younger patients, males and smokers [19] and higher in Asians [20]. A series of algorithms has been developed for the approximate prediction of clozapine levels according to patient factor [21]. Algorithms cannot account for other influences on clozapine plasma levels such as changes in adherence, inflammation [22] and infection [23].

The plasma level threshold for acute response to clozapine has been suggested to be 370 μg/L [24], 420 μg/L [25], 200 μg/L [26], 350 μg/L [27], 504 μg/L [28] and 550 μg/L [29]. Limited data series suggest that a level of at least 200 μg/L is required to prevent relapse [30]. In non-responders to clozapine, dose should be adjusted to give plasma levels in the range 350–500 μg/L. Those not tolerating clozapine may benefit from a reduction to a dose giving plasma levels in this range. An upper limit to the clozapine target range has not been defined. Plasma levels do seem to predict EEG changes [31] and seizures occur more frequently in patients with levels above 1000 μg/L [32], so levels should probably be kept well below this. Other non-neurological clozapine-related adverse effects also seem to be plasma level related [33] as might be expected. Owing to the complex metabolism of clozapine and its metabolites, plasma concentrations are influenced by smoking, gender, age, and the concomitant administration of other drugs.

Table 1. Atypical antipsychotic drug mechanisms of action

Genetic name	Pharmacodynamics
Clozapine	Antagonist at D1-3,5 receptors, with high affinity for D4 receptors. Also antagonist at serotonergic, adrenergic, cholinergic, and histaminergic receptors.
Quetiapine	Antagonist at D1-2, 5HT 1A-2A, norepinephrine transporter (NET), H1, M1, and α1b-2, receptors.
Olanzapine	Selective monaminergic antagonist with high affinity binding to 5-HT2A/2C, 5-HT6, D1-4, histamine H1, and α1-adrenergic receptors.
Amisulpride	Selectively dopamine D2 and D3 receptor antagonist. Potent antagonist at the 5-HT$_7$ receptor.
Aripiprazole	Partial agonist at D2 and 5-HT1A receptors, antagonist at 5-HT2A receptors. High affinity for D2, D3, 5-HT1A, and 5-HT2A receptors; moderate affinity for D4, 5-HT2C, 5-HT7, - α -adrenergic and H1 receptors. Moderate affinity for the serotonin reuptake site and no appreciable affinity for cholinergic muscarinic receptors.
Risperidone	Antagonist with high affinity binding to 5-HT2 and D2 receptors. Antagonist at H1, and α1-2 receptors.

The metabolism involves several P450 enzymes, in particular CYP1A2, with contributions from CYP3A4, and, to a lesser extent, CYP2D6. CYP1A2 enzyme accounts for approximately 70% of clozapine metabolism. It catalyzes the passage of clozapine to N-Demethyl-Clozapine in the liver, so that variations of the CYP1A2 activity has been related to drug clearance [34]. Considering these facts, a role of pharmacogenetic biomarker has been postulated for CYP1A2 in the treatment with clozapine [34, 35]. Note also that clozapine metabolism may become saturated at higher doses: the ratio of clozapine to norclozapine rises with increasing plasma levels, suggesting saturation [36]. Genotyping of the CYP enzymes has so far not been of any advantage in dosing of clozapine because the CYP1A2 remain the major metabolic pathway but genotyping of pharmacodynamic or pharmacokinetic mechanisms may be promising in the future. Unless intoxication is indicated, plasma levels should be obtained after steady-state concentration has been achieved (5-7 days) [37]. Blood sample should be drawn 12 ± 1 h postdose [38].

Quetiapine

The dose of quetiapine is weakly related to trough plasma levels [39, 40]. Mean levels reported within the dose range 150 mg/day to 800 mg/day range from 27 µg/L to 387 µg/L [41, 42], although the highest and lowest levels are not necessarily found at the lowest and highest doses. Age, gender and co-medication may contribute to the significant inter-individual variance observed in TDM studies, with female gender [42], older age and CYP3A4-inhibiting drugs [43, 44] likely to increase quetiapine concentration. Reports of these effects are conflicting [42] and not sufficient to support the routine use of plasma level monitoring based on these factors alone. Thresholds for clinical response have been proposed as 77 µg/L [39] and 50–100 µg/L (EPS has been observed in females with levels exceeding 210 µg/L. Despite the substantial variation in plasma levels at each dose, there is insufficient evidence to suggest a target therapeutic range, thus plasma level monitoring has little value. Current reports of quetiapine concentrations are from trough samples, because of the short half life of quetiapine, plasma levels tend to drop to within a relatively small range regardless of dose and previous peak level. Thus peak plasma levels may be more closely related to dose and clinical response, although monitoring is not currently justified in the absence of an established peak plasma target range. Quetiapine has an established dose–response relationship, and appears to be well tolerated at doses well beyond the licensed dose range. In practice, dose adjustment should be based on patient response and tolerability [45]. This drug similarly started out indicated for schizophrenia and bipolar mania comparable to risperidone and olanzapine. Similarly, higher doses (400–800 mg/d) are required to control the symptoms associated with these disorders [46], while very high doses of quetiapine (800 mg/d up to 2400 mg/d) have also reported [47]. Its D2 receptor antagonism is quite weak compared to all other second generation antipsychotics (SGA) and may be considered as a low potency or low affinity drug. This does not suggest it has low effectiveness, but rather requires more dosing milligrams to maintain at least 60% receptor occupancy to stop psychosis or mania. This low affinity may allow for quetiapine to maintaining a lower EPS side effect profile as a benefit [48]. A slow release, once daily version of quetiapine has been approved which may improve compliance. Absorption of the immediate and slow release products is predictable, though the slow release product achieves peak plasma levels, and likely sedating side effects, 3–4 h post dose [49]. This drug also is now approved as a monotherapy for bipolar depression and also as an augmentation strategy that is, added to selective serotonin reuptake inhibitors (SSRI's) or selective serotonin norepinephrine reuptake inhibitors (SNRI's) antidepressants, in unipolar major depressive disorder. Similar to the lower dose effectiveness potential in the off-label use of risperidone in depression, multiple, confirmative, regulatory studies have consistently shown that lower doses of quetiapine are quite effective in treating depressive states [50, 51].

Quetiapine is the only SGA approved as a monotherapy for bipolar depression. In theory it has very good antidepressant potential as such and observing its unique pharmacodynamic profile is worthy of discussion. Quetiapine has an active metabolite, norquetiapine, and between the parent drug and its metabolite many antidepressant and anxiolytic properties emerge [52]. This drug has remarkable H-1 receptor antagonism and similar to olanzapine may promote sedation and metabolic disorder onset [47]. H-1 receptor blockade can produce fatigue as a side effect but also somnolence as a bona fide clinical hypnotic effect [53]. Sometimes these side effects cause patients to stop taking this medication and sometimes these clinical effects improve sleep or agitation. Finally, the anticholinergic activity of quetiapine is quite low, so these side effects are largely avoided. Quetiapine has 5HT-2a and 2c antagonism, which lowers EPS rates and improves cognition likely as discussed for other SGAs.

Norquetiapine has two interesting features. First, it allows for 5HT-1a receptor agonism. Second, this metabolite has a very potent norepinephrine reuptake inhibitor (NRI) property which is similar to NRI properties possessed by FDA approved unipolar antidepressants such as venlafaxine, duloxetine, bupropion, nortryptiline, and desipramine [47]. Similar to these FDA approved agents in clinical application; one might expect improvements in cognition, energy, concentration, depression, and anxiety as a result. Again, it is likely that at lower doses of quetiapine, the drug is less effective at antagonizing and lowering dopamine activity resulting in an inability to treat psychosis and mania at low doses, but clinically has the potential to treat depression at low doses based on the serotonergic and noradrenergic pharmacodynamic properties noted above and per confirmatory regulatory trials showing clinical efficacy [54].

Olanzapine

Plasma levels of olanzapine are linearly related to daily dose, but there is substantial variation [55], with higher levels seen in women [56], non-smokers [57] and those on enzyme-inhibiting drugs [58]. With once-daily dosing, the threshold level for response in schizophrenia has been suggested to be 9.3 µg/L (trough sample) [59], 23.2 µg/L (12-hour post-dose sample) [56] and 23 µg/L at a mean of 13.5 hours postdose [60]. There is evidence to suggest that levels greater than 40 µg/L have no further therapeutic benefit [42]. Severe toxicity is uncommon but may be associated with levels above 100 µg/L, and death is occasionally seen at levels above 160 µg/L [61] (albeit when other drugs or physical factors are relevant). A target range for therapeutic use of 20–40 µg/L (12-hour post-dose sample) has been proposed [62] for schizophrenia (the range for mania is probably similar) [63]. Notably, significant weight gain seems most likely to occur in those with plasma levels above 20 µg/L. Constipation, dry mouth and tachycardia also seem to be plasma level related [64].

Olanzapine has a slightly more complicated pharmacodynamic profile when compared to risperidone and paliperidone. Along with D2 receptors has the ability to antagonize 5-HT2a receptors thus keeping EPS rates low when compared to FGAs. Olanzapine blocks 5-HT2c receptors as well. This action at 5-HT2c receptors may allow better norepinephrine and dopamine cortical activity through enhancing mesocortical pathways [65]. Enhancing dorsolateral prefrontal cortex DA activity through this 5-HT2c receptor antagonism, in theory, might enhance cognition, attention, concentration, and executive functioning. Olanzapine also has higher affinities to antagonize cholinergic muscarinic receptors and histamine-1 (H-1) receptors. Anticholinergic dry mouth, constipation, blurred vision, and memory problems, sedation, weight gain, and metabolic disorder side effects are likely to occur, respectively [66].

Amisulpride

Amisulpride plasma levels are closely related to dose with insufficient variation to recommend routine plasma level monitoring. Higher levels observed in women [67, 68] and older age [58] seem to have little significant clinical implication for either therapeutic response or adverse effects. A (trough) threshold for clinical response has been suggested to be approximately 100 µg/L and mean levels of 367 µg/L [58] noted in responders in individual studies. Adverse effects (notably EPS) have been observed at mean levels of 336 µg/L, 377 µg/L [69] and 395 µg/L [68].

A plasma level threshold of below 320µg/L has been found to predict avoidance of EPS [69]. Sparshatt et al. suggested that an approximate range of 200 µg/L to 320 µg/L leads to optimum clinical response and prevention of adverse effects [70]. In practice amisulpride plasma level monitoring is rarely undertaken and few laboratories offer amisulpride assays. The dose-response relationship is sufficiently robust to obviate the need for plasma sampling within the licensed dose range; adverse effects are well managed by dose adjustment alone. Plasma level monitoring is best reserved for those in whom clinical response is poor, adherence is questioned and in whom drug interactions or physical illness may make adverse effect more likely [71].

Aripiprazole

In practice plasma level monitoring of aripiprazole is rarely carried out. The dose–response relationship of aripiprazole is well established with a plateau in clinical response and D2 dopamine occupancy seen in doses above approximately 10 mg/day [72]. Plasma levels of aripiprazole, its metabolite, and the total moiety (parent plus metabolite) strongly relate linearly to dose, making it possible to predict, with some certainty, an approximate plasma level for a given dose.

Target plasma level ranges for optimal clinical response have been suggested as 146–254 µg/L and 150–300 µg/L, with adverse effects observed above 210 µg/L. Interindividual variation in aripiprazole plasma levels has been observed but not fully investigated, although gender appears to have little influence [73, 74]. Age, metabolic enzyme genotype and interacting medications seem likely causes of variation [74], however there are too few reports regarding their clinical implication to recommend specific monitoring in light of these factors. A putative range of between 150 μg/L and 210 μg/L, has been suggested as a target for patients taking aripiprazole who are showing little or no clinical response or intolerable EPS.

In regard to dosing, aripiprazole shows a difference depending upon which illness is being treated similar to other SGAs. Originally approved for treating psychosis from schizophrenia at doses starting from 15 mg up to 30 mg/d, this drug was secondarily approved to treat mania starting at 30 mg/d [75]. This higher dosing strategy uses aripiprazole's high D2 receptor affinity, despite partial D2 receptor agonism to lower dopamine neurotransmission. There is very little literature evidence showing super dosing above the approved limit of 30 mg/d. This agent was also approved for treating unipolar depression in those patients who failed to respond to initial antidepressant dosing. Aripiprazole was the first FDA approved drug for use as an augmentation strategy in major depressive disorder [75, 76].

Dosing in major depressive disorder is again low and ranges from 2 to 15 mg/d with the average dose being approximately 10 mg/d, which is much lower than doses used in schizophrenia or mania [77, 78]. At these doses, a reduction in dopamine transmission is not required. Instead, promoting dopamine, norepinephrine and serotonin likely occurs as the principal mechanism of action. More recently, this drug was approved for treating irritability due to autism in children in low doses of 2– 15 mg/d [78]. In regard to treating anxiety disorders, this drug contains robust activity partially agonizing 5HT-1a receptors similar to the mechanism of action for the FDA approved anxiolytic buspirone. Small open-label studies exist for generalized anxiety disorder (GAD) or panic disorder (PD) with suggested effectiveness in these patients at doses on average of 13.9 mg/d [79, 80]. Lower doses of aripiprazole seem to be effective in treating depression and anxiety where higher doses are required for mania and schizophrenia. From an adverse effect point of view, aripiprazole is known for its higher probability of inducing akathisia [75]. This may be due to its high D2 receptor affinity, but also may be due to its overall monoaminergic activity where restlessness and agitation may be confused with more traditional akathisa. This agent is felt to be more metabolically friendly in regards to minimizing weight gain. Finally, this drug is known to be a 2D6 liver enzyme substrate [71].

Risperidone

Risperidone plasma levels are rarely measured and very few laboratories have developed assay methods for its determination. The therapeutic range for risperidone is 20–60 μg/L of the active moiety (risperidone + 9-OH-risperidone) [81, 82]. Plasma levels of this magnitude are usually provided by oral doses of between 3 mg and 6 mg a day [81, 83]. Occupancy of striatal dopamine D2 receptors has been shown to be around 65% (the minimum required for therapeutic effect) at plasma levels of approximately 20 μg/L [82]. Risperidone long-acting injection (25 mg/2 weeks) appears to afford plasma levels averaging between 4.4 and 22.7 μg/L. Dopamine D2 occupancies at this dose have been variously estimated at between 25% and 71% [82, 84, 85], and there is considerable inter-individual variation around these mean values.

SIDE EFFECTS OF ANTIPSYCHOTIC TREATMENT

The majority of side-effects associated with antipsychotic treatment are dose-related. These include EPS, tardive dyskinesia, sedation, postural hypotension, anticholinergic effects, QTc prolongation and sudden cardiac death [1]. In addition, there are significant risks associated with first and second-generation antipsychotics: weight gain, diabetes, hyperlipidemia particularly with the second-generation drugs [2, 3, 4], movement disorders [5, 6], hyperprolactinemia and cardiovascular adverse effects. It is unknown if these risks compound when antipsychotics are prescribed in combinations [86]. Intolerable adverse effects and lack of efficacy contribute to a significant proportion of antipsychotic discontinuations [87]. Llerena et al [88] studied a sample of white Europeans treated with risperidone and demonstrated that the QTc interval was longer in the subjects with one active 2D6 gene compared with subject with two active genes. In their review, [89] describe that the number of 2D6 active genes was correlated with the QTc interval lengthening in patients treated with thioridazine and conclude that 2D6 phenotype and genotype must be taken into consideration in treatment with patients with other risk factors for long QT for example heart disease, congenital long QT, elderly. High-dose of antipsychotic treatment clearly worsens adverse effect incidence and severity [90], while polypharmacy (with the exception of augmentation strategies for clozapine) also seems to be ineffective [91, 92, 93] and to produce more severe adverse effects including increased mortality [1, 92]. A recent meta-analysis [94], revealed small but significant benefit for polypharmacy over single-drug treatment but this was in the context of poor-quality studies and publication bias. There is some evidence that dose reduction leads to improvements in cognition and negative symptoms [95]. The use of high-dose antipsychotics should be an exceptional clinical practice and only ever employed when standard treatments, including clozapine, have failed. Documentation of target symptoms, response and side-effects, ideally using validated rating scales, should be standard practice so that there is ongoing consideration of the risk–benefit ratio for the patient. In these cases, close physical monitoring is essential. The indications for drug monitoring have widened to include efficacy, compliance, drug-drug interactions, toxicity avoidance, and therapy cessation monitoring [96].

Extrapyramidal adverse effects of antipsychotics have been attributed to dopamine (D2) receptor blockade exceeding 80% [97]. Acute extrapyramidal effects including parkinsonism, dystonia and akathisia have been the subject of very few pharmacogenetic studies [98] and Kaiser et al. [99] found no association of D2 receptor polymorphisms with these side effects. Akathisia, described by Barnes et al. [100] as a subjective feeling of restlessness, urge to move constantly and dysphoria, is frequently present with first generation antipsychotic agents, but 7%–8% patients experience it with second generation agents like risperidone and aripiprazole [101, 102]. Akathisia has been regarded as a possible precursor of TD [103], which is a hyperkinetic, purposeless, repetitive, persistent drug induced movement disorder which occurs in 20%–30% of patients with prolonged antipsychotic treatment [104]. TD has been a major focus of antipsychotic pharmacogenetic studiesy [105]. CATIE study confirmed that the risk of tardive dyskinesia is associated to patient's age, duration of antipsychotic exposure, exposure to conventional antipsychotics, anticholinergic medications, substance abuse, presence of extrapyramidal side effects and akathisia [105]. In addition to these known predictors, it is believed that a genetic component contributes to development of TD. Based on animal studies, pathophysiology of TD was attributed to up-regulation of the dopamine receptors and their hypersensitivity due to dopamine blockade by antipsychotic drugs [106].

The dopamine D2-family of receptors have been the focus of pharmacogenetic studies, along with serotonin receptor polymorphisms and hepatic isoenzyme genes. Polymorphisms of metabolic enzymes like CYP450 genes 2D6, 1A2, 3A4, have studied to explore their potential association with TD [107, 108, 109] and [110]. In these studies, it was found that polymorphisms of 2D6 resulting in reduced activity of this enzyme correlated positively with higher AIMS [111] scores and the development of TD. Furthermore, a polymorphism of CYP1A2 gene was significantly associated with TD severity in a study by [112] with even more pronounced effect in the smoker group of the sample of Caucasians and African Americans, while [113] did not replicate these results in a German sample. Among the metabolic disturbances associated with the use of antipsychotic drugs, weight gain has come to the attention of patients, families, care providers and the general public especially with the development of second generation antipsychotic drugs. There is abundant information about the association of antipsychotic treatment with risk of obesity, cardiovascular disease and their dire consequences on general health and life expectancy [114, 115]. While risks of weight gain are defined for various antipsychotics [116] front line practitioners have limited tools to predict patients at risk. This individual variability can only lead one to suspect that the interaction of genes and environment is heavily illustrated in this area. [116].

Quetiapine's adverse effect profile shows remarkable sedation, favorable EPS rates, and a fair risk for metabolic disorders. Until recently, it was unclear if metabolic symptoms emerged in a dose-dependent fashion or if any exposure to quetiapine created risk for weight gain, hyperlipidemia, or hyperglucosemia. Quetiapine XR has now been studied from 50 to 600 mg/d in a myriad of psychiatric disorders and regulatory data would suggest that doses around 150 mg/d may be safer than those at 300 mg/d. For example, weight gain and hyperglycemia nearly comparable to placebo rates, whereas 300 mg nearly doubled these two side effects' prevalence in acute studies. This data was obtained when quetiapineXR was being studied for antidepressant augmentation in unipolar depression [71, 117]. The upper limit of dosage or plasma levels of clozapine has received scant attention in the literature. Risk of seizure seems to grow as a function of the plasma level [118, 119, 120], and dosages above 600 mg have thus been associated with an increased risk of seizure [121]. Likewise, cognitive functions, such as vigilance and memory, have been shown to deteriorate with rising plasma levels [122]. No dose relationship has been established in connection with other serious adverse events, such as myocarditis [123], cardiomyopathy, and agranulocytosis [124]. A Chinese study [125] found that concentrations above 700 ng / ml were associated with diminished rates of response, suggesting an inverted curvilinear concentration–response curve. A retrospective study by Ulrich et al. [126], found plasma levels above 900 ng /ml to be associated with intoxication. Other studies have failed to identify an upper limit of response [25, 27].

PHARMACOGENETICS AND AGE ASSOCIATED VARIABILITY

Pharmacogenetics is defined by the European Medicines Agency (EMEA) as the "study of interindividual variations in DNA sequence related to drug response" [127, 128]. These genetic variations may be due to the existence of: i) mutations or polymorphisms that affect one or very few nucleotides. The SNPs (single nucleotide polymorphisms) may be nonsynonymous (if they imply a change in any amino acid of the protein or modify promoter activity) or synomymous (if their alteration does not cause amino acid change; ii) variable number of tandem repeats (VNRT); and iii) events of increase or loss of large genoma regions, which is known as CNVs (Copy Number Variants), as occurs with the CYP2D6 gene. It has been postulated that other factors such as the epigenetics, fundamentally the variation in the methylation patterns, may also be involved in the variability of the drug response. For these reasons, pharmacogenetics appears to provide opportunities for informed decision-making along the pharmaceutical pipeline [129]. The ultimate aim of pharmacogenetic research is to introduce pre-treatment testing that would allow personalization of therapies in terms of drug choice or drug dose, and thereby improve clinical outcomes [130]. However, there is also increasing realization that testing will need to adhere to standards. To this end, the Analytic validity, Clinical validity, Clinical utility and Ethical, legal and social implications model has been developed to structure the assessment of pharmacogenetic diagnostic tests [131].

The pharmacokinetic genes contribute to the differences in plasma level or tissue distribution of drugs. Examples of pharmacokinetic genes are those coding for cytochrome P450 (CYP450), a set of enzymes involved in the first phase of metabolism of many antipsychotics. Some of CYP450 genes are highly polymorphic and it is thought that their variations can contribute to side effects of antipsychotics. The function of these genes is known, and the phenotypes resulted from their polymorphisms can be characterized by measuring drug metabolic ratios [132]. Four predictive phenotypes can be differentiated, depending on the combination of the alleles present in an individual. Extensive metabolizers (EM) are characterized the individuals with normal metabolism who have 1 to 2 active copies of the gene. It is clear that most of the population has this genotype. Intermediate metabolizers (IMs) are those individuals who have one inactive copy and another with reduced activity. Others reserve this term for those having a single active copy of the gene, (with which the EMs would be those having two active copies). Furthermore, it is believed that this category only has experimental interest, since phenotypically IMs do not seem to be distinguished from EMs. Thus, both phenotypes are generally grouped when clinically oriented genotyping is made.

Those individuals who have not inherited any active copy of the gene, either because they have two copies of a defective enzyme with decreased activity, or because they only have one copy of the gene (the other copy would be deleted) and this is defective or even because they totally lack the gene (both copies deleted, which is extremely rare), have very slow metabolism related to the normal one and they are called poor metabolizers (PM). This pattern is that which is most frequently associated with the appearance of adverse effects. On the contrary to the previous case, there is the possibility that the individual may have more than two active copies of the gene and they are called ultrarapid metabolizers (UM) [133]. Metabolic categories have variable distribution between ethnic groups for example 5%-10% of Caucasians are poor metabolizers while 29% of North Eastern Africans and Middle Easterners are ultrarapid metabolizers [134, 135, 136]. The traditional idea in pharmacogenetic studies of the cytochrome P450 (CYP) metabolic isoenzymes has been that the subjects called poor metabolizers (PMs) (who lack activity for that isoenzyme [135, 137] are the "problem patients" genetically speaking, because PMs using average doses may be more prone to adverse drug reactions (ADRs). Patients with 3 or more active copies including the so-called ultrarapid metabolizers (UMs) [135, 137] or even the extensive metabolizers (EMs) with 2 active alleles. These patients may be difficult to manage for genetic reasons, because of the potential for poor efficacy of the average doses of drugs. If this hypothesis is correct, the prevalence of these non-responders for genetic reasons may be much higher for drugs with wide therapeutic windows than for those with narrow therapeutic windows.

Four P450 enzymes are of particular importance for clinical psychopharmacology: CYP1A2, CYP2C19, CYP2D6 and CYP3A4 [138]. Numerous authors suggested that genotyping for families of CYP450 enzymes (2D6, 2C19) could potentially aid in prescribing antipsychotic drugs [7, 136, 139, 140]. Cytochrome P450 (CYP450) microsomal enzymes mediate approximately 80% of the oxidative drug metabolism. More than 50% of the drugs responsible for adverse drug reactions are metabolized by polymorphic phase-one metabolism enzymes and of these, 86% are CYP450 [135]. One or more CYP450 enzymes may contribute to the oxidative metabolism of a given drug. CYP2D6 metabolizes many psychotropic drugs, including antipsychotics like haloperidol, thioridazine, perphenazine, chlorpromazine, risperidone, aripiprazole [7, 140] and levomepromazine [141]. CYP2D6 is a highly polymorphic gene with more than 70 variants, resulting in four above mentioned phenotypes. CYP450 1A2 and 3A4 are important in metabolism of antipsychotics [7, 136] but individual genetic factors are yet to be clearly recognized in the activity of these enzymes [135]. CYP1A2 is the major enzyme involved in the metabolism of several psychotropic drugs, such as clozapine [142]. The CYP3A subfamily consists of four enzymes, and together they make up 30% of the total P450 liver content [138]. The major form in the human liver and in gut mucosa is CYP3A4. CYP3A4 catalyses the biotransformation of carbamazepine [143]. Regarding CYP2D6, approximately 7% of whites are CYP2D6 PMs, whereas 1% to 3% in other races are CYP2D6 PMs [135, 137]. Regarding CYP2C19, approximately one fourth of east Asians are CYP2C19 PMs, whereas less than 5% in other races are CYP2C19 PMs [137]. The extreme cases of CYP PMs, who are PMs for both CYP2D6 and CYP2C19, are rare subjects (<1% in all races) [144]. Webster and collegues indicated that current antipsychotics may be the ideal place for implementing pharmacogenetic techniques, since they are efficacious in only 30% of patients and tend to have a narrow therapeutic window [145]. Considering the above, Roses [129], correctly on the authors opinion, suggested that, the future may lead to recommendations that would determine the best drug and the best dose for a particular patient, which determination is called "efficacy pharmacogenetics".

THERAPEUTIC DRUG MONITORING

The term therapeutic drug monitoring (TDM) defines the laboratory measurement of a chemical parameter that, with appropriate clinical interpretation, will directly influence drug prescribing procedures [9]. Otherwise, TDM refers to the individualization of drug dosage by maintaining plasma or blood drug concentrations within a targeted therapeutic range [10]. By combining knowledge of pharmaceutics, pharmacokinetics, and pharmacodynamics, TDM enables the assessment of the efficacy and safety of a particular medication in a variety of clinical settings. The goal of this process is to individualize therapeutic regimens for optimal patient benefit [11]. TDM is used mainly for monitoring drugs with narrow therapeutic window, drugs with marked pharmacokinetic variability, medications which are difficult to monitor target concentrations, and drugs known to cause therapeutic and adverse effects. The process of TDM is predicated on the assumption that there is a definable relationship between dose and plasma or blood drug concentration, and, subsequently, between concentration and therapeutic effects. TDM begins when the drug is first prescribed, and involves determining an initial dosage regimen appropriate for the clinical condition and such patient characteristics as age, weight, organ function, concomitant drug therapy and gene variations. When interpreting concentration measurements, factors that need to be considered include the sampling time in relation to drug dose, dosage history, patient response, and the desired biological targets. The goal of TDM is to use appropriate concentrations of difficult-to-manage medications to optimize clinical outcomes in patients in various clinical conditions [11].

The monitoring of atypical antipsychotics (APs) in the blood of patients has been widely introduced in daily practice. Psychiatrists are becoming more and more aware of the beneficial effects of TDM [38, 146, 147] which is accepted for some of the antipsychotics such as clozapine [148] or haloperidol [149]. Antipsychotics tend to act in a slow, approximate manner. A few patients develop rapid, response, while most of them get better over time, and some do not respond at all. Due to the delayed and unstable response, clinicians may prescribe very high drug dosages early in the treatment that can increase the incidence of side effects and treatment drop-outs. Although there is no robust clinical benefit of TDM for the 2nd generation antipsychotics [56, 150], physicians are highly interested in TDM in cases of therapy resistance, side effects [151] or poor compliance. Thus, TDM of a number of psychotropic medications has proven to be of value, enabling minimization of the limitations of considerable genetic variability in their metabolism and the high rates of poor compliance with many psychiatric disorders. In summary, therapeutic drug monitoring of antipsychotic drugs has proven to be of notable value for determining poor compliance of patients and addressing the challenges associated with considerable genetic or developmental variability in their metabolism. It is essential to notice that, in order to conduct pharmacology and toxicology studies and clinical TDM of antipsychotics, as well as address the challenges associated with polypharmacy and drug metabolism, highly sensitive, selective and accurate bioanalytical methods are essential [152].

PERSONALIZED PRESCRIPTION

More than 100 years ago Dr. Abraham Jacobi, the father of American paediatrics, recognised the importance of and need for age-appropriate pharmacotherapy when he wrote, "Pediatrics does not deal with miniature men and women, with reduced doses and the same class of disease in smaller bodies, but ... has its own independent range and horizon [8]. The recognition that developmental changes profoundly affect the responses to medications (both efficacy and side effects) produced a need for age-dependent adjustment in doses. However, the selection of doses in paediatric patients requires a consideration of pharmacokinetic parameters, and warrants specific studies in children and adolescents. Personalized medicine is health care that tailors interventions to individual variation in risk and treatment response [153]. Drug marketing and all the studies related to drug registration are geared toward recommending an "average" dosage for an "average" patient. However, there are many patients who are not "average". Patients used by pharmaceutical companies to participate phase two or three clinical trials are relatively healthy patients with no comorbidities and few co-medications. In the "real" world, a lot of individuals do not meet the criteria of the "average patient", for genetic or environmental reasons. Moreover, an unavoidable environmental factor, polypharmacy, is becoming the norm in the Consultation-Liaison (C-L)/Med-Psych setting and in all psychiatric settings [154].

Until today, limited attempts have been performed to propose personalization dosing for psychiatric drugs. Kirchheiner et al. (2004) [139] investigated the personalization of dosing with studies of blood levels, assuming that these medications may follow linear kinetics. They proposed modifying some antipsychotic (AP) dosages based on the fact that some of them are metabolized by some polymorphic cytochrome P450 (CYP) enzymes. Any dosing personalization needs to be anchored in understanding of the pharmacologic response of each drug [155], it's pharmacodynamic and pharmacokinetic actions, and that they can be influenced by the environment, particularly drug-drug interactions, and by genetic variations. Environmental influences tend to be temporary, present only as long as the environmental factor is present, while genetic variations would tend to be longstanding and permanent. Information on the relative importance of genetic effects on AP response is limited by the difficulty of conducting twin and family studies in this area [156].

Although other studies suggest that only approximately half of patients may need "unusual" doses be cause of pharmacokinetic factors [157], it is obvious that there is a need to pay careful attention to personalizing dosing and that many patients need doses higher or lower than those usually recommended. The demonstration of a genetically determined metabolism of antipsychotics was one of the next steps. Consequently, this encouraged clinicians to use TDM in combination with pharmacogenetic tests [139, 158, 159]. In this direction, consensus guidelines aim to optimize the use of TDM of antipsychotics and to recommend when the combination of TDM and genotyping/phenotyping procedures, may improve therapeutic efficacy. Therefore, the indications for TDM, taking into account the different classes of drugs, had to be defined, the most relevant reports of the literature had to be selected, especially also with regard to reference values of plasma concentrations (therapeutic windows) and steady-state drug concentrations at clinically relevant doses. There was also a general need for recommendations regarding the practice of TDM in the clinical context and in the laboratory [159].

CHILD AND ADOLESCENT APS TREATMENT

The field of child and adolescent psychiatry attracts a significant attention during the last years, due to the increasing awareness of psychiatric disorders in these younger age groups, and increasing possibilities for treatment, including psychopharmacological treatment modalities. However, pharmacological treatment of children and adolescents is largely based on evidence from adults' studies that results in an increasing awareness that such evidence is not sufficient and does not always apply to children and adolescents, with subsequent failure of the treatment. APs are frequently prescribed in children and adolescents as first-line treatment for schizophrenia and other mental disorders despite the metabolic adverse side effects often reported. Unfortunately, most AP drugs used in these ages are applied "off label" with a direct risk of under- or overdosing and a delayed risk of long-term side effects. The selection of doses in paediatric psychiatric patients requires a consideration of pharmacokinetic parameters and the development of central nervous system (CNS), and warrants specific studies in children and adolescents [160].

Inadequate weight gain and obesity, hypertension, and lipid and glucose abnormalities are common metabolic side effects of great concern for the long lasting consequences of APs therapy. Moreover, the particular vulnerability of young people to these metabolic side effects seems to predict adult obesity, metabolic syndrome, and cardiovascular morbidity [161, 162]. Therefore, the evaluation of the long-term outcomes of early antipsychotic administration in animal models regarding endocrine and metabolic function becomes of increasing relevance. In addition, to the best of our knowledge few data on the cognitive consequences of antipsychotic treatment in children are currently available [163], and possible long-term effects have been scarcely investigated [164]. Studies in children are relatively rare, or are limited by design (open label, small group size and short duration) since they were not only difficult to carry out from a practical point of view [165, 166], but they were also considered, until recently, as ethically difficult to defend. Furthermore, evidence from studies in adults was considered applicable to children, with extrapolation consisting mostly of adjustment of the doses to suit children's lower body weight [167]. That means lack of knowledge regarding the efficacy of pharmacological treatment and its safety, particularly long-term safety [168, 169, 170]. Recently, however, there is an increasing awareness that children are not mere small adults, and that efficacy and safety established in adults, cannot be simply extrapolated to children without further investigation. Effective and safe use of medication in children and adolescents needs to be based on evidence that is specific for this age group [171, 172]. Considering the above, it can be clearly supported that clinical studies in children and adolescents, should be supported by PK and dose response studies. The following age classification is suggested in the ICH and CHMP guidelines: newborn infants (0 to 27 days), infants and toddlers (28 days to 23 month), children (2 to 11 years) and adolescents (12 to 17 years) [173]. The PK in children aged 2-4 years is the least predictable. However, pharmacological studies in children with psychiatric disorders below the age of 4 years are rare. The PK in adolescent patients is often similar to the PK in adults. Therefore, in many cases limited confirmatory pharmacokinetic data are sufficient in this group. Even less is known about pharmacodynamic changes in relation to development. Animal studies suggest that pharmacodynamic parameters (i.e. receptor sensitivity) in young animals may be different from that in adult animals [174, 175]. Such differences are also described at the level of susceptibility for side-effects [176]. Since such data are lacking for most of the psychotropic drugs applied in the child and adolescent and psychiatry, therapeutic drug monitoring is a valid tool to optimise pharmacotherapy and to enable to adjust the dosage of drugs according to the characteristics of the individual patient. Furthermore, genetic variability influences drug effects from absorption of the drug until its complete elimination [177].

Genetic variability exists both at the pharmacokinetic and pharmacodynamic side of drug action. Many enzymes involved in drug metabolism carry genetic variants (polymorphisms) which can decrease enzyme activity or even lead to complete deficiency [178]. Genetic variants in drug targets such as receptor molecules or intracellular structures of signal transduction and gene regulation directly and indirectly influence drug response. The prevalence of the different types of metabolizers varies a lot between ethnic groups [179]. In young patients, especially in smaller children, pharmacogenetics might gain a special importance since the enzyme activity changes over the time especially in early development. Thus, it might gain special importance in children when enzyme activities differ from those in adults. Developmental changes in physiology produce many of the age-associated changes in the absorption, distribution, metabolism, and excretion of psychotropic drugs that result in altered pharmacokinetics and thus serve as the determinants of age-specific dose requirements. Such changes might include a) the gastrointestinal function, b) body composition, c) Regional blood flow, d) Organ perfusion, e) Permeability of cell membranes, f) Acid-base balance, g) Passive diffusion of drugs into the central nervous system, h) metabolic capacity and i) renal function [8, 160, 180]. Gastric emptying, intestinal mobility or intestinal length, influence the available period for the drug presence at the site of absorption. Similarly, bile secretion rate influence the drug ability for reabsorption by the gastrointestinal tract and thus its PK profile. Furtehrmore, since the distribution of a drug is affected by its lipophilicity, extra-cellular and total-body water space and body fat, influence its distribution throuought the body. Changes also, in the composition and amount of circulating plasma proteins affects the amount of free drug while changes such as the liver size and renal function might affect the metabolism activity amd excretion, respectively.

> Although the above factors that potentially modify the PK profile of an AP drug, no systematic studies were carried out to show how each of these factors is changed over lifetime and whether there are gender dependent changes. These developmental changes in physiology have different effects on concentrations in the blood and most likely also at the target structures in the central nervous system (CNS). Therefore, the approach to extrapolate age-specific dosing regimes from adult data has limited value and the selection of doses in paediatric patients requires a consideration of pharmacokinetic parameters [181].

According to Mehler-Wex et al. [160], although it is generally accepted that development can alter the action of and response to a drug, little information exists about the effect of human ontogenesis on interactions between psychoactive drugs and biological target structures (i.e. the pharmacodynamics) and the consequence of these interactions (i.e. efficacy and side effects). Although, cell birth, neuronal differentiation and migration of neurons to target areas are almost complete within the first few years of life in humans, there is a lifelong change in the synaptogenesis and synapse elimination with changes in the density of neurotransmitter receptors, sensitivity of signal transduction pathways, activity of neurotransmitter metabolising enzymes and density of neurotransmitter re-uptake transporters. The ontogenesis of the CNS has an influence on the interaction of a psychotropic drug with biological structures in the CNS (e.g. neurotransmitter metabolism, neurotransmitter neurotransmitter receptors, neurotransmitter transporters, signal transduction) and the resulting therapeutic effect. These changes in the ontogenesis of pharmacodynamics indicate that there is a difference in the relationship between the blood concentration of a psychotropic drug and therapeutic response to a psychotropic drug in children, adolescents and adults [160]. Conclusively, in this younger age group TDM is a valid tool to optimise pharmacotherapy and enables the clinician to adjust the dosage of drugs according to the characteristics of the individual patient. Moreover, situations are defined when pharmacogenetic (phenotyping or genotyping) tests are informative in addition to TDM [159].

DISCUSSION AND PERSPECTIVES

The authors believe that any attempt to develop personalized dosing in youth, will have to take into account TDM and multiple complex variables, including genetic and developmental influences. The aim of TDM is to optimize pharmacotherapy by maximizing therapeutic efficacy, while minimizing adverse events, in those instances where the blood concentration of the drug is a better predictor of the desired effect than the dose. The reasons why these principles have gained wide acceptance include: (1) a better relationship between the effect of a given drug and its concentration in the blood than the dose of the drug and the effect; (2) a thorough understanding of pharmacokinetics, (3) the development of reliable and relatively easy to use drug-monitoring assays. In addition, TDM can also be useful in cases in which compliance is in question, where it is not clear if the right drug is being taken, where dosage adjustment is required as a result of drug–drug interactions, and where intoxication is suspected. Thus, adequate dosing in paediatric psychiatric patients requires a consideration of pharmacokinetic parameters and the development of the CNS, and warrants specific studies in children and adolescents. Conversely, TDM does not appear to be justified for all patients and all situations, and TDM cannot replace clinical judgment. The physician should be aware that TDM is not available for all drugs and that its benefit depends on their level of recommendation for TDM, on the availability of established plasma concentration ranges at fixed doses, and on the therapeutic window. He/she should also take into consideration the recommendations of the laboratory in regard to information on anticoagulants, the timing of blood sampling (steady-state conditions, trough levels, etc), and conditions for shipment to the laboratory before sampling blood for TDM [159]. TDM is thus one aspect of the therapeutic strategy. The results of TDM should be interpreted with expertise, especially in situations where pharmacogenomics and pharmacogenetic particularities, drug interactions, or comorbidity may influence the fate of the drug in the organism.

Admittedly, some important questions related to TDM are still waiting for an answer. In contrast to traditional TDM, which cannot be performed until after a drug is administered to the patient, pharmacogenetics-oriented TDM can be conducted even before treatment begins. Pharmacogenetic information can be applied a priori for initial dose stratification and identification of cases where certain drugs are simply not effective. However, traditional TDM will still be required for all of the reasons that we use it now. In current clinical practice, pharmacogenetic testing is performed for only a few drugs and in a limited number of teaching hospitals and specialist academic centres and we believe that other drugs (e.g. SGAs) are potential candidates for pharmacogenetics-oriented TDM. However, prospective studies of phaymacogenetics-oriented TDM must be performed to determine its efficacy and cost effectiveness in optimising therapeutic effects while minimising toxicity. In the future, in addition to targeting a patient's drug concentrations within a therapeutic range, pharmacists are likely to be making dosage recommendations for individual drugs on the basis of the individual patient's genotype. As we enter the era of personalised drug therapy, we will be able to identify not only the best drug to be administered to a particular patient, but also the most effective and safe dosage from the outset of therapy. According to the authors opinion, the combination of TDM and genotyping procedures wuld provide a significant tool for the management of psychiatric treatment of youth.

Of interest, experts invloved in the teatment of psychiatry treatment in children and adolescent, established on 2007, a multi-centre TDM network which includes twelve Departments of Child and Adolescent Psychiatry in Germany, Austria and Switzerland [182]. The network uses a multi-centre TDM system including both standardized measurements of blood concentrations of psychotropic drugs and the documentation of efficacy and side effects of the medication. Each data is systematically documented via an internet databse which simplifies their final evaluation. In this way, individuals with abnormal blood levels on the one hand or low drug efficacy or severe side effects, respectively, despite of normal plasma levels on the other hand, are detected easily and transferred to further genetic analyses. In the authors opinion, such multi-centre standardized TDM documentation will provide data for future research on psychopharmacological treatment in children and adolescents, as a baseline, for example, for clinically relevant interactions with various co-medications. Phycisians who are involved in the psychiatric treatment of youth, must be aware of the therapeutic failure and/or the risk for side effects, if factors that might influence the pharmacokinetic of the prescribed medications would not be considered. In such cases, TDM might be a usefull tool in order to reduce the risk factors and increase the safety and efficacy of the antipsychotic treatment.

REFERENCES

[1] Ray, W. A. (2009). Atypical antipsychotic drugs and the risk of sudden cardiac death. *N. Engl. J. Med.,* 360, 225–235.

[2] Haro, J. M., Novick, D., Suarez, D., Alonso, J., Lépine, J. P., Ratcliffe, M. (2006). Remission and relapse in the outpatient care of schizophrenia: three-year results from the Schizophrenia Outpatient Health Outcomes study. *J. Clin. Psychopharmacol.,* 26(6), 571-578.

[3] Lambert, M. T., Copeland, L. A., Sampson, N., Duffy, S. A. (2006). New-onset type-2 diabetes associated with atypical antipsychotic medications. *Prog. Neuropsychopharmacol. Biol. Psychiatry.,* 30(5), 919-923.

[4] Olfson, M., Marcus, S. C., Corey-Lisle, P., Tuomari, A. V., Hines, P., L'Italien, G. J. (2006). Hyperlipidemia following treatment with antipsychotic medications. *Am. J. Psychiatry.,* 163(10), 1821-1825.

[5] Joy, C. B., Adams, C. E., Lawrie, S. M. (2006). Haloperidol versus placebo for schizophrenia. *Cochrane Database Syst. Rev.,* 18(4), CD003082.

[6] Shirzadi, A. A., Ghaemi, S. N. (2006). Side effects of atypical antipsychotics: extrapyramidal symptoms and the metabolic syndrome. *Harv. Rev. Psychiatry,* 14(3), 152-164.

[7] Dahl, M. L. (2002). Cytochrome p450 phenotyping/genotyping in patients receiving antipsychotics: useful aid to prescribing? *Clin. Pharmacokinet.,* 41, 453–470.

[8] Kearns G., Abdel-Rahman S, Alander S, Blowey D, Leeder J, Kauffman R. (2003). Developmental pharmacology – Drug disposition, action, and therapy in infants and children. *N. Engl. J. Med.,* 349(12):1157-1167.

[9] Touw, D. J., Neef, C., Thomson, A. H., Vinks, A. A. (2005). Cost-Effectiveness of Therapeutic Drug Monitoring. A Systematic Review. *Ther Drug Monit,* 27 (1), 10-17.

[10] Birkett, D. J. (1997). Pharmacokinetics made easy: therapeutic drug monitoring. *Aust. Prescr.,* 20, 9-11.

[11] Kang, J. S., Lee M. H. (2009). Overview of Therapeutic Drug Monitoring. *The Korean Journal of Internal Medicine,* 24 (1), 1-10.

[12] Quitkin, F., Rifkin, A., Klein, D. F. (1975). Very high dosage vs standard dosage fluphenazine in schizophrenia. A double-blind study of nonchronic treatment-refractory patients. *Archives of General Psychiatry,* 32(10), 1276–1281.

[13] Kane, J. M., Rifkin, A., Woerner, M., Reardon, G., Sarantakos, S., Schiebel, D., Ramos-Lorenzi, J. (1983). Lowdose neuroleptic treatment of outpatient schizophrenics: I. Preliminary results for relapse rates. *Arch. Gen. Psychiatry,* 40, 893–896.

[14] Kane, J. M., Rifkin, A., Quitkin, F., Klein, D. F. (1976). Antipsychotic drug blood levels and clinical outcome. In: Klein, DF.; Gittelman-Klein, R., editors. *Progress in Psychiatric Drug Treatment. Brunner Mazel*; NY, 399-408

[15] Geddes, J., Freemantle, N., Harrison, P., Bebbington, P. (2000). Atypical antipsychotics in the treatment of schizophrenia: systematic overview and meta-regression analysis; *BMJ,* 321,1371-1376.

[16] Leucht, S., Wahlbeck, K., Hamann, J., Kissling, W. (2003). New generation antipsychotics versus low-potency conventional antipsychotics: a systematic review and meta-analysis. *Lancet,* 361(9369), 1581–1589.

[17] Leucht, S., Corves, C., Arbter, D., Engel, R. R., Li, C., Davis, J. M. (2009). Second-generation versus firstgeneration antipsychotic drugs for schizophrenia: a meta-analysis. *Lancet,* 373(9657), 31–41.

[18] Vardakou, I., Dona, A., Pistos, C., Alevisopoulos, G., Athanaselis, S., Maravelias, C., Spiliopoulou, C. (2010). Validated GC/MS method for the simultaneous determination of clozapine and norclozapine in human plasma. Application in psychiatric patients under clozapine treatment. *J. Chromatogr. B Analyt. Technol. Biomed Life Sci.,* 878(25), 2327-2332.

[19] Taylor, D. (1997). Doses of carbamazepine and valproate in bipolar affective disorder. *Psychiatr. Bull.,* 21, 221–223.

[20] Ng CH, Chong, S. A., Lambert, T., Fan, A., Hackett, L. P., Mahendran, R. (2005). An inter-ethnic comparison study of clozapine dosage, clinical response and plasma levels. *Int. Clin. Psychopharmacol.,* 20, 163–168.

[21] Rostami-Hodjegan, A. et al. (2004). Influence of dose, cigarette smoking, age, sex, and metabolic activity on plasma clozapine concentrations: a predictive model and nomograms to aid clozapine dose adjustment and to assess compliance in individual patients. *J. Clin. Psychopharmacol.,* 24, 70–78.

[22] Haack, M. J. et al. (2003). Toxic rise of clozapine plasma concentrations in relation to inflammation. *Eur. Neuropsychopharmacol.,* 13, 381–385.

[23] De Leon J et al. (2003). Serious respiratory infections can increase clozapine levels and contribute to side effects: a case report. *Prog. Neuropsychopharmacol. Biol. Psychiatry,* 27, 1059–1063.

[24] Hasegawa, M. et al. (1993). Relationship between clinical efficacy and clozapine concentrations in plasma in schizophrenia: effect of smoking. *J. Clin. Psychopharmacol.*, 13, 383–390.
[25] Potkin, S. G. et al. (1994). Plasma clozapine concentrations predict clinical response in treatment-resistant schizophrenia. *J. Clin. Psychiatry,* 55(B), 133–136.
[26] VanderZwaag, C. et al. (1996). Response of patients with treatment-refractory schizophrenia to clozapine within three serum level ranges. *Am. J. Psychiatry*, 153, 1579–1584.
[27] Spina, E. et al. (2000). Relationship between plasma concentrations of clozapine and norclozapine and therapeutic response in patients with schizophrenia resistant to conventional neuroleptics. *Psychopharmacology*, 148, 83–89.
[28] Perry, P. J. (2001). Therapeutic drug monitoring of antipsychotics. *Psychopharmacol. Bull.*, 35, 19–29.
[29] Llorca, P. M. et al. (2002). Effectiveness of clozapine in neuroleptic-resistant schizophrenia: clinical response and plasma concentrations. *J. Psychiatry Neurosci.*, 27, 30–37.
[30] Xiang, Y. Q. et al. (2006). Serum concentrations of clozapine and norclozapine in the prediction of relapse of patients with schizophrenia. *Schizophr. Res.*, 83, 201–210.
[31] Khan, A. Y. et al. (2005). Examining concentration-dependent toxicity of clozapine: role of therapeutic drug monitoring. *J. Psychiatr. Pract.*, 11, 289–301.
[32] Greenwood-Smith, C. et al. (2003). Serum clozapine levels: a review of their clinical utility. *J. Psychopharmacol.*, 17, 234–238.
[33] Yusufi, B. et al. (2007). Prevalence and nature of side effects during clozapine maintenance treatment and the relationship with clozapine dose and plasma concentration. *Int. Clin. Psychopharmacol.*, 22, 238–243.
[34] Van der Weide, J., Steijns, L. S., van Weelden, M. J. (2003). The effect of smoking and cytochrome P450 CYP1A2 genetic polymorphism on clozapine clearance and dose requirement. *Pharmacogenetics,* 13, 169-172.
[35] Doude van Troostwijk, L. J., Koopmans, R. P., Vermeulen, H. D., Guchelaar, H. J. (2003). CYP1A2 activity is an important determinant of clozapine dosage in schizophrenic patients. *Eur. J. of Pharm. Sci.,* 20, 451-457.
[36] Palego, L. et al. (2002). Clozapine, norclozapine plasma levels, their sum and ratio in 50 psychotic patients: influence of patient-related variables. *Prog. Neuropsychopharmacol. Biol. Psychiatry,* 26, 473–480.
[37] Bell, R., McLaren, A., Galanos, J., Copolov, D. (1998). The clinical use of plasma clozapine levels. *Aust. N. Z. J. Psychiatry.,* 32(4), 567-574.
[38] Raggi, M. A. (2004). Pharmacological Treatment of Schizophrenia: Recent Antipsychotic Drugs and New Therapeutic Strategies. Current Medicinal Chemistry, 11(3), DOI: http://dx.doi.org/10.2174/0929867043456106.
[39] Hiemke, C. et al. (2004). Therapeutic monitoring of new antipsychotic drugs. *Ther. Drug Monit.*, 26, 156–60.
[40] Gerlach, M. et al. (2007). Therapeutic drug monitoring of quetiapine in adolescents with psychotic disorders. *Pharmacopsychiatry*, 40, 72–6.
[41] Hasselstrom, J. et al. (2004). Quetiapine serum concentrations in psychiatric patients: the influence of comedication. *Ther. Drug Monit.*, 26, 486–91.

[42] Mauri, M. C. et al. (2005). Clinical outcome and olanzapine plasma levels in acute schizophrenia. *Eur. Psychiatry*, 20, 55–60.
[43] Castberg, I. et al. (2007). Quetiapine and drug interactions: evidence from a routine therapeutic drug monitoring service. *J. Clin. Psychiatry*, 68, 1540–5.
[44] Aichhorn, W. et al. (2006). Influence of age, gender, body weight and valproate comedication on quetiapine plasma concentrations. *Int. Clin. Psychopharmacol.*, 21, 81–5.
[45] Prescribe Guidelines 10th Edition, Taylor, Paton, Kapur. ISBN-13:9781841846996.
[46] Gaebel, W., Riesbeck, M., von Wilmsdorff, M., Burns, T., Derks, E. M., Kahn, R. S., Rössler, W., Fleischhacker, W. W. EUFEST Study Group. (2010). Drug attitude as predictor for effectiveness in first-episode schizophrenia: Results of an open randomized trial (EUFEST). *Eur. Neuropsychopharmacol.*, 20(5), 310-6.
[47] Citrome, L., Jaffe, A., Levine, J., Lindenmayer, J. P. (2005). Dosing of quetiapine in schizophrenia: how clinical practice differs from registration studies. *J. Clin. Psychiatry.*, 66(12), 1512-6.
[48] Stahl, S. M. Essential psychopharmacology: The prescriber's guide. 3rd ed. Cambridge University Press: Cambridge, 2009.
[49] Citrome, L., Jaffe, A., Levine, J. (2007). Datapoints: The ups and downs of dosing second-generation antipsychotics. *Psychiatr. Serv.*, 58(1), 11.
[50] Gao, K., Sheehan, D. V., Calabrese, J. R. (2009). Atypical antipsychotics in primary generalized anxiety disorder or comorbid with mood disorders. *Expert Rev. Neurother.*, 9(8), 1147-58.
[51] Wang, H. N., Peng, Y., Tan, Q. R., Chen, Y. C., Zhang, R. G., Qiao, Y. T., Wang, H. H., Liu, L., Kuang, F., Wang, B. R., Zhang, Z. J. (2010). Quetiapine ameliorates anxiety-like behavior and cognitive impairments in stressed rats: implications for the treatment of posttraumatic stress disorder. *Physiol. Res.*, 59(2), 263-71.
[52] Nybarg, S., Takano, A., Jucaite, A. (2008). PET-measured occupancy of the norepinephrine transporter by extended release quetiapine fumarate (quetiapine XR) in brains of healthy subjects. *Eur. Neuropsychopharmacol.*, 18(4), 270.
[53] Scharf, M., Rogowski, R., Hull, S., et al. (2008). Efficacy and safety of doxepin 1 mg, 3 mg, and 6 mg in elderly patients with primary insomnia: A randomized, double-blind, placebo-controlled crossover study. *J. Clin. Psychiatry*, 69, 1557–1564.
[54] Shajahan, P., Taylor, M. (2010). The uses and outcomes of quetiapine in depressive and bipolar mood disorders in clinical practice. *J. Psychopharmacol.*, 24(4), 565-72.
[55] Aravagiri, M. et al. (1997). Plasma level monitoring of olanzapine in patients with schizophrenia: determination by high-performance liquid chromatography with electrochemical detection. *Ther. Drug Monit.*, 19, 307–13.
[56] Perry, P. J. (2001). Therapeutic drug monitoring of antipsychotics. *Psychopharmacol. Bull.*, 35, 19–29.
[57] Gex-Fabry, M. et al. (2003). Therapeutic drug monitoring of olanzapine: the combined effect of age, gender, smoking, and comedication. *Ther. Drug. Monit.*, 25, 46–53.
[58] Bergemann, N. et al. (2004). Plasma amisulpride levels in schizophrenia or schizoaffective disorder. Eur. Neuropsychopharmacol., 14, 245–50.
[59] Perry, P. J. et al. (1997). Olanzapine plasma concentrations and clinical response in acutely ill schizophrenic patients. *J. Clin. Psychopharmacol.*, 6, 472–7.

[60] Fellows, L. et al. (2003). Investigation of target plasma concentration–effect relationships for olanzapine in schizophrenia. *Ther. Drug. Monit.*, 25, 682–9.
[61] Rao, M. L. et al. (2001). Olanzapine: pharmacology, pharmacokinetics and therapeutic drug monitoring. *Fortschr. Neurol. Psychiatr.*, 69, 510–17.
[62] Robertson, M. D. et al. (2000). Olanzapine concentrations in clinical serum and postmortem blood specimens – when does therapeutic become toxic? *J. Forensic Sci.*, 45, 418–21.
[63] Bech, P. et al. (2006). Olanzapine plasma level in relation to antimanic effect in the acute therapy of manic states. *Nord. J. Psychiatry*, 60, 181–2.
[64] Kelly, D. L. et al. (2006). Plasma concentrations of high-dose olanzapine in a double-blind crossover study. *Hum. Psychopharmacol.*, 21, 393–8.
[65] Stahl, S. M. (2008). Stahl's essential psychopharmacology: Neuroscientific basis and practical applications, 3rd ed. Cambridge:Cambridge University Press.
[66] Cutler, A., Ball, S., Stahl, S. M. (2008). *Dosing Atypical antipsychotics*. CNS Spectr., 13(5)(9), 1–16.
[67] Muller, M. J. et al. (2008). Amisulpride doses and plasma levels in different age groups of patients with schizophrenia or schizoaffective disorder. *J. Psychopharmacol.*, 23, 278–86.
[68] Muller, M. J. et al. (2006). Gender aspects in the clinical treatment of schizophrenic inpatients with amisulpride: a therapeutic drug monitoring study. *Pharmacopsychiatry*, 39, 41–6.
[69] Muller, M. J. et al. (2007). Therapeutic drug monitoring for optimizing amisulpride therapy in patients with schizophrenia. J. Psychiatr. Res., 41, 673–9.
[70] Sparshatt, A. et al. (2008). Quetiapine: dose–response relationship in schizophrenia. *CNS Drugs*, 22, 49–68.
[71] Schwartz, T. L., Stahl, S. M. (2011). Treatment Strategies for Dosing the Second Generation Antipsychotics. *CNS Neuroscience and Therapeutics*, 17, 110–117.
[72] Mace, S. et al. (2009). Aripiprazole: dose–response relationship in schizophrenia and schizoaffective disorder. *CNS Drugs*, 23(9), 773-780.
[73] Molden, E. et al. (2006). Pharmacokinetic variability of aripiprazole and the active metabolite dehydroaripiprazole in psychiatric patients. *Ther. Drug Monit.*, 28, 744–9.
[74] Bachmann, C. J. et al. (2008). Large variability of aripiprazole and dehydroaripiprazole serum concentrations in adolescent patients with schizophrenia. *Ther. Drug Monit.*, 30, 462–6.
[75] Aripiprazole (AbilifyTM) FDA Package Inser.
[76] Arbaizar, B., Dierssen-Sotos, T., Gomez-Acebo, I., Llorca, J. (2009). Aripiprazole in major depression and mania: Meta-analyses of randomized placebo-controlled trials. *Gen. Hosp. Psychiatry*, 31, 478–483.
[77] Nelson, J. C., Mankoski, R., Baker, R. A., Carlson, B. X., Eudicone, J. M., Pikalov, A., Tran, Q. V. (2010). Effects of aripiprazole adjunctive to standard antidepressant treatment on the core symptoms of depression: A post-hoc, pooled analysis of two large, placebo-controlled studies. Berman RM. *J. Affect Disord.*, 120, 133–140.
[78] Marcus, R. N., Owen, R., Kamen, L., Manos, G., McQuade, R. D., Carson, W. H., Aman, M. G. (2009). A placebo-controlled, fixed-dose study of aripiprazole in children and adolescents with irritability associated with autistic disorder. *J. Am. Acad. Child Adolesc. Psychiatry*, 48, 1110–1119.

[79] Hoge, E. A. Worthington, J. J., Kaufman, R. E., Delong, H. R., Pollack, M. H., Simon, N. M. (2008). Aripiprazole as augmentation treatment of refractory generalized anxiety disorder and panic disorder. *Cns. Spectrums*, 13, 522–527.
[80] Menza, M. A., Dobkin, R. D., Marin, H. (2007). An open-label trial of aripiprazole augmentation for treatment-resistant generalized anxiety disorder. *J. Clin. Psychopharmacol.*, 27, 207–210.
[81] Olesen, O. V. et al. (1998). Serum concentrations and side effects in psychiatric patients during risperidone therapy. *Ther. Drug Monit.*, 20, 380–4.
[82] Remington, G. et al. (2006). A PET study evaluating dopamine D2 receptor occupancy for long-acting injectable risperidone. *Am. J. Psychiatry*, 163, 396–401.
[83] Taylor, D. (2006). Risperidone long-acting injection in practice – more questions than answers? *Acta Psychiatr. Scand.*, 114, 1–2.
[84] Medori, R. et al. (2006). Plasma antipsychotic concentration and receptor occupancy, with special focus on risperidone long-acting injectable. *Eur. Neuropsychopharmacol.*, 16, 233–40.
[85] Gefvert, O. et al. (2005). Pharmacokinetics and D2 receptor occupancy of long-acting injectable risperidone (Risperdal ConstaTM) in patients with schizophrenia. *Int. J. Neuropsychopharmacol.*, 8, 27–36.
[86] Freudenreich, O., Goff, D. C. (2002). Antipsychotic combination therapy in schizophrenia: A review of efficacy and risks of current combinations. *Acta Psychiatrica Scandinavica.*, 106, 323–330.
[87] Lieberman, J. A., Stroup, T. S., McEvoy, J. P., Swartz, M. S., Rosenheck, R. A., Perkins, D. O., Keefe, R. S., Davis, S. M., Davis, C. E., Lebowitz, B. D., Severe, J., Hsiao, J. K. (2005). Effectiveness of antipsychotic drugs in patients with chronic schizophrenia. *N. Engl. J. Med.*, 353(12), 1209-1223.
[88] Llerena, A., Berecz, R., Dorado, P., et al. (2004). QTc interval, CYP2D6 and CYP2C9 genotypes and risperidone plasma concentrations. *J. Psychopharmacology*, 18, 189–193.
[89] Dorado, P., Berecz, R., Penas-Lledo, E. M., et al. (2006). Clinical implications of CYP2D6 genetic polymorphism during treatment with antipsychotic drugs. *Current Drug Targets*, 7, 1671–1680.
[90] Bollini, P. et al. (1994). Antipsychotic drugs: is more worse? A meta-analysis of the published randomized control trials. *Psychol. Med*, 24, 307–316.
[91] Taylor, D. M. (2002). Prolongation of QTc interval and antipsychotics. *Am. J. Psychiatry*, 159(6), 1062.
[92] Centorrino, F. et al. (2004). Multiple versus single antipsychotic agents for hospitalized psychiatric patients: case-control study of risks versus benefits. *Am. J. Psychiatry*, 161, 700–706.
[93] Kreyenbuhl, J. et al. (2007). Adding or switching antipsychotic medications in treatment-refractory schizophrenia. *Psychiatr. Serv.*, 58, 983–990.
[94] Correll, C. U. et al. (2009). Antipsychotic combinations vs monotherapy in schizophrenia: a meta-analysis of randomized controlled trials. *Schizophr. Bull.*, 35, 443–457.
[95] Kawai, N. et al. (2006). High-dose of multiple antipsychotics and cognitive function in schizophrenia: the effect of dose-reduction. Prog. Neuropsychopharmacol. *Biol. Psychiatry*, 30, 1009–1014.

[96] Reynolds, D. J., Aronson, J. K. (1993). ABC of monitoring drug therapy: making the most of plasma drug concentration measurements. *BMJ*, 306, 48-51.
[97] Kapur, S., Seeman, P. (2001). Does fast dissociation from the dopamine d(2) receptor explain the action of atypical antipsychotics?: A new hypothesis. *Am. J. Psychiatry*, 158(3), 360-369.
[98] Mihara, K., Kondo, T., Suzuki, A., Yasui, N., Ono, S., Otani, K., Kaneko, S. (2001). No relationship between--141C Ins/Del polymorphism in the promoter region of dopamine D2 receptor and extrapyramidal adverse effects of selective dopamine D2 antagonists in schizophrenic patients: a preliminary study. *Psychiatry Res.*, 101(1), 33-38.
[99] Kaiser, R., Tremblay, P. B., Klufmöller, F., Roots, I., Brockmöller, J. (2002). Relationship between adverse effects of antipsychotic treatment and dopamine D(2) receptor polymorphisms in patients with schizophrenia. *Mol. Psychiatry.*, 7(7), 695-705.
[100] Barnes TR, Halstead SM, Little PW. (1992). Relationship between iron status and chronic akathisia in an in-patient population with chronic schizophrenia. *Br. J. Psychiatry*, 161, 791-796.
[101] http://www.risperdal.com
[102] Swainston Harrison, T., Perry, C. M. (2004). Aripiprazole: a review of its use in schizophrenia and schizoaffective disorder. Drugs, 64(15), 1715-1736.
[103] Eichhammer, P., Albus, M., Borrmann-Hassenbach, M., Schoeler, A., Putzhammer, A., Frick, U., Klein, H. E., Rohrmeier, T. (2000). Association of dopamine D3-receptor gene variants with neuroleptic induced akathisia in schizophrenic patients: a generalization of Steen's study on DRD3 and tardive dyskinesia. *Am. J. Med. Genet.*, 96(2), 187-191.
[104] Chouinard, G., (2004). New nomenclature for drug-induced movement disorders including tardive dyskinesia. *J. Clin. Psychiatry*, 65(9), 9-15.
[105] Miller, D. D., McEvoy, J. P., Davis, S. M., Caroff, S. N., Saltz, B. L., Chakos, M. H., Swartz, M. S., Keefe, R. S., Rosenheck, R. A., Stroup, T. S., Lieberman, J. A. (2005). Clinical correlates of tardive dyskinesia in schizophrenia: baseline data from the CATIE schizophrenia trial. *Schizophr. Res.*, 80(1), 33-43.
[106] Casey, D. E., (2004). Pathophysiology of antipsychotic drug-induced movement disorders. *J. Clin. Psychiatry*, 65, (9), 25-28.
[107] Reynolds, G. P.,Hill, M. J., Kirk, S. L. (2006). The S-HT2Creceptor andantipsychotic-induced weight gain-mechanisms and genetics. *J. Psychopharmacol.*, 20(4), 15-18.
[108] Kapitany, T., Meszaros, K., Lenzinger, E., Schindler, S. D., Barnas, C., Fuchs, K., Sieghart, W., Aschauer, H. N., Kasper, S. (1998). Genetic polymorphisms for drug metabolism (CYP2D6) and tardive dyskinesia in schizophrenia. *Schizophr. Res.*, 32(2), 101-106.
[109] Ohmori, O., Suzuki, T., Kojima, H., Shinkai, T., Terao, T., Mita, T., Abe, K. (1998). Tardive dyskinesia and debrisoquine 4-hydroxylase (CYP2D6) genotype in Japanese schizophrenics. *Schizophr. Res.*, 32(2), 107-113.
[110] Ellingrod, V. L., Schultz, S. K., Arndt, S. (2000). Association between cytochrome P4502D6 (CYP2D6) genotype, antipsychotic exposure, and abnormal involuntary movement scale (AIMS) score. *Psychiatr. Genet.*, 10(1), 9-11.

[111] Guy, W. (1976). Abnormal involuntary movement scale. In: ECDEU assessment manual for psychopharmacology. Washington, DC: U.S. *Public Health Service*. 534–537.
[112] Basile, V. S., Ozdemir, V., Masellis, M., et al. (2000). A functional polymorphism of the cytochrome P450 1A2 (CYP1A2) gene: association with tardive dyskinesia in schizophrenia. *Mol. Psychiatry*, 5, 410–417.
[113] Schulze, T. G., Schumacher, J., Muller, D. J., et al. (2001). Lack of association between a functional polymorphism of the cytochrome P450 1A2 (CYP1A2) gene and tardive dyskinesia in schizophrenia. *Am. J. Med. Genet.*, 105, 498–501.
[114] Newcomer, J. W. (2006). Medical risk in patients with bipolar disorder and schizophrenia. *J. Clin. Psychiatry.*, 67(9), 25–30.
[115] Sipos, F. R., Kehoe, P. G., Burns, T., et al. (2006). The cardiovascular and respiratory health of people with schizophrenia. *Acta Psychiatrica Scandinavica*, 113, 245–246.
[116] Muller, D. J., Kennedy, J. L. (2006). Genetics of antipsychotic treatment emergent weight gain in schizophrenia. *Pharmacogenomics*, 7, 863–887.
[117] Quetiapine (SeroquelTM) FDA Package Insert.
[118] Dumortier G, Mahé V, Pons D, Zerrouk A, Januel D, Degrassat K. (2001). Clonic seizure associated with high clozapine plasma level. *J. Neuropsychiatry Clin. Neurosci.*, 13(2), 302-303.
[119] Simpson, G. M., Cooper, T. A. (1978). Clozapine plasma levels and convulsions. *Am. J. Psychiatry*, 135(1), 99-100.
[120] Pisani F, Oteri G, Costa C, Di Raimondo G, Di Perri R. (2002). Effects of psychotropic drugs on seizure threshold. *Drug Saf.*, 25(2), 91-110.
[121] Devinsky, O., Honigfeld, G., Patin, J. (1991). Clozapine-related seizures. *Neurology*, 41(3), 369-371.
[122] Rajji, T. K., Uchida, H., Ismail, Z., Ng, W., Mamo, D. C., Remington, G., Pollock, B. G., Mulsant, B. H. (2010). Clozapine and global cognition in schizophrenia. *J. Clin. Psychopharmacol.*, 30(4), 431-436.
[123] Ronaldson, K. J., Taylor, A. J., Fitzgerald, P. B., Topliss, D. J., Elsik, M., McNeil, J. J. (2010). Diagnostic characteristics of clozapine-induced myocarditis identified by an analysis of 38 cases and 47 controls. *J. Clin. Psychiatry*, 71(8), 976-981.
[124] Kilian, J. G., Kerr, K., Lawrence, C., Celermajer, D. S. (1999). Myocarditis and cardiomyopathy associated with clozapine. *Lancet*, 354(9193), 1841-5.
[125] Liu, H. C., Chang, W. H., Wie, F. C., Lin, S. K., Lin, S. K., Jann, M. W. (1996). Monitoring of plasma clozapine levels and its metabolites in refractory schizophrenic patients. *Ther. Drug Monit.*, 18(2), 200-7.
[126] Ulrich, S., Baumann, B., Wolf, R., Lehmann, D., Peters, B., Bogerts, B., Meyer, F. P. (2003). Therapeutic drug monitoring of clozapine and relapse--a retrospective study of routine clinical data. *Int. J. Clin. Pharmacol. Ther.*, 41(1), 3-13.
[127] Comittee for medicinal products for human use European Medicines Agency (CHMP). Refl ection paper on the use of pharmacogenetics in the pharmacokinetic evaluation of Medicinal Products. *European Medicines Agency* (EMEA) 2007.
[128] Gesteira, A., Barros, F., Martín, A., Pérez, V., Cortés, A., Baiget, M., Carracedo A. (2010). Pharmacogenetic studies on the antipsychotic treatment. Current status and perspectives. *Actas Esp. Psiquiatr.*, 38(5), 301-316.

[129] Roses, A. D. (2004). Pharmacogenetics and drug development: the path to safer and more effective drugs. *Nat. Rev. Genet.*, 5(9), 645-656.
[130] Grossman, I. (2007). Routine pharmacogenetic testing in clinical practice: dream or reality? *Pharmacogenomics,* 8, 1449–1459.
[131] Fleeman, N., Dundar, Y., Dickson, R., Jorgensen, A., Pushpakom, S., McLeod, C., Pirmohamed, M., Walley, T. (2011). Cytochrome P450 testing for prescribing antipsychotics in adults with schizophrenia: systematic review and meta-analyses. *The Pharmacogenomics Journal.*, 11, 1–14.
[132] Dahl, M. L. (2002). Cytochrome p450 phenotyping/genotyping in patients receiving antipsychotics: useful aid to prescribing? *Clin. Pharmacokinet.*, 41, 453–470.
[133] Gesteira, A., Barros, F., Martín, A., Pérez, V., Cortés, A., Baiget, M., Carracedo A. (2010). Pharmacogenetic studies on the antipsychotic treatment. Current status and perspectives. *Actas Esp. Psiquiatr.*, 38(5), 301-316.
[134] Bradford, L. D. (2002). CYP2D6 allele frequency in European Caucasians, Asians, Africans and their descendants. *Pharmacogenomics,* 3(2), 229-243.
[135] Sundberg, M. I. (2005). Genetic polymorphisms of cytochrome P450 2D6 (CYP2D6): clinical consequences, evolutionary aspects and functional diversity. *The Pharmacogenomics Journal*, 5, 6–13.
[136] De Leon, J., Armstrong, S. C., Cozza, K. L. (2006). Clinical Guidelines for Psychiatrists for the Use of Pharmacogenetic Testing for CYP450 2D6 and CYP450 2C19. *Psychosomatics*, 47(1), 75-85.
[137] Rogers, J. F., Nafziger, A. N., Bertino, J. S. (2002). Pharmacogenetics Affects Dosing, Efficacy, and Toxicity of Cytochrome P450– Metabolized Drugs. *The American Journal of Medicine*, 113, 746-750.
[138] Shimada, T., Gillam, E. M., Sandhu, P., Guo, Z., Tukey, R. H., Guengerich, F. P. (1994). Activation of procarcinogens by human cytochrome P450 enzymes expressed in Escherichia coli. Simplified bacterial systems for genotoxicity assays. *Carcinogenesis*, 15(11), 2523-2529.
[139] Kirchheiner, J., Nickchen, K., Bauer, M., (2004). Pharmacogenetics of antidepressants and antipsychotics: the contribution of allelic variations to the phenotype of drug response. *Mol. Psychiatry*, 9, 442–473.
[140] Murray, M. (2006). Role of CYP pharmacogenetics and drug-drug interactions in the efficacy and safety of atypical and other antipsychotic agents. *J. Pharm. Pharmacol.*, 58(7), 871-885.
[141] Brøsen, K. (1993). CYP2D6 genotype determination. *Ugeskr Laeger*, 15, 155(46), 3779-3780.
[142] Brøsen, K. (1995). Drug interactions and the cytochrome P450 system. The role of cytochrome P450 1A2. *Clin. Pharmacokinet.*, 29(1), 20-25.
[143] Brøsen, K,. Kragh-Sørensen, P. (1993). Concomitant intake of nortriptyline and carbamazepine. *Ther. Drug Monit.*, 15(3), 258-260.
[144] Johnson, M., Markham-Abedi, C., Susce, M. T., Murray-Carmichael, E., McCollum, S., de Leon, J. (2006). A poor metabolizer for cytochromes P450 2D6 and 2C19: a case report on antidepressant treatment. *CNS Spectr.*, 11(10), 757-760.
[145] Webster, A., Martin, P., Lewis, G. (2004). Integrating pharmacogenetics into society: in search of a model. *Nature,* 5, 663–669.

[146] Mitchell, P. B. (2001). Therapeutic drug monitoring of psychotropic medications. *Br. J. Clin. Pharmacol.*, 49, 303-312.
[147] Mauri, M. C. (2007). Two weeks' quetiapine treatment for schizophrenia, drug-induced psychosis and borderline personality disorder: a naturalistic study with drug plasma levels. *Expert. Opin. Pharmacother.*, 8, 2207–2213.
[148] Fabrazzo, M., La Pia, S., Monteleone, P., Esposito, G., Pinto, A., De Simone, L., Bencivenga, R., Maj, M. (2002). Is the time course of clozapine response correlated to the time course of clozapine plasma levels? A one-year prospective study in drug-resistant patients with schizophrenia. *Neuropsychopharmacology*, 27(6),1050-1055.
[149] Palao, D. J., Arauxo, A., Brunet, M., Bernando, M., Haro, J. M., Ferrer, J., Gonzalez-Monclus, E. (1994). Haloperidol: therapeutic window in schizophrenia. *J. Clin. Psychopharmacol.*, 14(5), 303-310.
[150] Preskorn, S. H., Burke, M. J., Fast, G. A. (1993). *Therapeutic Drug Monitoring. Psychiatr. Clin. North. Am.*, 16, 611-645.
[151] Heller, S., Hiemke, C., Stroba, G., Rieger-Gies, A., Daum-Kreysch, E., Sachse, J., Härtter, S. (2004). Assessment of Storage and Transport Stability of New Antidepressant and Antipsychotic Drugs for a Nationwide TDM Service. *Ther. Drug Monit.*, 26 (4), 459-461.
[152] Zhang, G., Terry A. V., Bartlett, M. G. (2008). Bioanalytical methods for the determination of antipsychotic drugs. *Biomed. Chromatogr.*, 22, 671–687.
[153] Conti, R., Veenstra, D. V., Armstrong, K., Lesko, L. J., Grosse, S. D. (2010). Personalized Medicine and Genomics: Challenges and Opportunities in Assessing Effectiveness, Cost-Effectiveness, and Future *Research Priorities. Medical Decision Making. DOI:* 10.1177/0272989X09347014.
[154] De Leon, J., Sandson, N. B., Cozza, K. L. (2008). A Preliminary Attempt to Personalize Risperidone Dosing Using Drug–Drug Interactions and Genetics: Part I. Psychosomatics, 49(3), 258 - 270.
[155] Preskorn, S. H. (1998). A message from the Titanic. *J. Pract. Psychiatry Behav. Health*, 4, 236–242.
[156] Arranz, M. J., de Leon J. (2007). Pharmacogenetics and pharmacogenomics of schizophrenia: a review of the last decade of research. *Mol. Psychiatry*, 12, 707–747.
[157] De Leon, J., Armstrong, S. C., Cozza, K. L. (2006). Clinical Guidelines for Psychiatrists for the Use of Pharmacogenetic Testing for CYP450 2D6 and CYP450 2C19. *Psychosomatics*, 47(1), 75-85.
[158] Dahl, M. L., Sjöqvist, F. (2000). Pharmacogenetic Methods as a Complement to Therapeutic Monitoring of Antidepressants and Neuroleptics. *Ther. Drug Monit.*, 22(1), 114-117.
[159] Baumann, P., Hiemke, C., Ulrich, S., Gaertner, I., Rao, M. L., Eckermann, G., Gerlach, M., Kuss, H. J., Laux, G., Müller-Oerlinghausen, B., Riederer, P., Zernig, G. (2004). Therapeutic Monitoring of Psychotropic Drugs. An Outline of the AGNP-TDM Expert Group Consensus Guideline. *Ther. Drug Monit.*, 26, 167–170.
[160] Mehler-Wex C., Kölch M., Kirchheiner J., Antony G., Fegert J.M. and Gerlach M. (2009) Drug monitoring in child and adolescent psychiatry for improved efficacy and safety of psychopharmacotherapy. *Child and Adolescent Psychiatry and Mental Health* 2009, 3:14 (doi:10.1186/1753-2000-3-14; (http://www.capmh.com/content/3/1/14).

[161] Findling, R. L., McNamara, N. K., Stansbrey, R. J., Feeny, N. C., Young, C. M., Peric, F. V., Youngstrom, E. A. (2006). The Relevance of Pharmacokinetic Studies in Designing Efficacy Trials in Juvenile Major Depression. *J. Child Adolesc. Psychopharmacol.,* 16(1– 2), 131-145.

[162] Vitiello, B., Correll, C., van Zwieten-Boot, B., Zuddas, A., Parellada, M., Arango, C. (2009). Antipsychotics in children and adolescents: increasing use, evidence for efficacy and safety concerns. *Eur. Neuropsychopharmacol.,* 19, 629 - 635.

[163] Aman, M. G., Hollway, J. A., McDougle, C. J., Scahill, L., Tierney, E., McCracken, J. T., Arnold, L. E., Vitiello, B., Ritz, L., Gavaletz, A., Cronin, P., Swiezy, N., Wheeler, C., Koenig, K., Ghuman, J. K., Posey, D. J. (2008). Cognitive effects of risperidone in children with autism and irritable behavior. *J. Child Adolesc. Psychopharmacol.,* 18, 227 - 236.

[164] Llorente-Berzal, A., Mela, V., Borcel, E., Valero, M., López-Gallardo, M., Viveros, M. P., Marco, E. M. (2011). Neurobehavioral and metabolic long-term consequences of neonatal maternal deprivation stress and adolescent olanzapine treatment in male and female rats. *Neuropharmacology,* 1-10.

[165] Greenhill, L. L., Vitiello, B., Riddle, M. A., Fisher, P., Shockey, E., March, J. S., Levine, J., Fried, J., Abikoff, H., Zito, J. M., McCracken, J. T., Findling, R. L., Robinson, J., Cooper, T. B., Davies, M., Varipatis, E., Labellarte, M. J., Scahill, L., Walkup, J. T., Capasso, L., Rosengarten, J. (2003). Review of safety assessment methods used in pediatric psychopharmacology. *J. Am. Acad. Child Adolesc. Psych.,* 42, 627–633.

[166] Greenhill, L. L., Vitiello, B., Fisher, P., Levine, J., Davies, M., Abikoff, H., Chrisman, A. K., Chuang, S., Findling, R. L., March, J., Scahill, L., Walkup, J., Riddle, M. A. (2004). Comparison of increasingly detailed elicitation methods for the assessment of adverse events in pediatric psychopharmacology. *J. Am. Acad. Child Adolesc. Psych.,* 43, 1488–1496.

[167] Schirm, E., Tobi, H., de Jong-van den Berg, L. T. (2002). Unlicensed and off label drug use by children in the community: cross sectional study. *BMJ,* 324, 1312–1313.

[168] Vitiello, B., Riddle, M. A., Greenhill, L. L., March, J. S., Levine, J., Schachar, R. J., Abikoff, H., Zito, J. M., McCracken, J. T., Walkup, J. T., Findling, R. L., Robinson, J., Cooper, T. B., Davies, M., Varipatis, E., Labellarte, M. J., Scahill, L., Capasso, L., (2003). How can we improve the assessment of safety in child and adolescent psychopharmacology? *J. Am. Acad. Child Adolesc. Psych.,* 42, 634–641.

[169] Correll, C. U., Carlson, H. E. (2006). Endocrine and metabolic adverse effects of psychotropic medications in children and adolescents. *J. Am. Acad. Child Adolesc. Psych.,* 45, 771–791.

[170] Rey, J. M., Martin, A. (2006). Selective serotonin reuptake inhibitors and suicidality in juveniles: review of the evidence and implications for clinical practice. *Child Adolesc. Psychiatr. Clin. N. Am.,* 15, 221–237.

[171] Clinical investigation of medicinal products in the paediatric population 2001 – CPMP/ICH/2711/99 (ICH11)

[172] Wohlfarth, T., Kalverdijk, L., Rademaker, C., Schothorst, P., Minderaa, R., Gispen-de Wied, C. (2009). Psychopharmacology for children: From off label use to registration. *Eur. Neuropsychopharmacol.,* 19, 603–608.

[173] CHMP guideline on the role of pharmacokinetics in the development of medicinal products in the paediatric population. London, 28 June 2006. Doc. Ref. EMEA/CHMP/EWP/147013/2004.(http://www.emea.europa.eu/pdfs/human/ewp/14701304en.pdf)

[174] Carrey, N., Dursun, S. M. (1997). Psychopharmacology across life span: focus on developmental pharmacodynamics. *Hum. Psychopharmacol.,* 12, 525–526.

[175] Carrey, N., Dursun, S., Clements, R., Renton, K., Waschbusch, D., Macmaster, F. P. (2002). Noradrenergic and serotonergic neuroendocrine responses in prepubertal, peripubertal, and postpubertal rats pretreated with desipramine and sertraline. *J. Am. Acad. Child Adolesc. Psych.*, 41(8), 999–1006.

[176] Keepers, G. A., Clappison, V. J., Casey, D. E. (1983). Initial anticholinergic prophylaxis for neuroleptic-induced extrapyramidal syndromes. *Arch. Gen. Psychiatry*, 40, 1113–1117.

[177] Evans, W., McLeod, H. (2003). Pharmacogenomics – drug disposition, drug targets, and side effects. *N. Engl. J. Med.*, 348(6), 538-549.

[178] Evans, W., Relling, M. (1999). Pharmacogenomics: translating functional genomics into rational therapeutics. *Science*, 286(5439), 487-491.

[179] Bertilsson, L. (1995). Geographical/interracial differences in polymorphic drug oxidation. Current state of knowledge of cyto chromes P450 (CYP) 2D6 and 2C19. *Clin. Pharmacokinet.*, 29(3), 192-209.

[180] Hiemke C, Härtter S, H W. (2000). Therapeutisches Drug Monitoring (TDM). In Laboruntersuchungen in der psychiatrischen Routin Edited by: Gastpar M, Banger M. Stuttgart: Thieme; 2000:106-133.

[181] Findling, R. L., McNamara, N. K., Stansbrey, R. J., Feeny, N. C., Young, C. M., Peric, F. V., Youngstrom, E. A. (2006). The Relevance of Pharmacokinetic Studies in Designing Efficacy Trials in Juvenile Major Depression. J. Child Adolesc. Psychopharmacol., 16(1– 2), 131-145. *Competence Network on TDM in Child and Adolescent Psychiatry* [http://tdm-kjp.de].

In: Youth: Practices, Perspectives and Challenges
Editor: Elizabeth Trejos-Castillo

ISBN: 978-1-62618-067-3
© 2013 Nova Science Publishers, Inc.

Chapter 4

THE ASSESSMENT OF SCHIZOTYPAL EXPERIENCES IN ADOLESCENT POPULATION

Eduardo Fonseca-Pedrero[1,3,*], *Mercedes Paino*[2,3], *Serafín Lemos-Giráldez*[2,3] *and José Muñiz*[2,3]
[1]Department of Educational Sciences, University of La Rioja, Spain
[2]Department of Psychology, University of Oviedo, Spain
[3]Center for Biomedical Research in the Mental Health Network (CIBERSAM), Spain

ABSTRACT

Schizotypal experiences represent the behavioural expression of liability for psychotic disorders in general population. Empirical evidence indicates that participants with high scores on schizotypal self-reports are at a heightened risk for the later development of psychotic disorders. In the literature, there are different measurement instruments for the assessment of schizotypal experiences in both adults and adolescents. There is no doubt that having a measuring instrument with adequate psychometric properties, reliability and sources of validity evidence, allow us to make well-founded decisions based on score profiles, for instance, screening participants at-risk for a more comprehensive psychological assessment. Within this research context, the main goal of this study was to analyze the rates of schizotypal experiences, the internal structure and reliability of the Oviedo Questionnaire for Schizotypy Assessment (ESQUIZO-Q) in nonclinical adolescents. The final sample consisted of 3,056 participants, 1,469 males, with a mean age of 15.9 years ($SD = 1.2$). The results indicated that schizotypal experiences are very common in this age group. The analysis of the underlying internal structure of the ESQUIZO-Q subscales revealed a three-factor solution specified in the following components: Reality Distortion, Anhedonia and Interpersonal Disorganization. The levels of internal consistency for the subscales of the ESQUIZO-Q were acceptable. The ESQUIZO-Q is a brief and easily administered self-report with adequate psychometric characteristics for the assessment of schizotypal experiences in nonclinical adolescents. Future studies should explore in more depth the psychometric properties of

---

[*] Corresponding of Author: Eduardo Fonseca-Pedrero, University of La Rioja, C/ Luis de Ulloa, s/n, Edificio VIVES; C.P.: 26002, Logroño, La Rioja, Spain, Tel: +34 941 299 309, Fax: +34 941 299 333, e-mail: eduardo.fonseca@unirioja.es.

the ESQUIZO-Q (e.g., predictive validity) as well as the development of computerized-adaptive versions.

Keywords: Schizoypal; Schizotypy, Assessment; Psychosis; Risk; Adolescent

1. INTRODUCTION

1.1. Schizophrenia and Schizotypy

Schizophrenia is a serious and devastating mental disorder characterized by symptoms such as hallucinatory experiences, delusional ideation, disorganized speech and behavior, which usually has its onset during late adolescence or early adulthood (American Psychiatric Association, 2000; van Os and Kapur, 2009). Epidemiological data indicates that the median lifetime prevalence estimated for schizophrenia is 4.0 per 1,000 persons (McGrath, Saha, Chant, and Welham, 2008). Also, schizophrenia and related disorders have a direct impact on the lives of individuals at the personal, educational, familiar and work levels. In fact, psychotic symptoms do not only have a clear repercussion on the health and quality of life of patients, but also on health care costs and society (Mangalore and Knapp, 2007; Wu et al., 2005). For example, patients with schizophrenia die, on average, 12-15 years earlier than the general population. The main reason for this mortality increase, in addition to suicide, is related to physical causes and the increase in the frequency of risk factors such as the lack of physical activity, obesity, diabetes, and tobacco addiction (Dixon et al., 2000; Lasser et al., 2000; Saha, Chant, and McGrath, 2007).

Since the beginning of the 20th century there has been an attempt to relate different personality typologies with schizophrenia (Kendler, 1985). There are two main hypotheses which were originally very different, but that currently can be seen as complementary. The first hypothesis holds that personality traits, or any of their components, could be considered as a specific predisposing factor for psychosis and not as a manifestation of it. The second hypothesis holds that personality traits could be conceived as precursors or behaviors that precede the onset of psychosis. This set of personality characteristics which attempts to predict the onset of psychosis, as well as define and identify the at-risk clinical state for its development, can be included in what is commonly known as schizotypy.

Schizotypy is a complex construct which is intimately related at historical, conceptual, genetic, neurodevelopmental, neurocognitive, and psychophysiological levels to schizophrenia-spectrum disorders, such as schizophrenia, psychotic affective disorders and schizoid, schizotypal and paranoid personality disorders (Kwapil and Barrantes-Vidal, in press; Lenzenweger, 2010; Raine, 2006). Arriving at an operative and concise definition of the current meaning of schizotypy is a difficult task given that this construct can be associated to a wide heterogeneity of meanings. In this regard, some authors employ the term schizotypy to make reference to an attenuated form of schizophrenia, thus, representing a premorbid or prodromal phase of the disorder (Raine, 2006). Other authors define it as a personality organization that represents genetic vulnerability toward psychosis (Meehl, 1962). On the other hand, from a dimensional point of view, schizotypy can be understood as a set of personality traits and experiences (cognitive, emotional and behavioral) which are expressed along a dynamic continuum of adjustment ranging from psychological well-being to schizophrenia-spectrum personality disorders and full-blown schizophrenia (Claridge, 1997). These traits are present in the general population, are not necessarily associated to a mental disorder, and are configured as an indicator of vulnerability for psychosis in general, and schizophrenia in particular. However, despite the divergence in the conceptual delimitation of schizotypy, all these conceptions explicitly or implicitly assume the following: a) the necessity of the confluence or interaction of multiple neurodevelopmental (e.g., problems during labor and delivery), genetic (e.g., first degree relatives of patients with schizophrenia) and/or psychosocial factors (e.g., stressful situations, urbanicity or depression) for the development of a clinical condition of functional psychosis; and b) the possibility of finding individuals with "intermediate" phenotypic expressions at some point of the dynamic continuum of adjustment that, although they may never evolve into clinical psychosis, can exhibit emotional, cognitive, affective, neuropsychological and interpersonal deficits which are qualitatively similar, but less severe, than those found in patients with schizophrenia (Armando et al., 2010; Fonseca-Pedrero, Paino, Lemos-Giraldez et al., 2011; Kwapil, Barrantes Vidal, and Silvia, 2008; Raine, 2006; van Os, Linscott, Myin-Germeys, Delespaul, and Krabbendam, 2009; Wigman et al., 2011).

1.2. Psychometric High-Risk Paradigm: The Assessment of Schizotypal Experiences

A current line of research in the field is based on the idea of early detection, prevention and intervention in individuals at-risk for psychosis with the aim of mitigating or reducing the impact the disorder can cause on the personal, familial and social spheres (McGorry, Killackey, and Yung, 2008; Yung et al., 2007). This fact has propeled, among other aspects, the construction and validation of measurement instruments for the assessment of schizotypy, or more generically, psychosis proneness (Fonseca-Pedrero et al., 2008).

The aim of the "psychometric high-risk" paradigm is the detection, by means of self-reports and based on their score profiles, of those participants with a higher theoretical risk of transiting toward a psychotic disorder in the future (Lenzenweger, 1994). This method allows, in combination with other methods (e.g., genetic high-risk), the analysis of possible etiopathogenetic mechanisms that are at the basis of these types of disorders (Kwapil et al., 2008). The "psychometric high-risk" paradigm is considered a reliable, valid and useful method for the psychometric detection of individuals at-risk for schizophrenia-spectrum disorders. The use of these tools constitutes, in comparison to other techniques, a rapid, efficient and noninvasive method of assessment (Gooding, Tallent, and Matts, 2005; Kelleher, Harley, Murtagh, and Cannon, 2011; Kwapil et al., 2008). Moreover, it allows the study of symptoms that are similar to those found in patients with schizophrenia while avoiding the confounding effects frequently found in these individuals (e.g., medication or stigmatization).

The cornerstone of this research paradigm is founded on data from predictive validity analyses. Independent longitudinal studies indicate that individuals from the general population who report schizotypal experiences such as magical thinking, hallucinatory experiences, delusional ideation and/or anhedonia have a greater risk of transiting toward a schizophrenia-spectrum disorder (Chapman, Chapman, Raulin, and Eckblad, 1994; Dominguez, Saka, Lieb, Wittchen, and van Os, 2010; Dominguez, Wichers, Lieb, Wittchen, and van Os, 2011; Gooding et al., 2005; Poulton et al., 2000; Welham et al., 2009). For example, Poulton et al., (2000) in a longitudinal study carried out in New Zealand in a sample of children, found that more than 25% of the participants who reported these experiences at the age of 11 years developed a schizophreniform disorder at the age of 26 years. In this regard, schizotypal experiences could be considered an exophenotypic risk marker for schizophrenia (Raine, 2006) or a behavioral expression of liability for psychosis (van Os et al., 2009).

The detection of these types of individuals at-risk for psychosis, whether in the clinical or educational settings, requires having adequate measurement instruments that allow us to make solid and well-founded decisions based on the data. Among the most used tools in the literature for the asessment of this construct in adult populations we find the Wisconsin Schizotypy Scales (Chapman, Chapman, and Kwapil, 1995), the Schizotypal Personality Questionnaire (SPQ) (Raine, 1991) and the Thinking and Perceptual Style Questionnaire (TPSQ) (Linscott and Knight, 2004). Likewise, and given that adolescence is a developmental period of special risk for schizophrenia-spectrum disorders (Walker and Bollini, 2002), efforts have also been directed at the assessment of schizotypal experiences in this age group. Good example of these self-reports are: the Junior Schizotypy Scales (JSS) (Rawlings and MacFarlane, 1994), the Schizotypy Traits Questionnaire (STA) for children (Cyhlarova and Claridge, 2005), and the Oviedo Questionnaire for Schizotypy Assessment (ESQUIZO-Q) (Fonseca-Pedrero, Muñiz, Lemos-Giráldez, Paino, and Villazón-García, 2010). Regarding the last mentioned, the ESQUIZO-Q, it is a brief and easy measurement instrument specifically designed for the assessment of schizotypal traits and experiences in adolescents. The construction and validation of the ESQUIZO-Q was carried out including the advances in psychological and educational measurement (e.g., differential item functioning) in a sample of 1,683 Spanish adolescents. The results showed that the ESQUIZO-Q presented adequate psychometric properties. The levels of internal consistency for the 10 subscales that comprised it ranged from .62 to .90. Likewise, none of the 51 items showed differential functioning as a function of gender of the adolescents (Fonseca-Pedrero, Lemos-Giráldez, Paino, and Muñiz, 2011; Fonseca-Pedrero, Lemos-Giráldez, Paino et al., 2011; Fonseca-Pedrero, Paino, Lemos-Giráldez et al., 2011).

It should be mentioned that the different measurement instruments originally developed for their use in adult populations have also been used in youth (e. g., SPQ or TPSQ) (Chen, Hsiao, and Lin, 1997; Fonseca-Pedrero, Linscott, Lemos-Giráldez, Paino, and Muñiz, 2010; Fossati, Raine, Carretta, Leonardi, and Maffei, 2003; Venables and Bailes, 1994). It is well known that this practice implies limitations, although it is equally true that the psychometric characteristics of these self-reports in children and adolescents are quite acceptable. Thus, the validation of self-reports which have not been specifically designed for the assessment of schizotypy in this age group may also be an interesting practice wherever it is supported by the data.

The number of available self-reports for the assessment of schizotypal experiences and traits in adolescents is quite limited and their psychometric qualites have been barely examined. Moreover, it is necessary to have measurement instruments specifically designed for their use in this age group available, as well as an exhaustive and well-founded study of their metric quality in reference to their reliability and different sources of validity evidence. By way of example, it would not be of much use to employ an instrument for the assessment of schizotypal experiences in adolescents with the aim of identifying participants at-risk for schizophrenia if, for instance, the psychometric characteristics of the instrument were unknown, as the inferences (e.g., whether an adolescent is at-risk or not) and the decisions (e.g., whether a more exhaustive psychological evaluation or a preventive intervention must be performed) extracted from the data would be completely ambiguous and unfounded, and would lead to a significant impact on the participants.

1.3. Epidemiology of Schizotypal Experiences in Non Clinical Adolescents

Schizotypal experiences -also known as psychotic-like experiences- represent the behavioral expression of vulnerability for psychotic disorders in general population (van Os et al., 2009). In this sense, a continuous dose-response risk function exists between these kind of experiences and later clinical disorder (Dominguez et al., 2011; Kelleher and Cannon, 2011). Psychotic symptoms are reported not only by patients with schizophrenia but also by healthy members of the general population. In this sense, clinical cases of psychosis represent only a small proportion of the phenotypic continuum of psychosis. The mean prevalence rate of these experiences in general population are of around 5% (Nuevo et al., in press; Scott et al., 2008; van Os et al., 2009). For instance, Nuevo and colleagues (in press) conducted a Worldwide Health Survey in a sample of 256,445 participants, from nationally representative samples of 52 countries. The results showed that the overall prevalence for specific psychotic symptoms ranged from 4.8% for delusions of control to 8.4% for delusions of reference and persecution. Also, the nonclinical expression of the psychosis phenotype has been associated with the same risk factors related to schizophrenia (e.g., cannabis, neurodevelopmental, genetic, urbanicity, etc.) conferring aetiological validity on this construct and suggesting a possible continuity between the clinical and the nonclinical psychosis phenotypes (Kelleher and Cannon, 2011).

In particular, the percentage of self-reported positive schizopytal experiences in adolescents is higher than that found in studies with adults in both clinical and general population samples. The prevalence of positive schizotypal experiences varies considerably across epidemiological studies. It must be mentioned that strict comparison among studies is limited by the type of measurement instrument and the characteristics of the sample used as well as by the statistical criteria employed to determine the prevalence of these experiences (Fonseca-Pedrero, Lemos-Giráldez, Paino, and Sierra-Baigrie, 2011). This consideration must be kept in mind when interpreting and comparing the results obtained in different investigations. In this regard, Yung et al. (2009), using a sample of 875 Australian adolescents, found that around 28% of the assessed participants reported having heard voices sometimes, and 1.9% reported always or nearly always having experienced this. In another study, Scott et al. (2009), analyzing a sample of 1,261 Australian adolescents, found that 8.4% of these reported having had some visual or auditory hallucinatory experience. In another investigation by De Loore and cols. (2008) conducted in a sample of 1,903 Dutch adolescents, the results showed that 5.3% of the participants reported some hallucinatory experience. Higher percentages were found in the study by Horwood et al. (2008), who, using a sample of 6,455 English adolescents, found that 38.9% scored positively on more than one item regarding psychotic experiences, although when these experiences were assessed through an observer-rated method, the percentage decreased to 13.7%. Wigman et al. (2011), in two representative samples of Dutch adolescents (N = 5422; N = 2230) using the Community Assessment of Psychic Experiences-42 (CAPE-42), found that approximately 95% of both samples endorsed at least one positive psychotic experience at level "sometimes" and between 39-43% endorsed at least one experience at level "often" or "nearly always".

Recently, our research team has conducted an empirical study with the aim of examining the distribution of psychotic-like experiences in a representative sample of the adolescent general population (Fonseca-Pedrero, Lemos-Giráldez, Paino et al., 2011). In this research, a total of 1,438 students participated (691 males). The mean age was 15.9 years ($SD = 1.2$), ranging from 14 to 18 years. Ten items included in the ESQUIZO-Q that assess aspects related to magical thinking, unusual perceptual experiences and paranoid ideation were used. The results indicated that psychotic-like experiences are a very common phenomenon in this age group. Between 3.2 and 7.2% of the adolescents reported symptoms related to magical thinking; between 1.2 and 8.8% reported having experienced some unusual perceptual experience; finally, between 1.3 and 13.2% of the nonclinical adolescents were found to report paranoid ideation symptoms.

1.4. Multidimensionality of Schizotypy in Adolescent Population

The understanding of the structure and content of schizotypy in adolescent populations has considerably advanced in the last decade. When the dimensional structure underlying the measurement instruments which assess schizotypal experiences in this age group is analyzed, it can be observed that the construct is of a multidimensional nature (Cyhlarova and Claridge, 2005; Chen et al., 1997; Fonseca-Pedrero, Linscott et al., 2010; Fossati et al., 2003; Venables and Bailes, 1994), phenotypically similar to that found in the general adult population (Bora and Arabaci, 2009; Mason and Claridge, 2006; Wuthrich and Bates, 2006) and in patients with schizophrenia (Liddle, 1987). The number, structure and content of the dimensions found depend greatly on the measurement instrument used, the sample analyzed and the statistical analyses conducted. Nevertheless, although there is no unanimous agreement on the number of dimensions, the results of the different studies taken as a whole allow us to assert that schizotypy in adolescent populations is composed of three or four factors or dimensions, namely Positive (Cognitive-Perceptual, Reality Distortion or Unusual Perceptual Experiences), Negative (Anhedonia or Interpersonal), Disorganized (Cognitive Disorganization) and Impulsive Non-conformity. The Positive factor makes reference to an excessive or distorted functioning of a normal process and includes facets of the type of hallucinatory experiences, paranoid ideation, ideas of reference, and magical thinking. The Negative dimension refers to the reduction or deficit in the normal behavior, and includes facets regarding difficulties to experience pleasure at a physical (physical anhedonia) and social level (social anhedonia), blunted affect, lack of close friends and difficulties in personal relationships. The Disorganized dimension describes thought problems, and odd speech and behavior. The Impulsive Non-conformity dimension includes aspects related to rebelliousness, impulsiveness, and extravagance.

The three-factor model, also known as the Disorganized model (Raine, 1991), composed by the Positive, Interpersonal and Disorganized dimensions, is possibly one of the most replicable and consistent models. It has been found in nonclinical and outpatient adolescents from different cultures, across different statistical techniques (Axelrod, Grilo, Sanislow, and

McGlashan, 2001; Chen et al., 1997; Fonseca-Pedrero, Lemos-Giráldez, Paino, Villazón-García, and Muñiz, 2009; Fossati et al., 2003) and these dimensions have been shown to be invariant across gender and age (Fonseca-Pedrero, Paino, Lemos-Giráldez, Sierra-Baigrie, and Muñiz, 2011; Fossati et al., 2003). Other dimensional models of schizotypy are equally plausible. For example, in some studies, the third dimension of Disorganization could be substituted by a dimension of Impulsive Non-conformity (Fonseca-Pedrero, Linscott et al., 2010; Rawlings and MacFarlane, 1994) or by a more general dimension of Social Disorganization (Fonseca-Pedrero, Linscott et al., 2010). However, other studies posit a different three-factor model composed by the Positive, Paranoid Ideation/Social Anxiety, and Magical Thinking dimensions (Cyhlarova and Claridge, 2005) or by the factors of Magical Ideation/Perceptual Experiences, Ideas of Reference/Social Anxiety, and Suspiciousness (Wolfradt and Straube, 1998). Specifically, with respect to ESQUIZO-Q, the internal structure analysis yielded three second-order factors: Distortion of Reality (Unusual Perceptual Experiences, Paranoid Ideation, Magical Thinking and Ideas of Reference), Negative (Physical and Social Anhedonia) and Interpersonal Disorganization (Excessive Social Anxiety, Odd Behavior, Lack of Close Friends, Odd Thinking and Language) (Fonseca-Pedrero, Muñiz et al., 2010). This internal structure has been replicated in an independent study in a sample of nonclinical Spanish adolescents (Fonseca-Pedrero, Lemos-Giráldez, Paino et al., 2011).

1.5. Aims of Current Study

The ESQUIZO-Q is a self-report of recent construction and therefore it is necessary to carry out new studies that continue to examine its metric quality in a representative sample of adolescents. It is also important to improve our understanding of the psychopathological experiences among youth and develop early detection and intervention strategies in this sector of population in order to mitigate the potential impact of the disease at multiple levels (e.g., family, work, school). Within this research context, the main goal of this study was to analyze the rates of positive schizotypal experiences, as well as the internal structure and reliability of the ESQUIZO-Q in a large sample of Spanish adolescents from the general population. These goals would allow us to: a) deepen current knowledge regarding the psychometric characteristics of a self-report that can be used as a screening tool for the detection of individuals at-risk for psychosis; b) improve comprehension of schizotypal experiences in a developmental stage of special risk for psychosis such as adolescence; and c) advance the field by further understanding the expression of the extended psychosis phenotype in the general population.

2. METHOD

2.1. Participants

Two stratified random cluster sampling were carried out at the classroom level, in a population of approximately 37,000 students selected from the Principality of Asturias (a region in northern Spain) during two academic years (2008/2009 and 2009/2010). Previous data from this research has been published elsewhere (Fonseca-Pedrero, Lemos-Giráldez, Paino et al., 2011; Fonseca-Pedrero, Muñiz et al., 2010). The students were from various public and state-subsidized secondary schools and vocational training centres, as well as from a wide range of socio-economic levels.

The strata were created on the basis of geographical zone (East, West, Centre and Mining area) and educational stage (compulsory – to age 16 – and post-compulsory). The likelihood of the inclusion of a school was directly porportional to the number of students in it. The final sample was made up of N = 3,056 participants, 1,496 boys (48.1%).

The mean age was 15.9 years (SD = 1.2), with an age range of 14 to 18 years. The sample distribution according to age was the following: 14 year olds (N = 400; 13.1%), 15 year olds (N = 780; 25.5%), 16 year olds (N = 885; 29%), 17 year olds (N = 703; 23%) and 18 year olds (N = 288; 9.4%).

2.2. Instruments

The Oviedo Questionnaire for Schizotypy Assessment (ESQUIZO-Q) (Fonseca-Pedrero, Muñiz et al., 2010) is a self-report composed of 51 items in a 5-point Likert-type response format (1= "*completely disagree*"; 5= "*completely agree*") designed to assess schizotypal traits in Spanish adolescents. The ESQUIZO-Q is based on the diagnostic criteria proposed in the DSM-IV-TR (American Psychiatric Association, 2000) and on Meehl's schizotaxia model (1962) regarding genetic predisposition to schizophrenia.

The items of ESQUIZO-Q were selected on the basis of an exhaustive review of the literature on schizotypy (Fonseca-Pedrero et al., 2008). Its construction was conducted following the proposed steps for the construction of measurement instruments (Schmeiser and Welch, 2006) and the guidelines for multiple-choice item construction (Moreno, Martínez, and Muñiz, 2006). The ESQUIZO-Q comprises a total of 10 subscales derived empirically by means of factor analysis: Ideas of Reference, Magical Thinking, Unusual Perceptual Experiences, Odd Thinking and Language, Paranoid Ideation, Physical Anhedonia, Social Anhedonia, Odd Behavior, Lack of Close Friends and Excessive Social Anxiety. These subscales are grouped into three general dimensions: Reality Distortion, Anhedonia, and Interpersonal Disorganization.

Internal consistency levels for the ESQUIZO-Q subscales ranged from .62 to .90 and different sources of validity evidence were obtained (Fonseca-Pedrero, Lemos-Giráldez et al., 2011; Fonseca-Pedrero, Lemos-Giráldez, Paino et al., 2011; Fonseca-Pedrero, Paino, Lemos-Girádez et al., 2011).

The Oviedo Infrequency Scale (INF-OV) (Fonseca-Pedrero et al., 2009) is a 12-item self-report with a 5-point Likert-type rating scale format (1= "*totally disagree*"; 5= "*totally agree*"). Its goal is to detect participants who respond randomly, pseudorandomly or dishonestly on self-reports (e.g., "*The distance between Madrid and Barcelona is greater than between Madrid and New York*"). This type of self-report is frequently used in studies on psychosis proneness. Students with more than 2 incorrect responses on this test were removed from the study.

2.3. Procedure

The administration of the questionnaires was conducted in a collective manner in groups of 10 - 35 students during the school schedule and in a room prepared for this purpose.

The study was presented to participants as an investigation regarding diverse personality characteristics, assuring participants of the confidentiality of their answers as well as the voluntary nature of their participation.

The completion of the questionnaires was conducted under the supervision of a researcher at all times. In cases where necessary, parental informed consent was obtained. The study is part of a wider investigation on the detection and early intervention in psychological disorders in adolescence (www.p3-info.es).

The study was approved by the Research and Ethics Committees at the University of Oviedo, and the Department of Education of the Principality of Asturias.

2.4. Data Analysis

First, the descriptive statistics for the ESQUIZO-Q subscales and second-order dimensions were calculated. Second, the Pearson correlations among the subscales of the ESQUIZO-Q were examined.

In addition, rates of positive schizotypal experiences were analyzed using ten items of the self-report. Next, the dimensional structure underlying the ESQUIZO-Q subscales was analyzed by means of a Principal Components Analysis with posterior Oblimin rotation. Fourth, the reliability for both subscales and general dimensions of the ESQUIZO-Q were estimated using Cronbach´s Alpha coefficient.

For the statistical analyses we used the SPSS 15.0 program (Statistical Package for the Social Sciences, 2006).

3. RESULTS

3.1. Descriptive Statistics

Table 1 shows the descriptive statistics for the total sample referring to the number of items, mean, standard deviation, asymmetry and kurtosis values, score range and levels of internal consistency for the ESQUIZO-Q subscales as well as for the second-order dimensions. As can be observed, the asymmetry and kurtosis values for the subscales fell within the normality range. The Pearson correlations among the ESQUIZO-Q subscales are displayed in Table 2. It can observed that: a) there was a positive correlation among the Ideas of Reference, Magical Thinking and Unusual Perceptual Experiences subscales; b) there were also strong correlations among the subscales Odd Thinking and Language, Excessive Social Anxiety, Lack of Close Friends and Odd Behavior; c) the Physical Anhedonia subscale correlated negatively with the remaining subscales and positively with the Social Anhedonia subscale; and d) the Social Anhedonia subscale correlated significantly, although weakly, with the remaining subscales.

Table 1. Descriptive statistics for the subscales and the dimensions of the Oviedo Questionnaire for Schizotypy Assessment (ESQUIZO-Q)

Subscales	N° items	M	SD	Asymmetry	Kurtosis	Range	Alpha Cronbach
REF	4	6.16	2.61	1.42	2.00	4-20	.70
MAG	5	7.69	3.04	1.36	1.88	5-25	.67
EXP	7	10.38	4.36	1.84	4.06	7-35	.79
PA	5	8.10	3.31	1.30	1.77	5-25	.74
PhysAnh	4	7.82	2.64	0.70	0.61	4-20	.60
SocAnh	5	7.62	2.42	1.09	1.27	5-19	.61
OTL	6	13.96	4.71	0.39	-0.27	6-30	.77
OB	4	6.93	2.88	1.27	1.70	4-20	.68
LCF	4	9.57	3.71	0.39	-0.45	4-20	.63
ANX	7	15.09	5.19	0.71	0.41	7-35	.78
Dimensions							
Reality Distortion	21	32.34	10.39	1.39	2.76	21-97	.84
Anhedonia	9	15.43	4.10	0.78	0.95	9-35	.66
Interpersonal Disorganization	21	45.56	11.83	0.45	0.10	21-93	.87

Note: REF: Ideas of Reference; MAG: Magical Thinking; EXP: Unusual Perceptual Experiences; PA: Paranoid Ideation; PhysAnh: Physical Anhedonia; SocAnh: Social Anhedonia; OTL: Odd Thinking and Language OB: Odd behavior; LCF: Lack of Close Friends; ANX: Excessive Social Anxiety.

3.2. Rates of Positive Schizotypal Experiences

The number and percentage of participants who answered "*I agree quite a bit*" (4) or "*Completely agree*" (5) in the response categories of the 10 selected items in the ESQUIZO-Q are presented in Table 3. As can be seen, between 4.7 and 8.8% of the adolescents reported symptoms related to magical thinking (items 1 to 3); between 2.7 and 10% of the participants reported having experienced some unusual perceptual experience (items 4 to 7); finally, between 2 and 14.5% of the adolescents were found to report paranoid ideation symptoms (items 8 to 10). Moreover, 36.7% of adolescents reported at least one or more positive schizotypal experiences.

3.3. Validity Evidence Based on Internal Structure

A Principal Components Analysis was conducted with posterior Oblimin rotation using the ESQUIZO-Q subscales.

Table 2. Pearson correlations among the subscales of the Oviedo Questionnaire for Schizotypy Assessment (ESQUIZO-Q)

	REF	MAG	EXP	PA	PhysAnh	SocAnh	OTL	OB	LCF	ANX
REF										
MAG	.49*									
EXP	.54*	.54*								
PA	.40*	.38*	.45*							
PhysAnh	-.11*	-.10*	-.14*	-.05*						
SocAnh	.09*	.02	.09*	.16*	.31*					
OTL	.32*	.33*	.41*	.40*	-.12*	.09*				
OB	.37*	.28*	.42*	.48*	.10*	.17*	.33*			
LCF	.21*	.17*	.27*	.37*	-.06*	.15*	.32*	.36*		
ANX	.25*	.25*	.28*	.32*	-.11*	.10*	.41*	.32*	.30*	

*$p < .01$.

Note: REF: Ideas of Reference; MAG: Magical Thinking; EXP: Unusual Perceptual Experiences; PA: Paranoid Ideation; PhysAnh: Physical Anhedonia; SocAnh: Social Anhedonia; OTL: Odd Thinking and Language OB: Odd behavior; LCF: Lack of Close Friends; ANX: Excessive Social Anxiety.

Table 3. Number (and percentage) of participants who obtained high scores (values of 4 or 5 on the Likert scale) on ten selected items of the Oviedo Questionnaire for Schizotypy Assessment (ESQUIZO-Q) relative to positive schizotypal experiences

Selected items of the ESQUIZO-Q (positive schizotypal experiences)	Total sample (N = 3,056) N (%)
1. "I believe that the things that are on the radio or television have a special meaning to me, that my friends don't understand"	143 (4.7)
2. "I think that there are some people who can read other people's minds"	270 (8.8)
3. "I believe there are people who can control the thoughts of others"	197 (6.4)
4. "Being alone at home, I have had the feeling that someone was talking to me"	260 (8.5)
5. "I hear voices that others can't hear"	81 (2.7)
6. "When I am alone, I have the feeling that someone is whispering my name"	103 (3.4)
7. "I have thoughts which are so real that it seems as if someone was talking to me"	306 (10.0)
8. "I think that someone is planning something against me"	236 (7.7)
9. "Somebody has it in for me"	444 (14.5)
10. "My classmates are against me"	62 (2.0)

Table 4. Principal Components Analysis of the Oviedo Questionnaire for Schizotypy Assessment (ESQUIZO-Q) subscales

Subscales	Components		
	I	II	III
Lack of Close Friends	.80		
Excessive Social Anxiety	.72		
Odd Thinking and Language	.59		
Odd Behavior	.54		
Paranoid Ideation	.47		
Physical Anhedonia		.81	
Social Anhedonia		.79	
Magical Thinking			.85
Ideas of Reference			.81
Unusual Perceptual Experiences			.76
Eigenvalue	3.58	1.35	1.04
% Explained variance	35.75	13.48	10.43
% Accumulated explained variance	35.75	49.23	59.66

Note: factorial loadings inferior to .30 have been eliminated.

Table 4 shows the factorial loadings and the percentage of explained and accumulated variance by the three obtained components. The sampling adequacy measure was 7245.86 ($p < .001$), being the KMO index .84. The first component corresponded to the subscales Lack of Close Friends, Excessive Social Anxiety, Odd Thinking and Language, Odd Behavior and Paranoid Ideation, and was denominated Interpersonal Disorganization. The second component corresponded to the Physical and Social Anhedonia subscales and was denominated Anhedonia. Finally, the third component grouped the subscales Magical Thinking, Ideas of Reference, Unusual Perceptual Experiences and Paranoid Ideation and was named Reality Distortion. The Paranoid Ideation facet saturated both in the Interpersonal Disorganization and Reality Distortion components. The correlation between the three dimensions was the following. FI-FII: .05; FI-FIII: .43; FII-FIII: -.01.

3.4. Analysis of Internal Consistency

As can be observed in Table 1, the levels of internal consistency for the ESQUIZO-Q subscales ranged from .60 (Physical Anhedonia) to .79 (Unusual Perceptual Experiences). The levels of internal consistency for the general dimensions of the ESQUIZO-Q ranged from .66 (Anhedonia) to .87 (Interpersonal Disorganization).

DISCUSSION

Adolescence is an interesting period for the early detection of serious mental disorders, such as is the case of psychosis, as well as for the study of risk and protection markers. Both from a clinical and a research perspective, it is of great importance to have at our disposal measurement instruments that are brief, easy and of rapid application to use as screening methods for the detection and posterior preventive intervention of participants who are at-risk for psychosis. Thus, the main goal of the present study was to analyze the rates of positive schizotypal experiences, the internal structure and reliability of the Oviedo Questionnaire for Schizotypy Assessment (ESQUIZO-Q) (Fonseca-Pedrero, Muñiz et al., 2010) in a community sample of Spanish adolescents. The results showed that the ESQUIZO-Q is a self-report with an adequate psychometric characteristic that can be used for schizotypy assessment in adolescents.

The levels of internal consistency for the subscales and the general dimensions of the ESQUIZO-Q ranged from .60 to .87. Some of the reliabilities estimated were inferior to .70; however, it must be taken into account that certain subscales that constitute the ESQUIZO-Q are composed of a reduced number of items. The obtained results are completely convergent with those found in previous studies. For example, Fonseca-Pedrero et al. (2010) had found that the levels of internal consistency for the ESQUIZO-Q subscales ranged from .62 to .90, whereas for the second-order dimensions, they ranged from .67 to .88. Undoubtedly, in future studies, it would be interesting to incorporate a greater number of items in the Anhedonia dimension of the ESQUIZO-Q to improve its internal consistency.

The analysis of the internal structure of the ESQUIZO-Q subscales reflected that schizotypy is a three-factor structure specified in the following factors: Reality Distortion, Anhedonia and Interpersonal Disorganization. This three-factor model is completely convergent with the previous studies conducted with the ESQUIZO-Q and these data also support the underlying structure of this self-report (Fonseca-Pedrero, Lemos-Giráldez, Paino et al., 2011; Fonseca-Pedrero, Muñiz et al., 2010). In previous studies that have used other self-reports (e.g., SPQ, Wisconsin Schizotypy Scales), a factorial structure similar to the one in this study is found (Bora and Arabaci, 2009; Fonseca-Pedrero et al., 2009; Fossati et al., 2003; Kwapil et al., 2008; Wuthrich and Bates, 2006), although we must keep in mind the difficulties inherent to the comparison between studies (e.g., cultural origin or sampling). For example, Fonseca-Pedrero et al. (2010), using the TPSQ in a sample of Spanish adolescents, obtained a three-factor structure composed of the dimensions: Aberrant Information Processing, Anhedonia, and Social Disorganization. Other studies using the SPQ by Raine (1991) consistently replicate the disorganized model of schizotypal personality composed of the Positive, Interpersonal and Disorganized dimensions (Bora and Arabaci, 2009; Fonseca-Pedrero et al., 2009; Fossati et al., 2003; Wuthrich and Bates, 2006). These data indicate that schizotypy seems to be a multifactorial structure specified in three correlated factors similar to that found in the young adults and in patients with schizophrenia.

The ESQUIZO-Q can also be used as a measurement instrument for the assessment of the rate of positive schizotypal experiences in adolescent populations. The results of this study show that between 2 and 14.5% of the adolescents, reported some positive schizotypal experience. These data are also convergent with those found in other previous studies conducted with the ESQUIZO-Q (Fonseca-Pedrero, Lemos-Giráldez, Paino et al., 2011) and with nonclinical adolescents from different cultures (Armando et al., 2010; Wigman et al., 2011; Yung et al., 2009). Likewise, previous studies indicate that this group of experiences are frequent in this developmental stage and that their frequency and intensity are greater than that reported by adults from the general population (Nuevo et al., in press; Scott et al., 2008; van Os et al., 2009). Moreover, previous investigations indicate that a continuous dose-response risk function exists between subclinical psychotic experiences and later clinical disorder (Dominguez et al., 2011; van Os et al., 2009). However, it is equally true that most of the participants who report positive schizotypal experiences may be experiencing a transitory state or may never progress to clinical psychotic disorder. Specifically, between 10 and 35% of these subclinical psychotic experiences can interact synergetically or additively with other environmental (i.e., genetic, trauma, cannabis, urbanicity, victimization, etc.) or genetic factors, increasing the persistence of psychotic experiences and consequently becoming abnormally persistent, clinically relevant and need of care (Cougnard et al., 2007; De Loore et al., 2011; van Os et al., 2009). In addition, these individuals who report schizotypal experiences present a greater degree of affective, social, interpersonal and behavioral deficits (Armando et al., 2010; Fonseca-Pedrero, Paino, Lemos-Girádez et al., 2011; Kwapil et al., 2008; Lenzenweger, McLachlan, and Rubin, 2007; Raine, 2006; Wigman et al., 2011; Yung et al., 2009). These data seem to reflect that the alterations characteristic of patients with schizophrenia can also be found in samples of the general population below the clinical threshold supporting the continuity between clinical and nonclinical psychosis phenotype. According to this theory, schizotypal experiences are situated at some point of this continuum and could be seen as an "intermediate" phenotype, qualitatively similar and quantitatively less severe than the symptomatology found in patients with schizophrenia presenting itself with a lesser intensity, persistence, frequency and associated disability (Dominguez et al., 2011; van Os et al., 2009; Wigman et al., 2011).

The results obtained from studies on the psychometric high-risk paradigm have important practical implications. Measuring instruments such as ESQUIZO-Q can be used as screening tools in educational settings. The assessment of uncommon beliefs and thoughts, such as schizotypal experiences, could be carried out within a multi-step process. In the first phase we would detect those participants with a hypothetical liability to schizophrenia spectrum disorders, based on the self-report scores. Then, in a second step, there would be a more comprehensive psychological assessment. In this phase, the certainty and the distress of the psychotic-like experiences and the symptoms of depression would be assessed; other risk factors of psychosis such as genetic background (e.g. first-degree relatives of patients), cannabis use, or coping strategies would be evaluated as well. At this stage, information from other sources close to the individual, such as parents, close friends or teachers can also be gathered, in a multi-informant assessment. In third place, participants could be sent to a specialized mental health care center to receive a prophylactic treatment. This multi-step process is just one of the possible ways, as it may be the case of a participant who is sent directly to the mental health care center due to the severity of his/her psychopathological symptoms and signs.

Issues like those raised above open the debate on the possibility of early interventions before the development of psychotics symptoms, which is related to the Attenuated Psychotic Symptoms Risk Syndrome, recently proposed in the DSM-V. From our point of view, assessing the risk of psychosis requires reliable and rigorous data, allowing a precise and accurate detection of individuals at high risk, in order to make sound decisions, for instance, whether to use psychopharmacological treatments or not when psychotic symptoms are below the critical threshold. This requires: a) rigorous assessments which collect information from different sources, not only self-report; and b) standardized testing protocols, both nationally and internationally, must be developed. To this end it is necessary to create multidisciplinary teams composed of psychologists, physicians, neuropsychologists, social workers, and other health professionals. Current research going in this direction, and although we are still in a development phase, everything suggests that we have a promising future in this area of study. The psychometric high-risk paradigm is only a small part of the different action lines that currently exist (e.g. first episode psychosis, clinical high-risk studies), however we believe that they are generating very interesting clues. We should not forget that the main goal of this research is to mitigate the potential impact of psychotic disorder in the individual.

The results found in the present study should be interpreted in light of the following limitations. First, the extracted conclusions are founded exclusively on a self-report and there is no doubt that the use of external informants such as parents or teachers via hetero-reports would have been interesting. Second, it is frequent that the questions on these self-reports can cause some kind of stigma on participants. Third, the schizotypal experiences must always be analyzed within a biopsicosocial model. The additive or synergic interactions between schizotypal experiences and genetic, chemical, cognitive and social factors are relevant and interesting with a view to understanding and explaining the transition to the clinical state. Fourth, no information was gathered regarding the participants´ psychiatric morbidity or the use or abuse of substances, aspects which may be partially modulating the obtained results.

Future lines of research should continue to examine the psychometric properties of ESQUIZO-Q in other samples of interest, such as adolescents or young adults with prodromes ("clinical high-risk" studies). It is specifically relevant to determine the predictive validity of this self-report (e.g., sensitivity and specificity) in longitudinal studies. Finally, integration of schizotypy within dimensional models of personality and the study of measurement invariance across cultures are interesting lines of study for the near future.

Acknowledgments

This research was funded by the Spanish Ministry of Science and Innovation (MICINN) and by the Instituto Carlos III, Center for Biomedical Research in the Mental Health Network (CIBERSAM). Project references: BES 2006-12797, SEJ 2008-03934, PSI2011-28638 and PSI 2008-06220.

References

American Psychiatric Association. (2000). *Diagnostic and Statistical Manual of Mental Disorders* (4 th ed revised). Washington, DC: American Psychiatric Association.

Armando, M., Nelson, B., Yung, A. R., Ross, M., Birchwood, M., Girardi, P., and Nastro, P. F. (2010). Psychotic-like experiences and correlation with distress and depressive symptoms in a community sample of adolescents and young adults. *Schizophrenia Research*, 119, 258-265.

Axelrod, S. R., Grilo, M. C., Sanislow, C., and McGlashan, T. H. (2001). Schizotypal Personality Questionnaire-Brief: Factor structure and convergent validity in inpatient adolescent. *Journal of Personality Disorders*, 15(2), 168-179.

Bora, E., and Arabaci, L. A. (2009). Effect of age and gender on schizotypal personality traits in the normal population. *Psychiatry and Clinical Neurosciences*, 63, 663-669.

Claridge, G. (1997). Schizotypy: Implications for illness and health. Oxford: Oxford University Press.
Cougnard, A., Marcelis, M., Myin-Germeys, I., De Graaf, R., Vollebergh, W., Krabbendam, L., Lieb, R., Wittchen, H. U., Henquet, C., Spauwen, J., and Van Os, J. (2007). Does normal developmental expression of psychosis combine with environmental risk to cause persistence of psychosis? A psychosis proneness-persistence model. *Psychological Medicine*, 37, 513-527.
Cyhlarova, E., and Claridge, G. (2005). Development of a version of the Schizotypy Traits Questionnaire (STA) for screening children. *Schizophrenia Research*, 80 (2-3), 253-261.
Chapman, J. P., Chapman, L. J., and Kwapil, T. R. (1995). Scales for the measurement of schizotypy. In A. Raine, T. Lencz and S. A. Mednick (Eds.), *Schizotypal Personality* (pp. 79-106). New York: Cambridge University Press.
Chapman, J. P., Chapman, L. J., Raulin, M. L., and Eckblad, M. (1994). Putatively psychosis-prone subjects 10 years later. *Journal of Abnormal Psychology*, 87, 399-407.
Chen, W. J., Hsiao, C. K., and Lin, C. C. H. (1997). Schizotypy in community samples: The three-factor structure and correlation with sustained attention. *Journal of Abnormal Psychology*, 106(4), 649-654.
De Loore, E., Gunther, N., Drukker, M., Feron, F., Sabbe, B., Deboutte, D., van Os, J., and Myin-Germeys, I. (2008). Auditory hallucinations in adolescence: A longitudinal general population study. *Schizophrenia Research*, 102, 229-230.
De Loore, E., Gunther, N., Drukker, M., Feron, F., Sabbe, B., Deboutte, D., van Os, J., and Myin-Germeys, I. (2011). Persistence and outcome of auditory hallucinations in adolescence: a longitudinal general population study of 1800 individuals. *Schizophrenia Research*, 127, 252-256.
Dixon, L., Weiden, P., Delahanty, J., Goldberg, R., Postrado, L., Lucksted, A., and Lehman, A. (2000). Prevalence and correlates of diabetes in national schizophrenia samples. *Schizophrenia Bulletin*, 26, 903-912.
Dominguez, M. D., Saka, M. C., Lieb, R., Wittchen, H. U., and van Os, J. (2010). Early expression of negative/disorganized symptoms predicting psychotic experiences and subsequent clinical psychosis: a 10-year study. *American Journal of Psychiatry*, 167, 1075-1082.
Dominguez, M. G., Wichers, M., Lieb, R., Wittchen, H.-U., and van Os, J. (2011). Evidence that onset of clinical psychosis is an outcome of progressively more persistent subclinical psychotic experiences: An 8-Year Cohort Study. *Schizophrenia Bulletin*, 37, 84-93.
Fonseca-Pedrero, E., Lemos-Giráldez, E., Paino, M., and Sierra-Baigrie, S. (2011). Psychotic-like experiences in nonclinical adolescents. In M. S. Payne (Ed.), *Hallucinations: Types, stages, and treatments* (pp. 131-146). New York: Nova Science Publishers.
Fonseca-Pedrero, E., Lemos-Giráldez, S., Paino, M., and Muñiz, J. (2011). Schizotypy, emotional-behavioural problems and personality disorder traits in a non-clinical adolescent population. *Psychiatry Research*, 190, 316-321
Fonseca-Pedrero, E., Lemos-Giráldez, S., Paino, M., Sierra-Baigrie, S., Santarén-Rosell, M., and Muñiz, J. (2011). Internal structure and reliability of the Oviedo Schizotypy Assessment Questionnaire (ESQUIZO-Q). *International Journal of Clinical and Health Psychology*, 11, 385-402.

Fonseca-Pedrero, E., Lemos-Giráldez, S., Paino, M., Villazón-García, U., and Muñiz, J. (2009). Validation of the Schizotypal Personality Questionnaire Brief form in adolescents. *Schizophrenia Research*, 111, 53-60.

Fonseca-Pedrero, E., Linscott, R. J., Lemos-Giráldez, S., Paino, M., and Muñiz, J. (2010). Psychometric properties of two measures for the assessment of schizotypy in adolescents. *Psychiatry Research*, 179, 165–170.

Fonseca-Pedrero, E., Muñiz, J., Lemos-Giráldez, S., Paino, M., and Villazón-García, U. (2010). ESQUIZO-Q: Cuestionario Oviedo para la Evaluación de la Esquizotipia [ESQUIZO-Q: Oviedo Questionnaire for Schizotypy Assessment]. Madrid: TEA ediciones.

Fonseca-Pedrero, E., Paino, M., Lemos-Girádez, S., Sierra-Baigrie, S., Ordóñez, N., and Muñiz, J. (2011). Early psychopathological features in Spanish adolescents. *Psicothema*, 23, 87-93.

Fonseca-Pedrero, E., Paino, M., Lemos-Giráldez, S., García-Cueto, E., Campillo-Álvarez, A., Villazón-García, U., and Muñiz, J. (2008). Schizotypy assessment: State of the art and future prospects. *International Journal of Clinical and Health Psychology*, 8, 577-593.

Fonseca-Pedrero, E., Paino, M., Lemos-Giráldez, S., Sierra-Baigrie, S., and Muñiz, J. (2011). Measurement invariance of the Schizotypal Personality Questionnaire-Brief across gender and age. *Psychiatry Research*, 190, 309-315.

Fossati, A., Raine, A., Carretta, I., Leonardi, B., and Maffei, C. (2003). The three-factor model of schizotypal personality: Invariance across age and gender. *Personality and Individual Differences*, 35, 1007-1019.

Gooding, D. C., Tallent, K. A., and Matts, C. W. (2005). Clinical status of at-risk individuals 5 years later: Further validation of the psychometric high-risk strategy. *Journal of Abnormal Psychology*, 114, 170-175.

Horwood, J., Salvi, G., Thomas, K., Duffy, L., Gunnell, D., Hollis, C., Lewis, G., Menezes, P., Thompson, A., Wolke, D., Zammit, S., and Harrison, G. (2008). IQ and non-clinical psychotic symptoms in 12-year-olds: results from the ALSPAC birth cohort. *British Journal of Psychiatry*, 193, 185-191.

Kelleher, I., and Cannon, M. (2011). Psychotic-like experiences in the general population: characterizing a high-risk group for psychosis. *Psychological Medicine*, 41, 1-6.

Kelleher, I., Harley, M., Murtagh, A., and Cannon, M. (2011). Are screening instruments valid for psychotic-Like experiences? A validation study of screening questions for psychotic-like experiences using in-depth clinical interview. *Schizophrenia Bulletin*, 7, 362-369.

Kendler, K. S. (1985). Diagnostic approaches to schizotypal personality disorder: A historical perspective. *Schizophrenia Bulletin*, 11, 538-553.

Kwapil, T. R., and Barrantes-Vidal, N. (in press). Schizotypal Personality Disorder: An Integrative Review. In T. A. Widiger (Ed.), The Oxford Handbook of Personality Disorders. New York: Oxford University Press.

Kwapil, T. R., Barrantes Vidal, N., and Silvia, P. J. (2008). The dimensional structure of the Wisconsin schizotypy scales: Factor identification and construct validity. *Schizophrenia Bulletin*, 34, 444-457.

Lasser, K., Boyd, J. W., Woolhandler, S., Himmelstein, D. U., McCormick, D., and Bor, D. H. (2000). Smoking and mental illness: a population-based prevalence study. *JAMA*, 284, 2606-2610.

Lenzenweger, M. F. (1994). Psychometric high-risk paradigm, perceptual aberrations, and schizotypy: An update. *Schizophrenia Bulletin*, 20, 121-135.

Lenzenweger, M. F. (2010). Schizotypy and schizophrenia: The view from experimental psychopathology. New York: Guilford Press.

Lenzenweger, M. F., McLachlan, G., and Rubin, D. B. (2007). Resolving the latent structure of schizophrenia endophenotypes using expectation-maximization-based finite mixture modeling. *Journal of Abnormal Psychology*, 116, 16-29.

Liddle, P. (1987). The symptoms of chronic schizophrenia: A re-examination of the positive-negative dichotomy. *British Journal of Psychiatry*, 151, 145-151.

Linscott, R. J., and Knight, R. G. (2004). Potentiated automatic memory in schizotypy. *Personality and Individual Differences*, 37, 1503-1517.

Mangalore, R., and Knapp, M. (2007). Cost of schizophrenia in England. *The Journal of Mental Health Policy and Economics*, 10, 23-41.

Mason, O., and Claridge, G. (2006). The Oxford-Liverpool Inventory of Feelings and Experiences (O-LIFE): Further description and extended norms. *Schizophrenia Research*, 82(2), 203-211.

McGorry, P. D., Killackey, E., and Yung, A. (2008). Early intervention in psychosis: concepts, evidence and future directions. *World Psychiatry*, 7, 148-156.

McGrath, J., Saha, S., Chant, D., and Welham, J. (2008). Schizophrenia: a concise overview of incidence, prevalence, and mortality. *Epidemiologic Reviews*, 30, 67-76.

Meehl, P. E. (1962). Schizotaxia, schizotypy, schizophrenia. *American Psychologist*, 17(12), 827-838.

Moreno, R., Martínez, R., and Muñiz, J. (2006). New guidelines for developing multiple-choice items. *Methodology*, 2, 65-72.

Nuevo, R., Chatterji, S., Verdes, E., Naidoo, N., Arango, C., and Ayuso-Mateos, J. L. (in press). The continuum of psychotic symptoms in the general population: A cross-national study. Schizophrenia Bulletin.doi: 10.1093/schbul/sbq099.

Poulton, R., Caspi, A., Moffitt, T. E., Cannon, M., Murray, R., and Harrington, H. (2000). Children's self-reported psychotic symptoms and adult schizophreniform disorder: a 15-year longitudinal study. *Archives of General Psychiatry*, 57, 1053-1058.

Raine, A. (1991). The SPQ: A scale for the assessment of schizotypal personality based on DSM-III-R criteria. *Schizophrenia Bulletin*, 17, 555-564.

Raine, A. (2006). Schizotypal personality: Neurodevelopmental and psychosocial trajectories. *Annual Review of Clinical Psychology*, 2, 291-326.

Rawlings, D., and MacFarlane, C. (1994). A multidimensional schizotypal traits questionnaire for young adolescents. *Personality and Individual Differences*, 17, 489-496.

Saha, S., Chant, D., and McGrath, J. (2007). A systematic review of mortality in schizophrenia: is the diff erential mortality gap worsening over time? *Archives of General Psychiatry*, 64, 1123-1131.

Scott, J., Martin, G., Bor, W., Sawyer, M., Clark, J., and McGrath, J. (2009). The prevalence and correlates of hallucinations in Australian adolescents: Results from a national survey. *Schizophrenia Research*, 109, 179-185.

Scott, J., Welham, J., Martin, G., Bor, W., Najman, J., O' Callaghan, M., Williams, G., Aird, R., and McGrath, J. (2008). Demographic correlates of psychotic-like experiences in young Australian adults. *Acta Psychiatrica Scandinavica*, 118, 230-237.

Schmeiser, C. B., and Welch, C. (2006). Test development. In R. L. Brennan (Ed.), Educational Measurement (4th ed.) (pp. 307-353). Westport, CT: American Council on Education/Praeger.

Statistical Package for the Social Sciences. (2006). SPSS Base 15.0 User's Guide. Chicago, IL: SPSS Inc.

van Os, J., and Kapur, S. (2009). Schizophrenia. *Lancet*, 374, 635-645.

van Os, J., Linscott, R. J., Myin-Germeys, I., Delespaul, P., and Krabbendam, L. (2009). A systematic review and meta-analysis of the psychosis continuum: Evidence for a psychosis proneness-persistence-impairment model of psychotic disorder. *Psychological Medicine*, 39, 179-195.

Venables, P. H., and Bailes, K. (1994). The structure of schizotypy, its relation to subdiagnoses of schizophrenia and to sex and age. *British Journal of Clinical Psychology*, 33, 277-294.

Walker, E., and Bollini, A. (2002). Pubertal neurodevelopmental and the emergence of psychotic symptons. *Schizophrenia Research*, 54, 17-23.

Welham, J., Scott, J., Williams, G., Najman, J., Bor, W., O'Callaghan, M., and McGrath, J. (2009). Emotional and behavioural antecedents of young adults who screen positive for non-affective psychosis: a 21-year birth cohort study. *Psychological Medicine*, 39, 625-634.

Wigman, J. T., van Winkel, R., Raaijmakers, Q. A., Ormel, J., Verhulst, F. C., Reijneveld, S. A., van Os, J., and Vollebergh, W. A. (2011). Evidence for a persistent, environment-dependent and deteriorating subtype of subclinical psychotic experiences: a 6-year longitudinal general population study. *Psychological Medicine*, 41, 2317-2329.

Wigman, J. T., Vollebergh, W. A., Raaijmakers, Q. A., Iedema, J., van Dorsselaer, S., Ormel, J., Verhulst, F. C., and van Os, J. (2011). The structure of the extended psychosis phenotype in early adolescence--A cross-sample replication. *Schizophrenia Bulletin*, 37, 850-860.

Wolfradt, U., and Straube, E. R. (1998). Factor structure of schizotypal traits among adolescents. *Personality and Individual Differences*, 24, 201-206.

Wu, E. Q., Birnbaum, H. G., Shi, L., Ball, D. E., Kessler, R. C., Moulis, M., and Aggarwal, J. (2005). The economic burden of schizophrenia in the United States in 2002. *Journal of Clinical Psychiatry*, 66, 1122-1129.

Wuthrich, V., and Bates, T. C. (2006). Confirmatory factor analysis of the three-factor structure of the schizotypal personality questionnaire and Chapman schizotypy scales. *Journal of Personality Assessment*, 87, 292-304.

Yung, A. R., Killackey, E., Hetrick, S. E., Parker, A. G., Schultze-Lutter, F., Klosterkoetter, J., Purcell, R., and Mcgorry, P. D. (2007). The prevention of schizophrenia. *International Review of Psychiatry*, 19, 633-646.

Yung, A. R., Nelson, B., Baker, K., Buckby, J. A., Baksheev, G., and Cosgrave, E. M. (2009). Psychotic-like experiences in a community sample of adolescents: implications for the continuum model of psychosis and prediction of schizophrenia. *Australian and New Zealand Journal of Psychiatry*, 43, 118-128.

Section 2. Contextual Effects and Socialization Processes

In: Youth: Practices, Perspectives and Challenges
Editor: Elizabeth Trejos-Castillo

ISBN: 978-1-62618-067-3
© 2013 Nova Science Publishers, Inc.

Chapter 5

YOUTH VIOLENCE: RISKS, CAUSES, MANAGEMENT STRATEGIES AND DIRECTIONS FOR FUTURE INQUIRY

Suman Sarkar[*]
Birbal Sahni Institute of Palaeobotany, India

ABSTRACT

Youth forms a vital component of the social pyramid. This domain of the society refers to people who are too young to be classified as adults and simultaneously older than the category of children. It plays a pivotal role in laying the foundation of a nation's future but at the same time this group is very vulnerable to a number of negative factors prevailing in the society. The demon of youth violence is rapidly spreading its wings across the world in the present era leading to a rise in fear. This apprehensiveness is not restricted to those living in the most disadvantaged neighborhoods in larger cities, but extending to the residents of prosperous suburban communities, and even small towns and villages irrespective of the state, country and continent involved.

Youth violence is a high-priority issue gradually developing into a social epidemic with several risk factors, including individual beliefs and behaviors such as early aggression and use of alcohol and drugs, family characteristics like lack of proper parental supervision, peer and school influences such as associating with miscreant friends, and environmental factors such as access to firearms, increasing exposure to pornography on the internet and video games displaying acts of violence. Youth violence has reached a critical point in the world scenario, affecting the health of the society, quality of life, and economic development of the global communities. Rising gang violence involving youth, school shootings, teacher abuse and children injured/killed by youth-committed violence is a real concern. Suppression is certainly not a permanent solution and unsustainable in the long-run. Active prevention policies on the other hand effectively increase the opportunity for positive, long-term outcomes for youth and communities as a whole.

Research into the prevalence of violence and delinquency among youth has proliferated all across the world in the last couple of decades as a result of a manifold rise

---
[*] Email: suman763@gmail.com.

in cases of youth indulgence in violence. The aim of this current study is to analyze the trend of increasing youth violence and analyze the status of youth as being victimized or actually committing violence themselves? An attempt has been made to gain more insight into the social epidemic of youth violence along with the roles played by parents, family, various socio-cognitive policies and other preventive strategies to control the evil of youth violence. While social issues such as homelessness and poverty have long been recognized in urban communities, the very important factor of youth violence has recently been acknowledged as community concern as a whole in the world and it is a social imperative to not only analyze this evil but propose a preventive or decisive solution to pave way for a stronger social framework leading to a happier and peaceful future.

INTRODUCTION

Youth violence is progressively becoming a global public health epidemic affecting the livability of the society quite strongly, adding to the criminal efficiency of the world as a whole and plaguing the communities irrespective of their social status and structure. No country or community on the earth is unscathed by violence. There is indignation for change but is it as deep as the pockets of the very issue of youth violence? Going the other way round, it may be another instance where the axis of blame is so wide angle that we fail to see our own casual complicity. The subject of youth violence is actually very broad and requires specific handling of various aspects harnessing the problem. Quite sadly, children and teenagers in our society are not spared from the evil of violence. Some of the important factors that deserve urgent attention from us include sensitive issues like incarceration, parent counseling, neighborhood monitoring, peer behavior, home detention, rehabilitation camps and the role of media, police and judicial system in controlling youth violence. As per the recent trend, a lot of attention is being given to awareness regarding gang activities and their prevention policies that have become the virtual symbol of global youth violence. Unfortunately a large number of major issues such as lack of proper attention from parents, bullying during school days, endemic violence existing in the neighborhood and absence of positive role models are not being addressed properly. Every day we wake up to the obscene reports of violence viz., school shootings, teacher abuse, rapes and molestation involving young fellows, children injured/killed by rowdy activities in their neighborhood or homes that force us to ask ourselves what exactly is going wrong and where has the society failed in veraciously nurturing the future of tomorrow? In our society, violence is bursting. It is crossing all the social classes, genders and racial lines. It is becoming a legacy being passed on from one generation to another. Comprehensive research for initiating violence prevention and improving the overall outcomes in local communities as well as international circles has been prompted lately by practically proven issues such as criminal justice procedure costs, rising number of cases involving children uninterested in going to school and increasing percentage of uneducated, unemployed and ruthless youth in the global population (Goede and Spruijt, 1996).

This chapter discusses some distinct strategies for combating the problem of youth violence and offers some recommendations on the basis of various social, psychological and scientific evidences available. These practices do have the potential for designing and developing a better paradigm that includes perfect goals and objectives for our target of preventing youth violence. In order to obtain the best possible results, we need to engage the entire community in our mission and locate the right resources as well as task-partners. We have to keep the future perspectives in mind, determine a suitable time frame for various steps of the work and arrange for regular monitoring of the progress and outcome of the mission.

YOUTH VIOLENCE A MAJOR CONCERN: SITUATION GETTING BAD TO WORSE

Youth violence is a complex problem associated with several risk factors, some staying limited to individuals and their families, whereas others having wider implications. These include aggression at an early age, lack of parental supervision, use of alcohol or drugs, spousal abuse, coming in touch with delinquent friends, easier access to firearms, gambling and so on (Barnes et al., 1999; Howard et al., 1999). Unfolding this complex puzzle is actually the real challenge for researchers and volunteers concerned with the betterment of youth.

With ever increasing population rates, the state of youth violence is indeed getting more and more pathetic. The present generation youth are not only becoming the frequent victims of serious violence but getting equally involved as criminals at the same time. One important dimension of youth violence has however clearly changed in the present world that on overall basis it has gained in lethality. This accounts for a large number of serious injuries and mortality resulting due to the acts of hostility. A great increase in adolescent homicide rate over the last couple of decades is a grim evidence of this increased lethality. Easier availability and use of guns and other weapons in these violent exchanges is largely responsibly for this gain in the lethality measure. A dramatic decline in the commitment of most young persons to responsible, lawful behavior is adding the maximum weight to the negativity of youth violence (Mitchell et al., 2007). We must shift our focus on what has happened in the lives of these violent young people that they are losing the respect for human life. Reports of physical abuse of children and youth suggest that many are assaulted by family members and caretakers if assessed on an annual basis. Among children and youth, preschoolers have been found most likely to be the victims of physical assault, followed by elementary school-aged children, teenagers and infants. A small but significant percentage of youth are victims of a violent personal assault each year while at school. Overall, teenagers are more likely to be victims of an assault than persons above the age of 20. Suicide is now the third leading cause of death for youth. Clearly the danger bell of violence has struck the chord for our children and teenagers. If observed on basis of personal characteristics, young violent offenders and victims share many similarities. This is due to the involvement of victims in violent acts themselves or existence of high risk in those victims becoming violent during their adolescent years. Grouping of the young offenders on basis of their sex, caste, income and family-background can be deceptive. There is little evidence from the conducted studies for any difference in inclination towards violence by race, once social class is taken into account (Barnes et al., 1999). Therefore youth violence is a widespread social problem not just for the poor or minorities living in large cities but crosses all class, race, gender and residence boundaries.

With changing time and scenario in the international coliseum, a large percentage of youth find violence to be the only or most effective means of achieving status and respect in the society along with other basic personal luxuries (Checkoway, 2011). Unfortunately, violence like money and knowledge, has gained popularity as a form of power. For some youth, it is the only form of power available. With this mentality of limited alternatives combining with a weak commitment to internally controlled moral norms and lack of monitoring or supervision coming from parents/seniors in the family/neighborhood, violent behavior becomes coherent. Early exposure to violence in the family may involve either witnessing violence or physical abuse. Research suggests that these forms of exposure to violence during childhood increase the risk of violent behavior during adolescence by as much as 40 percent. Still, most youth who are victims of physical abuse do not go on to become serious violent offenders. While exposure to real violence and physical abuse on the part of family members have stronger modeling effects, heavy exposure to violence on television and movies is also causally linked to later violence. In many homes, television is the real babysitter, with little or no monitoring or supervision of content. When there is strong family bonding, effective teaching of moral values and norms, and efficient monitoring of behavior, the effect of exposure to violence on TV is probably negligible. In absence of this control measure, its effect can be quite strong. What is learned is not only how to do violence, but desensitization to violence and rationalizations for disengaging one's moral obligations to others. Even if violence is not modeled in the home, absence of effective social bonds and controls, together with a failure of parents to teach (and children to internalize) conventional norms and values, puts children at risk of violence later on in their lives.

In fact, parental neglect may have an even stronger impact than physical abuse, as it appears to be more damaging to the subsequent course of youth development (Howard et al. 1999).

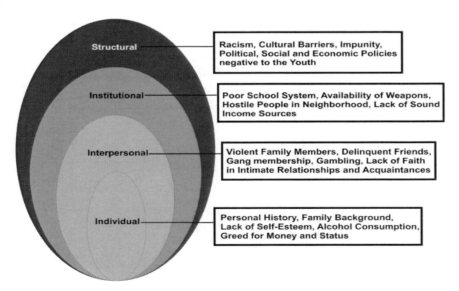

Figure. The Integrated Model For Aiolance Applied to Youth Violance.

Certain individual temperaments and acquired biological deficits may complicate or interfere with parents' efforts to develop good internal controls in their children. Factors like antisocial personality and attention shortage disorders, a fearless and impulsive temperament, exposure to lead and other neurotoxins may make it difficult for even the best parents to develop strong family bonding and provide effective monitoring of their children. Violence has four interrelated levels if seen on a general basis in terms of impact and intervention i.e., individual, interpersonal, institutional and structural (see Figure).

In context with the analysis of youth violence, a debatable question that comes to our mind is whether the present status of youth violence epidemic reflects a true picture of the behavior of the youth group or just a distortion resulting from excessive media coverage. Going by what we are seeing around us in everyday lives, the newspaper reports and television analyses in the current scenario, the former status sounds truer. Over the past few years, there has been a substantial rise in violence victimization rates for adolescents (especially the 12-15 year olds) and those involved in some violent activities as active offenders.

> Safety and security don't just happen; they are the result of collective consensus and public investment. We owe our children, the vulnerable citizens in our society, a life free of violence and fear – *Nelson Mandela.*

STATUS OF YOUTH VIOLENCE IN INDIA: THE PICTURE LOOKS FRIGHTENING

In India there are over 320 million people in the age category of 10-24 years, representing about 30 percent of the country's population. This cohort is healthier, better educated and more urbanized than the previous generations but at the same time face certain significant problems. A lack of knowledge and power needed to make informed choices pertaining to several crucial decisions in their lives keep them in a confused state of mind on several occasions. These vulnerabilities remain poorly understood and served, and it has been only since the mid-1990s that researchers and policymakers have started investigating these issues. There is still a deficit of evidences to identify the factors that protect the youth's abilities to ensure their health and autonomy to make desired choices. For effective youth protection, we need to identify key transitions facing young people, including education and livelihood opportunities, provide evidence at the state level on the magnitude and patterns of sexual and reproductive practices (in and outside of marriage), and related knowledge, decision-making practices and attitudes among youth. 41% children of the 5-12 age groups are sexually harassed in India according to a report of the Ministry of Women and Child Development. At least 21% children are sexually harassed by being kissed by their relatives against their will. According to the law, if someone powerfully kisses a child against his/her will then this is a kind of sexual abuse. 95% of such cases go unreported and no complaint is lodged by parents or children. At least 45% of boys and 55% of girls suffer the pain of sexual harassment. In 31.5% of such cases, family members, neighbors or friends are responsible for the harassment. 21% of these cases take place at home and 18.50% of such cases occur in schools. In last few years, states of Bihar, Maharashtra and Uttar Pradesh have been the leaders in reports of sexual harassment of children.

There is a lot of variation in the form of youth violence in urban and rural areas along with the upper/middle and lower class families in India. In the urban domain, it is more private and concealed within the four walls of homes. According to the recent surveys conducted across the Indian cities, most common reasons are disobeying parental advises and orders, lagging behind at the academic level, not being at par with children in neighborhood, debating with parents or speaking ill about other family members and not returning to home on time. In rural areas, frontline reasons are harassment for child labor, physical abuse or harm for not following family traditions, forcing kids (especially girls) to stay at home and carry out domestic activities, thus depriving them from going to school etc. Despite being in the modern 21st century, girls in India are getting victimized by a number of malpractices such as child marriage in a number of rural areas, dowry harassment both at the urban as well as rural level and enforced prostitution. As the common mob mentality of India still prefers at least one male child after marriage, the girls in most cases are cursed or assaulted for having taken birth in the home.

Large number of reported cases of paedophilia makes the picture even more frightening. Since last few years, the number of rape cases of pre-matured girls has been ascending. A survey of teens and college students has found rape to account for 70 percent of sexual assault cases in girls. It is largely due to the inadequate laws pertaining to rape conviction that rape victims are reluctant to report the matter to police or even disclose the fact before their parents. Apart from sexual abuse and rape, pushing, slapping, punching, stalking and emotional abuse are other forms of violence against children. Adding to the above cases, violence against physically/mentally challenged children is also very much prevalent in the Indian society. Instead of treating them with kindness and care, these children are beaten and harassed for being in such a handicapped state. In poor families, reports of selling body organs of the retarded children for the sake of money reflect height of cruelty and violence against innocent children.

RISK FACTORS ASSOCIATED WITH YOUTH VIOLENCE

The consequences of youth violence are very drastic and its effect is long lived. Children are very sensitive and not mature enough to realize the incidents of violence. In their juvenile phase, very often they try to imitate the things happening around them. In the process of following their parent's advice/instructions, mostly they become rigid in their opinion and approach towards life. If the attitude of parents itself is negative, the children are bound to get negatively influenced by it (Goede and Spruijt, 1996). Some risk factors involved with the parents are dramatic and obvious, such as unlawful and violent behavior, alcohol and drug abuse, child abuse and neglect etc. Other, more subtle predictors include harsh/inconsistent discipline, lack of emotional interaction with the child, and lack of proper supervision. Many other behaviors, although not related directly to parenting, are also associated with children's violent behavior. Examples include lack of communication between spouses, marital conflict and divorce, social isolation, and parental depression or stress.

Some children are considered to be at high risk for developing violent behaviors. These children already exhibit clear behavioral markers of violent activity, including factors like bullying other children or themselves being the target of bullies, exhibiting aggressive behavior or totally withdrawn, being truant from school and getting arrested before the age of 14, belonging to delinquent peer groups, abusing in general, getting used to alcohol or drugs and engaging in antisocial behavior such as treating animals cruelly (Barnes et al., 1999).

Children are likely to develop a hostile approach in life and adopt the bad traits they see around themselves. If a child is beaten for under performing at school, he may do the same to his children with the mindset that it is the perfect way to make a person work harder and succeed in life. Whenever a child is dropped out of school or forcefully engaged in child labor, there is a sudden leap which the child tries to take from his childhood to adulthood (Webster-Stratton, 1993). In this process, he misses out on many values and morals that must be inculcated in him at this stage of life for making him a good human being. He fails to develop a vision to see things from an unbiased point of view. All these factors make a child insensitive towards the society and the societal demands. Many children are traumatized and psychologically disturbed to such an extent that they start finding it unsustainable and eventually lose out their mental soundness. Sometime the children victimized by physical violence become handicapped as well. In a few cases, children do run away from their homes and try to become self-dependent while some commit suicide too. Children who run away from their homes indulge in malpractices due to improper education and bad company they become part of after leaving their homes (Gharabaghi and Stuart, 2010). Some even reciprocate the violence by harming the family members who inflicted harm to them. A girl child from a violent background usually withdraws from the society and becomes completely depressed.

Children subjected to violence usually become aggressive in order to solve their problems. Harshly treated adolescents may succumb to drugs and alcohol use. In India, a lot of helpless and abandoned children are picked up by gangs who sell their organs for making money. In most of the cities, the groups of beggars at traffic lights or railway platforms are the abandoned children who are physically deformed forcefully for begging. The children who escape being a part of such hostile circles are looked after by children welfare organizations like Indian Child Welfare Association (ICWA), CRY (Child Relief and You) and ChildLine India etc.

The rise in the cases of juvenile crime in the world as a whole has forced experts to lay thrust on inculcating values by the family members to ensure that the child does not deviate and resort to shortcuts in life. Psychologists blame it on mass media, society and family. Actually the children are getting what we are giving. Adding to the reducing tolerance power among the children is mass media, be it internet or television. These mediums actually provoke them towards costly mobile phones, latest model bikes, date culture and so on. When there are shortcuts in the form of crime to achieve these goals why will these children resist the easy way out? Nothing more than family is responsible for children moving towards negativity. Increasing pressure on the child to perform or be at par with role models envisaged by the parents confuses and frustrates them. Unable to bear the pressure, they either end up committing suicide or indulging in unlawful acts.

Increasing communication gap between the children and the family is the root cause of reducing tolerance power among them. All this has led to increase in the date culture among the children in the past few years or so. To fulfill the requirements and demands of their partners, these children have no option but to go for shortcuts. Contents of movies, television serials or at times even serious stuffs like newspapers has only acted as a supplement as far as what is being given to the children is concerned. If the children get to hear abusive languages in the movies and television without suitable guidance from the parents or other seniors, nobody should expect them to move on a right path.

The figures pertaining to youth violence can be brought down only if the family and the society wake up to give what should be given by it for reducing the communication gap and putting a check on contents in movies and internet. Opportunities for learning and engaging in violence are also provided by some neighborhoods. The presence of gangs and illegal markets in the neighborhood such as those of drugs not only provide the foundation for exposure to brutality but violent role models and misinterpretation of positive rewards for serious violent activity. Single parent families, ineffective parenting, violent behavior at schools, and high dropout, adolescent pregnancy and unemployment rates are all concentrated in such neighborhoods. While these violence-inducing neighborhoods are mostly the areas with high rates of concentrated poverty and negligent parents, the critical feature of such neighborhoods is the absence of any effective social or cultural organization. High transiency levels make it difficult for establishment of common values and norms, informal support networks and effective social controls. Soaring levels of chronic unemployment results in social isolation and undermines the relevance of completing school. Illegitimate enterprises and gangs find for themselves a perfect breeding ground in these conditions, partly because of a lack of suitable resistance means in such a neighborhood and in part as a means of providing some stable social organization and source of economy for youth and also the neighborhood as a whole. It is wrong to rate all the poor neighborhoods as disorganized but those with effective organization show lower rates of violent behavior, crime and substance use.

Living in such neighborhoods can be devastating for the universal approach of a family to provide a healthy, conservative upbringing for their children. The conventional opportunities for supporting this sort of positive parenting have few social reinforcements and also limited by racism, discrimination and social isolation from the labor market etc. The risks associated with participation in gangs and illicit economy matters are often negated by the possibility of gaining quick and substantial rewards. Involvement in these types of activities bring the youth at high risk of getting connected to violence both as victims as well as perpetrators. Such youth frequently become vulnerable to harmful social consequences and lose the pursuit of more conventional goals, drop out of school, get pregnant, and get trapped in health compromising and dysfunctional lifestyles which obstruct the normal course of adolescent development. This makes them ill-prepared to enter the usual adult roles and endanger the future of the world as a whole.

Although the violent behavioral patterns learned in early childhood has definite influence in the school life, a huge potential lies in the school itself for generating conflict and frustration among the youth amidst a wide array of harmful situations. A non-violent social adjustment at home does increase the likelihood of a successful adjustment to school and peers. Success of this cannot be guaranteed though. These are novel and negotiable social systems, where one must locate his or her niche. Both of these have their own performance demands and development tasks to complete. Failure to meet these expectations like success at the academic front, peer approval, personal competence and independence, self-efficacy and development of interpersonal relationships and intimacy creates stress and conflict. If these situations combine with reduced levels of monitoring and effective supervision, it increases the likelihood that violence will probably be the only answer resting with the youth as an answer to these problems. During the school phase, a large fraction of violence is related to competition and confrontations related to status (Checkoway, 2011). Grouping of academically poor students and aggressive troublemakers by use of ability tracking contributes to a collective adaptation to school failure and peer rejection. Notorious peer groups tend to come out of their classes and downbeat feelings of anger, rejection and alienation are mutually reinforced in these groups. It is clearly observable here that getting involved with a delinquent peer group is the most immediate and strongest cause of the actual onset of serious violent behavior. Actually at this point, violence is modeled, encouraged and rewarded. Reinforcement of the justifications for disengaging one's moral obligation to others can also be expected here. Effects of early exposure to violence, weak internal and family controls and aggressive behavior patterns developed in childhood all influence the selection of friends, and the type of friends largely determine what behavior patterns will be modeled, established and reinforced during adolescence. In this case strong bonding with parents can prove to be a protective factor which insulates youth from the influence of delinquent friends (Webster-Stratton, 1993). This can hold well only in case the friendship network is not dominated by such youth.

Gangs are a subtype of adolescent peer group, with a more formal uniqueness quotient and membership requirements. They tend to involve more delinquent youth of homogenous nature, often going for active recruitment of persons for their fighting skills or street smarts (Gretton and Clift, 2011). Membership entails violent behavior as an initiation ritual in most instances. It is wrong to say that all gangs are involved in serious violent behavior or drug distribution. Sometimes they serve a few positive functions, particularly in disorganized neighborhoods. They not only provide youth a sense of acceptance and personal worth (best character of friendship), but also a safe place to stay, food, clothing and protection from abusive parents. On an overall basis joining a gang greatly increases the risk of serious violence from both perpetration and victimization point of view.

The relationship between substance use and violence has lots of complications. Alcohol is implicated in over half of all homicides and assault cases occurring around the world. Parents used to alcohol abuse and illicit drugs are often seen to be neglectful regarding their children and become susceptible to violent acts. While alcohol addicts and gamblers are more likely to have a history of violent behavior, they have a more proportional representation among violent offenders as compared to the non-violent offenders (Barnes et al., 1999). Pharmacological studies have not found a conclusive relationship between alcohol use and violent behavior. Alcohol and psychoactive drugs definitely increase violent behavior but the exact mechanism has not yet been established. Drugs like marijuana and opium actually appears to inhibit violence, although withdrawal may precipitate an increase in risk of violence. It has not been a rare phenomenon for drug addicts and gamblers to commit violent crimes for supporting their drug habit. The commonest drug-violence is for selling drugs as the drug distribution network is extremely violent.

In the last two decades, firearm-related homicide rate for adolescents has more than doubled and firearms now account for nearly three-fourths of all homicides. Involvement of guns multiplies the cases of deaths resulting from youth violence incidents by 3 to 5 times. This is followed by use of knives, the next most lethal weapon. Nowadays, the trend of carrying guns is getting widespread among youth. Although concrete evidences are not available regarding the reason behind this development but subjective facts suggests it is to 'show off', to insure 'respect' and acceptance from others, and lastly for self-defense in light of growing violence all around (Gretton and Clift, 2011). Partly, it appears to be a response to the common perception that public authorities don't have the capacity to protect youth and maintain good sense of law and order in their neighborhoods or at school. School dropouts, drug dealers and youth with previous records of violence/anti-social activities are more likely to possess a gun than other adolescents. Majority of firearms used in various range of crimes are obtained by theft and other illegal means.

IS THE YOUTH CAUSING VIOLENCE OR GETTING VICTIMIZED THEMSELVES?

A tricky question that comes to our mind while talking about youth violence is whether the children and teenagers are actually acting as the culprits or at the receiving end of violent behavior coming from different sectors of the society. Some case studies from India (names and locations related to the incident not mentioned due to the sensitivity of the issues) are presented here to look into this significant matter.

Case 1 – A child aged 12 and from an urban-based family was brutally tortured by his step-father for nearly 3 years. The child lost interest in studies, went into a nutshell and became totally depressed. He started behaving abruptly with his friends of school and neighborhood. Finally one day, the extent of torture crossed every limit and the child died following a session of over-beating.

Case 2 - A teenage girl studying in 9th standard was constantly pressurized by her parents for scoring >95% marks in the school exams and regular comparisons were made with her classmate who lived in her neighborhood too and used to score better marks than her. The stress of studies reached to an extent that the poor girl committed suicide as she found no other way out to get away from the regular trauma.

Case 3 – A talented and bright young fellow committed suicide after a string of insults as a result of humiliating ragging by his seniors at the college. In spite of several anti-ragging campaigns and rules imposed by the government of India as well as the college authorities, ragging is continuing to be a menace for teenagers all over the country.

Case 4 – A 10 year old kid got negatively inspired by violent video games and tried to enact the same at his home by beating his younger brother with a steel bar and seriously injuring him in the process.

Case 5 – A college student shot at his fellow classmate when she declined his proposal of love. The girl was rushed to the hospital immediately but the doctors failed to rescue her.

Inference – Here in all the cases, the fate with which the victims met could have been different had the social structure, attitude and awareness quotient been different. In case 1, had the victim's mother and other family members tried for saving the child and interfered at the right time, he could have been saved. The offender i.e., the step-father should have been advised to go for parental counseling and perhaps the child would not have gone into depression and met his eventual fate.

In case 2, unnecessary comparisons with neighbor's child brought the victim into horrifying pressure which she could not handle and found no other way to get out of the trouble except suicide. The parents should have understood that every child is unique in his/her own way and it is harsh to compare them to anybody else.

Case 3 is difficult to assess from youth's point-of-view as the offender and sufferer both belong to the same category of youth. In such cases lack of good and friendly upbringing by parents, and environment of the school/college that breed negative features like ragging are the real culprits.

Case 4 brings the ball in the court of media that plays a vital role in the shape of the society that includes youth as an important section. Video games, television programs and movies showcasing violence as a symbol of supremacy and power are showing the wrong path to millions of school going kids and teenagers all around the world resulting in harm induced on youth as a whole.

Case 5 displays two aspects of violence. Firstly, it shows that in today's world the value for life has got downgraded severely. Petty quarrels and fights are leading to murder and hardcore cruelty. Secondly, availability of guns and various sorts of weapons are easily accessible to young fellows who still have not developed the kind of responsibility that is needed for using them in a suitable manner. Arms that are meant for self-defense are being used for settling minor matters and adding to the magnitude of aggression in the present world.

THE ADOLESCENCE-ADULTHOOD TRANSITION: A CRITICALLY VITAL PHASE

Involvement in violent behavior is reduced well enough by successful transitions into adult roles (work, marriage and parenting). Nearly 80 percent of the adolescents having a record of serious offences during their juvenile stages showed drastic reduction in violent output once they reached adulthood and faced more responsibilities. Race and economic conditions however prove to bring in exceptions regarding this matter. Race, in particular, can be related to finding and holding a job, and to marriage and stable cohabiting rates. The reservation policies existing in India are directly related to this facet of inducing possible frustration in youth who fail to get job or admission in good colleges due to restriction imposed by the reservation scheme.

Growing up in poor families and disorganized neighborhoods induces two major effects directly related to violent behavior. These factors limit the opportunities for employment which in turn, reduces the chances of marriage at the desired time and starting a family life (Miller and Porter, 2007). Employment and marriage are undoubtedly two basic symbols of adult status. Secondly, a normal course of adolescent development is seriously hampered by growing up in poor, disorganized neighborhoods. Levels of personal competences, self-efficacy, social skills and self-discipline are severely low in youth coming from such surroundings. Preparation for entering the job arena stays unfinished in case of such people and they fail to grab the right opportunity even if jobs are available. In this way, they are trapped in a phase of extended adolescence and continue to engage in adolescent behavior even when they rightly should be more responsible towards their family, community and country.

MANAGING YOUTH VIOLENCE: A TOUGH NUT TO CRACK?

A large number of complicated factors surround the identification of the best practices for youth violence prevention. These complications include the diversity in law policies, fundamentals of culture, education and employment, economic stability, and effectiveness of strategy implementations at the inter-societal, inter-regional, international and intercontinental levels. As youth violence is such a high-priority public health concern, majority of practices presented here are based on the empirical observations rather than purely theoretical viewpoints.

Since a large proportion of violent behavior is learned behavior, the general strategy for prevention and treatment interventions should be: 1) To reduce the modeling and reinforcement of violence as a means of solving problems and manipulating or controlling the behavior of others, and 2) To restructure those social conditions which generate and support violent lifestyles. The most effective strategy for accomplishing this is to assure a healthy course of child and adolescent development for all youth, so they are prepared to enter productive, responsible adult roles that are accessible in nature.

APPARENT GOALS AND OBJECTIVES FOR INTERVENTION OUTCOMES AND IMPLEMENTATION

Each intervention program requires a clear and specific set of observable goals and objectives that sets the platform for, and accelerates its successful accomplishment and effectiveness. The goals and objectives need to be behavior-based and outcome-oriented. If model of an intervention is being set up after an already established one, we need to use the original intervention's evaluation scaffold to frame up the new goals and objectives. Parents must be involved in setting up the objectives of the program by outlining their family's potential achievements in a certain time period under the practitioner's guidance. An initiative of this kind may seem overwhelming for parents involved because they face a healthy change regarding to their parenting technique and even the way they conduct their daily affairs. This leads to an enhancement of parents' sense of control and accountability.

Role of Parents in Managing Youth Violence

Role of parents hold a monumental value in managing youth violence. Emotionally distressed parents are very likely to pass on their insensitive manners to the kids who most probably develop a number of conduct disorders and antisocial behaviors. Parent- and family-based interventions are very necessary to check future youth violence. Evidences support the fact that if these interventions are started at an early phase, they can have substantial positive and long-term effects in reducing violent behavior by children and subsequently by teenagers too (Howard et al., 1999). These interventions must include features such as training provided for improvement in parenting skills e.g., better communication with their children using non-violent ways of resolving conflict, educating the people regarding fundamentals of child development and the factors that predispose children to violent behavior. This type of intervention is ideal for families with very young children and parents planning for children in the future. More evaluation research is needed for parent and family interventions. These interventions have to take into consideration measured reductions in conduct disorders, delinquent behaviors or drug use, all of which are considered precursors to violence. Parenting interventions are generally more successful if they are implemented with the unique characteristics and particular needs of the individual participants. It becomes very important to identify factors within the family unit that puts a child at risk for developing violent behaviors. These factors may be related to behaviors and characteristics of either the parents or the child or both of them.

The effectiveness of parenting interventions seems to increase exponentially in cases of very young children i.e., before the onset of antisocial or aggressive behaviors (Howard et al., 1999). As the child becomes adolescent, both the child and the parents are following well-established patterns and become resistant to long-term changes. Intervening with a mother during the latter part of pregnancy and continuing with intervention activities during the first few years of her motherhood can significantly reduce the risk of conduct disorder and violence that can influence the child in the future.

Parents with the tendency of regularly abusing their children need to develop better nurturing skills as alternatives to their depressing parenting behaviors and attitudes comprising of abusive, slang language. In these serious cases, the family-centered interventions based on a re-parenting philosophy have the best potential in teaching the required skills to such irresponsible parents. In such interventions, cognitive and affective activities are needed to be designed for building self-awareness, sense of positive self-esteem and empathy; alternatives to common harmful activities like yelling and hitting are to be taught with a sense of importance; family communication and awareness regarding needs should be enhanced; abusive behavior must be replaced with kind fostering; healthy physical and emotional development must be promoted; and lastly appropriate roles and developmental expectations must be taught with a sense of diligence.

It is a common observation for many parents of delinquent children using fruitless corrective techniques to bring them on the right path. For example, inadequate involvement of parents with delinquent children in monitoring their child's day-to-day activities, staying inconsistent in applying discipline, and failing to display good levels of participation in areas like monitoring the child's academic progress. This leads to a destructive pattern of "coercive interaction" existing between the child and the parents, characterized by a cycle of misbehavior from the child and parents replying in form of threatening the child. This reaction coming from the parents may be successful in the short-term but in the long run, harms the child by promoting further aggression. Parents need to take the initiative in breaking this cycle and change their tactics for teaching the children discipline and effectively dealing with the negative actions.

Effective parenting revolves around the fundamental principle of empowering the parents to effectively deal with their children regardless of their age. Parents, especially those of felonious children sometimes tend to lose control in many aspects of their lives. A sense of demoralization, frustration or depression creeps in their lives due to their inability to establish themselves as successful parents. Interventions should aim to increase the sense of self-control and self-efficacy in parents, provide them the confidence in their interactions with the children and make them accountable in an affirmative way for improvements in their children's behavior.

A way of empowering parents is to give them the required information that will help them understand and react appropriately to their children's behavior with respect to proper time and situation. Interventions should train the parents on how to nurture and communicate effectively with their children, praising and rewarding them for their prosocial behavior and confer family rules and consequences, without use of any violent means. In case punishment is the only alternative visible for a terribly notorious child, the intervention program should teach the parents effective means, such as 'time outs' and loss of privileges that do not promote any aggressive interactions between parents and the child.

It is necessary to involve the organizations sponsoring parents- and family- based interventions to themselves get engaged in the program and hold themselves accountable for the intervention impacts. This will bring them closer to the intervention and give more commitment to its objectives and outcome evaluation. Participation of parents is also very important as it will provide them a greater sense of empowerment and accountability both during and after the intervention. This will also help the practitioners tailor the participants' needs and priorities in a closer and better mode.

Role of the Neighborhood or Community

Management strategy involving the neighborhood can prove to be a comprehensive one which attempts to bring together all of the primary institutions that serve youth, e.g., families, health agencies, schools, employment, and justice, in an integrated, coordinated effort to develop an effective neighborhood organization and deliver the full range of needed services at a single site under a single administrative structure. Such schemes cover programs like family support, community development corporations, and school-based clinics. Unfortunately, there are few good evaluations of these neighborhood level approaches. In too many cases, neighborhood programs fail to develop a broad range of services or a cohesive neighborhood organization which is an essential to this approach. However, when such programs are implemented in a well defined way, they improve the emotional welfare of families, expand and develop informal social networks, and facilitate a successful course of youth development (Nissen et al., 2011). Theoretically, if sustained over five years or more, this approach should have the greatest payoff in reducing violence, crime and drug abuse, and facilitating a successful course of child and adolescent development.

CONSIDERATION OF CHIDLREN'S AGES IN DETERMINING THE INTERVENTION PROGRAM

Right from subjects of proper nurturing to infliction of discipline, a child's age influences several factors of parenting.

Parents of a young child must set up certain limits for their child's behavior, but with an older child under consideration, those limits have to be negotiated as demands for suitable parenting change with the mental growth of the child.

Young Children (Ages 10 and under)

In case of children aged 10 and below, intervention programs often have successful long-term and positive impact since the behavior patterns of both parents and children stay in a nascent stage and very much flexible (Taylor and Biglan, 1998).

An overview of the child development must be included in the intervention program designed for pre-school and elementary school children in order to let the participating parents set realistic and age-appropriate expectations about development of their child's behavior.

Some other possible tactics used in such intervention programs that tend to be useful for parents are to behave with their children as friends and not some strict guardian. This can be achieved by playing with the child against giving regular directions and praising the child for positive behavior with suitable gifts. In order to bring a successful transformation in a child's behavior, positive reinforcement must be accompanied by appropriate, consistent and measured acts of discipline but not in a harsh manner (Taylor and Biglan, 1998).

Parents of young children must uptake non-violent ways and a consistent set of rules for effectively implementing discipline in them when they commit some wrong activity. Parents must accompany their kids while watching movies and television programs so that they can provide on-spot counseling regarding violence while watching fights and bloodshed via these modern media elements.

Even if the parents themselves are not interested in those programs for e.g., cartoon movies (showing violence as a mode of comedy or fun like the protagonist hitting the negative characters), still they must sit with their children and guide them against any negative impact stuff shown in those programs.

Adolescents and Teens

In case of adolescents and teens, an intervention program for parents should explain important and apposite developmental issues critical to this vital phase of a person's life. This includes sexuality, growing independence and the high possibility of a rebellious behavior. Programs for parents with older children must have a curriculum that includes matters like application of non-depreciatory terms like competence, engaging the teenagers in constructive activities and reduction of fear etc. for reframing the underlying motives for a teenager's particular behavior, increasing positive and decreasing negative communication patterns among the immediate family members, extended members in case of joint families (common in India) and peers (Paterson and Panessa, 2008). Apart from these, improving parents' ability to identify positive role models for their sons and daughters is important and so is minimizing the negative influences.

TARGET HIGH-RISK FAMILIES: NO NEED TO SHY AWAY OR HESITATE

Families with a high risk for child abuse are those with parents or caretakers who have limited problem solving skills, poor impulse control and a history of violent behavior during adolescence. These caretakers are frequently young, low income, single parent, minority women with four or more children in the household. Fathers, when present, tend to be part-time employed and have a limited education.

These families have few resources and are experiencing both social isolation and economic stress. They have few alternatives and limited social supports from extended family or friendship networks which might provide social controls on their behavior and non-violent alternatives for managing their children (Lai, 2009).

Irrespective of their social and economic status, a lot of parents having children with record of antisocial behavior or delinquent acts live in a traumatic and isolated environment. Such parents are mostly distressed and socially cut off, with little access to social or psychological support. According to the general belief it's extremely difficult to implement effective parent-training programs for disadvantaged parents, particularly low-income single mothers.

This perception is totally misleading. Positive results have been obtained in a lot of cases involving low-income parents in planning, recruitment, group leadership and priority settings (Olds and Kitzman, 1990).

These programs have resulted in encouraging parenting behaviors and also enhanced family and community support networks (Campbell and Taylor, 1996).

The main target of violence-preventive intervention programs must be the low-income parents, single mothers and people with a history of abuse (Le and Stockdale, 2008). Unless these vulnerable groups of the society are looked at with special care and attention, it is useless to introduce fresh projects pertaining to youth violence and its prevention. This is because of the number of socioeconomic and psychological factors associated with them that put them at an increased risk for raising violent, antisocial children and need urgent focus.

CONSIDERATION OF CULTURAL AND DEMOGRAPHIC ISSUES A BIG NECESSITY

Some participant groups possess cultural values or behaviors that present unique challenges for the practitioners involved in the intervention. In such cases identification of cultural issues up front and designing of intervention materials for an appropriate address to the concerned audience are a prime necessity (Lai, 2009). Culture is a very important component of any social structure and relevant content promotes a strong sense of group ownership, ethnic identity, community-building and advancing one's group as a whole.

The traditional communication channels can prove to be ineffective in some families of low-socioeconomic status and parents harboring low level of education. In order to address this challenge, intervention managers need to de-emphasize written materials and verbal teaching methods. Role-playing and modeling techniques must be opted for instead to bring out successful results. For several groups, interactive teaching techniques are most effective.

These techniques incorporate not only moralistic teaching but also role-playing and problem-solving exercises. In some cases however, parents prefer didactic authority figures and show a lack of trust on exceedingly sociable strangers. As chances of being viewed as disrespectful are high, a practitioner would want to begin with a more formal style and ease into interactive teaching methods.

ADDRESSING THE ENVIRONMENTAL AND FINANCIAL CONCERNS

Suitable results expected from the intervention programs may not be obtained solely from interventions that focus solely on parents' behavior that fails to sustain in the environment outside the intervention. For long-term effects, context in which parenting takes place must also be addressed. In the present world, the interventions that have been expanded to focus on multiple issues like helping the parents improve their "life skills" and assist them in dealing with issues such as social isolation, stress, depression, marital conflict, housing, and money matters have been the most successful. The simple rule to be followed behind these broad interventions is that parents who are better able to manage everyday life issues will have the physical, psychological, and social resources to parent more effectively.

EFFECTIVE AND PLANNED IMPLEMENTATION OF THE INTERVENTION

Implementing the intervention depends on many factors, including the activities planned and the participants involved. Some general principles applicable to any parenting intervention are:

1) Convenience of the parents must be given top priority while setting the time and locations of activities.
2) Extract the best possible knowledge from the parents through sound counseling sessions that provide a suitable foundation for further actions.
3) Maximize interactive teaching opportunities with greater impact and minimize simple lectures that tend to be less effective.
4) Staffers should definitely make serious attempts to model the behaviors being taught (e.g., effective listening skills, non-aggressive reactions to conflict).
5) Giving appropriate opportunities to the parents for asking questions, offering their feedbacks, and practice the skills taught to them.
6) Implementing all the components of an effective intervention. Applying only the selected components may not produce the results of the original intervention.

Setting up a Realistic Time Frame for the Intervention

Parenting patterns are slightly hard to amend and there is a lack of quick fixes in this regard. Any intervention with a target of modifying parenting methods is expected to take few-several months to produce any significant results. Around 20-25 sessions are needed for interventions targeting high-risk families, whereas in case of the comparatively happier, no-risk families around 8-10 sessions are sufficient.

In most of the cases, intervention program sessions should occur regularly like weekly or biweekly and also need to be short like no more than two hours. Longer sessions can be successful but only if they are implemented with frequent breaks like those for refreshments. Formats involving away-from home group sessions should be convenient in terms of childcare, transportation and the availability of food (Olds and Kitzman, 1993). If they don't satisfy such norms, proper cooperation from parents is likely to go down after few such sessions.

Take Care of Intervention Staff to Prevent Exhaustion

Providing the staff members and intervention program managers with good support and encouragement is critically important for attaining success as the parent- and family-based interventions can be very challenging and emotionally draining. Regular training and consultation is needed by the staff members along with plenty of opportunities to talk with a supervisor about the progress of their fulfilling of the intervention objectives as well as the personal, job-related objectives. Hiring staff on a part-time basis or giving good workers a nice pay package can prevent staff burnouts. It is also beneficial to provide staff members with flexible schedules.

Regular Encouragement for the Participants to Stay Involved

Parent- and family-based interventions can carry on for several months with very subtle and gradual results. The interest of the participants needs to be maintained throughout and they must proceed towards the long-term goal. In addition to offering incentives like free food, transportation and childcare, planning events for persuading the parents to complete the intervention are expected to be particularly helpful. Good examples can be organizing graduation ceremonies or providing gift certificates as a reward for program/course completion.

Monitoring of the Progress and Quality of the Implementation

With the progress of the intervention, monitoring of the activities is vital to ensure that the activities are going on as per the planned schedule. Effective monitoring is important for implementing an evaluated intervention. All the steps are to be followed sequentially in order to achieve similar results.

The monitoring must begin with deciding upon the staff supervision based on the delivered outcomes. The accomplishments of the program should be recorded as they occur. Attendance records of the sessions must be tracked on regular basis.

Persons not involved directly in the intervention program but members of the project must be assigned the duty of performing spot-checks of the activities. Parents must be encouraged to maintain a record of what kinds of activities and information were delivered and lastly additional feedback from the parents and staffers needs to be collected for improving upon the outcome of the intervention.

Outcome Evaluation Having Value in Intervention Success Assessment

Evaluation of the intervention outcome has to be kept in mind from the very beginning of the program initiation. Participants must assess the gradual changes in self-behavior as well as that of their children.

These changes must also be observed and evaluated on parallel basis by the intervention staffers. A third party opinion can always be taken for identifying the changes properly and in a more refined manner. A review of the school records to check reduction in delinquent behavior or absenteeism can be made for those children whose families participated in the intervention programs.

Setbacks are to be Expected

Changes in the behavior of a person are gradual and not drastic happening overnight. A single treatment has remote chances of curing long-standing family issues, crises, and disciplinary problems. We need to set realistic expectations for any intervention and the parents must know that obstacles and setbacks are going to occur along the way (Taylor and Biglan 1998).

Informing parents beforehand regarding the possibility of resistance and recurring behavior problems from their children will better prepare them for these difficulties and keep them committed to the intervention.

Link Parent- and Family- Based Interventions with other Strategies

Although the parent-based interventions have been proven to be effective in terms of preventing violence by children and adolescents, children in the school age require additional strategies involving the consideration of factors outside the home as they are prone to be influenced by several of such factors that cannot be controlled by parents alone (Brestan and Eyberg 1998; Taylor and Biglan 1998; Tweed et al., 2011). Negative academic and social experiences in school can result in a development of violent behavior or associated risk factors in a child.

Evidences have demonstrated that when parents and school join hands to prevent youth violence, they are better placed than parent-based strategies alone (Coleman 1997; Webster-Stratton, 1993).

A coordinated effort among parents, teachers, school psychologists, and school nurses can identify problems at an early stage and in a better way to give the practitioners a better base for intervening with their programs and teach problem-solving, develop conflict-resolution skills and enhance academic skills (Tweed et al., 2011).

Gun Control Policies: Call for Stricter Legislation

In today's world, guns are being actively used in various crimes and compared to the situation few years back, availability of guns is much easier and accessible at very cheap rates. This brings them in the reach of even the poor people who under various socio-economical stresses make use of this for carrying out crimes and violent activities. There has been relatively little rigorous research on the effectiveness of various gun control policies. However, some evidence does exist for the effectiveness of restrictive handgun laws and mandatory sentences for firearm offenses. In the case of restrictive handgun laws, several studies have found significant declines in homicide rates. However no suitable evidences have been found for use of other weapons as a substitute. It cannot be ruled out that other weapons like knives are also being used in various incidents of violence. Stricter legislation with regard to sale of guns is urgently required. More research is needed in this area to establish the effects of various gun control measures.

Responses from the Judiciary System

In the last two decades, there has been a significant rise in the number of crimes involving the youth and justice response system across the world too has undergone several changes. In spite of the best efforts by the governments to install effective law policies, still we come across delays in processing time and pre-trial detention for juvenile cases, higher conviction rates and longer sentences, disproportionate use of government funds allocated for youth development and also a substantially lower probability of good medical treatment while in custody. The last two findings raise serious questions about the use of funds waived by the governments for bringing in effective justice system responses. It is hard to derive a proper theory pertinent to whether increases in sentence length or confinement in adult institutions have any significant deterrent effect over shorter sentences and confinement in juvenile institutions. In case of drug-related offenses, research demonstrates that best results for reducing adolescent drug use can only be obtained by educational awareness programs and community-based prevention programs. On the other hand, drug enforcement policies involving mandatory sentences and stronger sanctions appear to have very lesser deterrent effects and may induce further negative impacts. It is true that the prevention programs do take a lot of time and also difficult to implement, but at the same time violence reduction effects of such prevention programs are substantially greater and probably does not costs much too.

CONCLUSION

Youth violence is a pervasive, serious problem with long lasting consequences; it's not at all a natural module of the society. The widespread culture of violence that seems to have taken root in the world as a whole, particularly in disadvantaged areas must be explored in a more concise manner for achieving better results pertaining to prevention of youth violence. It is a complex social phenomenon that has only recently been recognized as not only a criminal justice issue, but also a developmental problem covering the entire globe. The nature and scope of violence among youth should be understood from point of view of both victims and perpetrators. A more refined analysis of the profiles of the youth perpetrators is needed to identify the risk factors that threaten the youth as well as the possible resilience factors which might protect them. Undoubtedly large-scale government-designed interventions fail if they have insufficient input from the local communities.

The societal production of criminals has to be checked applying a paradigm shift towards a more whole-societal, developmental, ecological and integrated plan of action. The problems of youth violence are not just the errant youth, but also the symptoms of societal problems. We need to rethink the way that we raise, nurture and provide for youth. The effort must be broad based and link schools, families, communities, government departments and support agencies in a common effort. All these bodies must be the simultaneous targets of the intervention programs.

While long-term efforts are vital for a successful outcome, it is important for the policymakers to make some immediate short-term efforts at the basic school level to protect the children against the rising rate of violence. This accentuates the use of human resources in situations where material resources are in short supply. Greater analytical work is needed, particularly in integrating the fields of youth development and violence and in understanding the issues that youth face, with the prime focus on their needs and perceptions.

> If we are to teach real peace in this world, and if we are to carry on a real war against war, we shall have to begin with the children – *Mahatma Gandhi*.

ACKNOWLEDGMENTS

I wish to express my sincere thanks and gratitude to the president of Nova Science Publishers Inc., Dr. Nadya Gotsiridze-Columbus for inviting me to send this paper. I am grateful to Dr. Elizabeth Trejos-Castillo, the editor of this volume for her appreciable guidance during the paper preparation. Thanks are due to Dr. N.C. Mehrotra, Director, Birbal Sahni Institute of Palaeobotany and Dr. Amit K. Ghosh for their kind encouragement. I would also like to thank the Council of Scientific and Industrial Research India for the NET fellowship (CSIR Grant No. 09/528(0016)/2009-EMR-I).

REFERENCES

Barnes, G.M., Welte, J.W., Hoffman, J.H., and Dintcheff, B.A. (1999). Gambling and alcohol use among youth: Influences of demographic, socialization, and individual factors. Addictive Behaviors, 24, 749-767.

Brestan, E.V., and Eyberg, S.M. (1998). Effective Psychosocial Treatments of Conduct-Disordered Children and Adolescents: 29 Years, 82 Studies, and 5,272 kids. *Journal of Clinical Child Psychology,* 27, 180-189.

Campbell, F.A., and Taylor, K. (1996). Early Childhood Programs that Work for Children from Economically Disadvantaged Families. *Young Children,* 51, 74-80.

Checkoway, B. (2011). What is youth participation? *Children and Youth Services Review,* 33, 340-345.

Coleman, M. (1997). Families and School: *In Search of Common Ground. Young Children,* 52, 14-21.

Gharabaghi, K., and Stuart, C. (2010). Voices from the periphery: Prospects and challenges for the homeless youth service sector. *Children and Youth Services Review,* 32, 1683-1689.

Goede, M.D., and Spruijt, E. (1996). Effects of parental divorce and youth unemployment on adolescent health. *Patient Education and Counseling,* 29, 269-276.

Gretton, H.M., and Clift, R.J.W. (2011). The mental health needs of incarcerated youth in British Columbia, Canada. *International Journal of Law and Psychiatry,* 34, 109-115.

Howard, D.E., Cross, S.I., Li, X., Huang, W. (1999). Parent-youth concordance regarding violence exposure: relationship to youth psychosocial functioning. *Journal of Adolescent Health,* 25, 396-406.

Lai, M.H. (2009). Toward an integrative and collaborative approach to Asian American and Pacific Islander youth violence research, practice and policy. *Aggression and Violent Behavior,* 14, 454-460.

Le, T.N., and Stockdale, G. (2008). Acculturative Dissonance, Ethnic Identity, and Youth Violence. *Cultural Diversity and Ethnic Minority Psychology,* 14, 1-9.

Miller, C., and Porter, K.E. (2007). Barriers to employment among out-of-school youth. *Children and Youth Services Review,* 29, 572-587.

Mitchell, K.J., Wolak, J., and Finkelhor, D. (2007). Trends in Youth Reports of Sexual Solicitations, Harassment and Unwanted Exposure to Pornography on the Internet. *Journal of Adolescent Health,* 40, 116-126.

Nissen, L.B. (2011). Community-directed engagement and positive youth development: Developing positive and progressive pathways between youth and their communities in Reclaiming Futures. *Children and Youth Services Review,* 33, S23-S28.

Olds, K.L., and Kitzman, H. (1990). Can Home Visitation Improve the Health of Women and Children at Environmental Risk? *Pediatrics,* 86, 108-116.

Olds, K.L., and Kitzman, H. (1993). Review of Research on Home Visiting for Pregnant Women and Parents of Young Children. *Future of Children,* 3, 53-92.

Paterson, B.L., and Panessa, C. (2008). Engagement as an ethical imperative in harm reduction involving at-risk youth. *International Journal of Drug Policy,* 19, 24-32.

Taylor, T.K., and Biglan, A. (1998). Behavioral Family Interventions for Improving Childrearing: A Review of the Literature for Clinicians and Policy Makers. *Clinical Child and Family Psychology Review,* 1, 41-60.

Tweed, R.G., Bhatt, G., Dooley, S., Spindler, A., Douglas, K.S., and Viljoen, J.L. (2011). Youth Violence and Positive Psychology: Research Potential Through Integration. *Canadian Psychology,* 52, 111-121.

Webster-Stratton, C. (1993). Strategies for Helping Early School-Aged Children With Oppositional Defiant and Conduct Disorders: The Importance of Home-School Partnerships. *School Psychology Review,* 22, 437-457.

In: Youth: Practices, Perspectives and Challenges
Editor: Elizabeth Trejos-Castillo

ISBN: 978-1-62618-067-3
© 2013 Nova Science Publishers, Inc.

Chapter 6

DETERMINING ADOLESCENTS' RISK FOR INVOLVEMENT IN BULLYING OR CYBERBULLYING: A REVIEW OF TWO STUDIES

Elizabeth L. W. McKenney[*], *Amanda M. Cole, Lisa M. Young, Emily J. Krohn, Stephen D. A. Hupp and Jeremy D. Jewell*
Southern Illinois University, Edwardsville, IL, US

ABSTRACT

As increasing attention is paid to the issue of bullying and cyberbullying in school-age populations, additional knowledge is needed regarding groups of students who are most likely to be involved in bullying. Involvement in bullying can include traditional forms of physical and verbal aggression, or can include cyberbullying. This chapter summarizes a series of studies investigating the role of gender, time spent online, time spent sending and receiving text messages ("texting"), parenting styles, and relationship dynamics within families in predicting involvement in bullying either as a bully or as a victim. Traditional bullying and cyberbullying were examined, and some important differences between bullying formats were observed regarding risk factors. Engaging in cyberbullying as a bully was more common among male, high school or college students; overall bullying (either traditional or digital) was associated with an authoritarian parenting style. Implications of these findings for practitioners include the need to attend to demographic characteristics in identifying targeted groups for prevention programs, and the potential importance of parent training as part of intervention with students who are already engaged in bullying. With regard to victimization, frequency of digital communication via instant messaging and text messaging predicted cybervictim status, with frequency of text messaging being the most significant predictor of cybervictimization. Family interaction patterns characterized by conflict within the family environment were predictive of victimization both traditionally and digitally. Finally, cohesion among family members was negatively correlated with both bullying

---

[*] Address Correspondence to: Elizabeth L. W. McKenney, Ph. D., NCSP Assistant Professor, Department of Psychology, Southern Illinois University Edwardsville. Email: elmcken @siue. edu.

and victimization in both formats. This finding indicates that there may be important skills taught in either emotional regulation or social interaction within cohesive families that serve to reduce adolescents' involvement in bullying. Implications for future research into school- and community-based interventions targeting family interaction patterns and important skills in preventing or reducing bullying are discussed.

INTRODUCTION

The issue of bullying is one of the fastest growing areas of educational policy-making and research. Due to several high profile incidences of student suicide related to bullying or cyberbullying in recent years, increasing attention has been paid to this issue at all levels including state legislation, educational and psychological research, and school-based intervention programs. Bullying is perhaps best defined as, "... aggressive behavior or "harm doing" by one person or a group, generally carried out repeatedly and over time, and which involves a power differential," (Hinduja & Patchin, 2010, p. 207). Cyberbullying expands on this definition by specifying the use of computers, cell phones, and other electronic forms of communication in a similar pattern of "willful and repeated harm," (Hinduja & Patchin, 2010, p. 208). Nationally representative studies of prevalence indicate that bullying peaks in early to mid-adolescence, during the middle and high school years (McKenna, Hawk, Mullen, & Hertz, 2011; Ybarra & Mitchell, 2004). Thus, both bullying and cyberbullying pervade throughout adolescence and can inflict serious emotional harm upon students throughout middle and high school.

In contrast with traditional popular beliefs that bullying is a predominantly male behavior involving physical harm and aggression toward others, it is now widely accepted that bullying occurs among both male and female peer groups. Although generally females are more likely to engage in relational aggression (gossiping, spreading rumors, excluding victims from socially desirable activities or groups; Li, 2005), males may also engage in relational forms of aggression, and female adolescents can and are at times physically aggressive toward their victims. Given the indirect nature of cyberbullying, relational aggression in particular is of rising concern among both male and female adolescent groups (Li, 2005).

PREVALENCE

An expansion of research into bullying has yielded new knowledge about the frequency of both bullying and cyberbullying among adolescents in many countries throughout the world. Upon looking across the prevalence rates reported by numerous researchers investigating the prevalence of cyberbullying among U. S., Canadian, and Chinese populations, Hinduja and Patchin (2010) determined that approximately 15 - 35% of students studied report cybervictimization, while 10 - 20% report cyberbullying others. A recent investigation with Taiwanese junior high school students (7th through 9th grades) yielded similar findings: 34.9% of those studied reported ever having experienced cybervictimization (Li, 2010).

Recent investigations into the prevalence of bullying on school campuses, which is considered to primarily reflect traditional forms of bullying, reveal similar results. In 2005,

Due et al. studied the prevalence of bullying among adolescents in Israel, Russia, the United States, Canada, and 24 European countries. In their study, the prevalence of bullying ranged from a low of 6.3% of 11, 13, and 15 year old girls in Sweden to a high of 41.4% of 11, 13, and 15 year old boys in Lithuania. Dinkes, Cataldi, and Lin-Kelly (2007), reporting on multiple surveys and databases collected by public health and justice agencies in the United States, found that an average of 28% of youth ages 12 - 18 reported being bullied in 2005, approximately 8% of whom reported being bullied almost daily. All studies described above included a roughly equal number of male and female participants, and the literature remains inconclusive as to whether male or female students engage in higher rates of bullying and cyberbullying (Li, 2010).

SEQUELAE

The consequences of bullying range from more mild forms of emotional distress to severe mental health problems, including depression, suicidal ideation, and attempted and completed suicide. A considerable body of research has demonstrated that involvement in bullying is related to several psychological indicators of distress. As summarized by Hinduja and Patchin (2010, p. 207), "... experience with peer harassment (most often as a victim but also as a perpetrator) contributes to depression, decreased self-worth, hopelessness, and loneliness - all of which are precursors to suicidal thoughts and behavior." While suicide related to bullying and cyberbullying is certainly of greatest concern, its incidence among students who are involved in some form of bullying remains relatively rare. Nevertheless, international research summarized by Hinduja and Patchin (2010) indicates that students who are bullied experience rates of suicidal ideation somewhere in the ranges of 4 - 18%, and are three to four times more likely to have suicidal ideation that their non-bullied or bullying peers.

In a study conducted in the Netherlands, a slightly larger percentage of boys who were bullied indirectly reported suicidal ideation than those who were bullied directly (18% versus 13%, respectively; van der Wal, de Wit, and Hirasing, 2003). Although an early study with respect to the rise of cyberbullying, these effects may indicate that the emotional sequelae of cyberbullying can be more pervasive and devastating than those typically produced by bullying. A recent analysis of survey data collected in 2005 revealed that middle school students involved in cyberbullying, either as victims or as bully victims, reported higher levels of depression than students who only reported involvement in traditional bullying (Wang, Nansel, & Iannotti, 2010). Researchers have posited that the greater reports of emotional distress as a result of being victimized by cyberbullying may be due to the seemingly inescapable nature of the bullying (i.e., it can be experienced at home, school, or any other location) and the permanence of the bullying acts themselves, as they can be repeatedly accessed via electronic communication devices and websites. Given several high-profile incidences of suicide related to cyberbullying in recent years, or cyberbullicide, the apparently stronger link between cyberbullying victimization and more severe forms of depression merits particular attention (Hinduja and Patchin, 2010).

The act of bullying itself may also be linked to more severe forms of aggression in later adolescence or adulthood. Espelage, Basille, and Hamburger (2012) recently reported on early results in a longitudinal study examining the degree to which perpetuating bullying is linked to homophobic bullying and sexually harassing statements to peers. They posit that a link between bullying, homophobic bullying, and sexual harassment may result in a higher perpetuation of sexual violence among students who engage in bullying when in middle school. Their results indicate strong correlations between bullying and homophobic teasing and between bullying and sexually harassing statements, providing initial support for their proposed model of developing sexual violence. As more data is gathered and reported, additional attention should be paid to the extent to which bullying may predict sexual violence later in adolescence and adulthood. The possibility of a link between the two behaviors underscores the need to more thoroughly understand bullying and cyberbullying, and to develop effective intervention protocols that strengthen alternate forms of adolescent peer interactions.

INTERVENTIONS ADDRESSING BULLYING AND CYBERBULLYING

In response to the continuing need to respond to and attempt to prevent bullying within the school context, several programs have been developed at all levels of the K-12 curriculum that can be effective at preventing bullying and cyberbullying, and decreasing participation in both forms of aggression when they are already present. Programs targeting youth violence, including bullying and cyberbullying, are evaluated via a cooperative effort under the direction of the United States Department of Justice to identify those programs that demonstrate the strongest and most consistent evidence of efficacy in preventing and decreasing bullying in schools (Evidence-Based Program Directory). Prevention programs are evaluated on a scale of one to three, on which Level 1 is characterized by consistently high fidelity in implementation, robust empirical findings, and sophisticated experimental evaluation procedures. Programs classified at Level 2 feature adequate fidelity, empirical findings, and sufficiently strong experimental procedures (e.g., quasi-experimental designs). Programs placed at Level 3 have demonstrated generally positive results, but often with minimal fidelity, mixed empirical findings, and limited experimental procedures (Evidence-Based Program Directory). Of those programs evaluated for their potential to decrease school violence, three are specific to bullying and have demonstrated evidence of efficacy at a classification of Level 2. No programs specific to bullying have been classified at Level 1.

The three programs at Level 2 are Steps to Respect®: A Bullying Prevention Program, Olweus Bullying Prevention Program, and Success in Stages®. While the Olweus program was initially developed in Norway and extensively researched in Europe before being applied to the United States, both the Steps to Respect® and Success in Stages® programs were developed and researched in the United States. Details regarding each program, including the intended age range, general procedures for implementation, and evidence of efficacy, are provided below. Generally, each program emphasizes increasing adult awareness of bullying, and increasing both student and adult awareness of how bullying negatively impacts others and the school environment. The Olweus and Steps to Respect® programs emphasize increasing student skill in recognizing and responding to bullying, while the Success in Stages® programs focus greater attention on individual recognition of the need to change one's behavior (i.e., bullying) and the steps necessary to effectively navigate that change.

The Olweus program has undergone the most attempts at replication and has consistently demonstrated encouraging results. The program emphasizes intervention at the school, classroom and individual levels via increased adult awareness of bullying and engagement in changing bullying within the school environment. Intervention and prevention components are specifically designed for students between the ages of six and 14; indicating that the program is primarily designed for elementary and middle school populations. The program begins with an assessment of the extent of bullying within a school via a questionnaire distributed to students. Program components include developing specific rules regarding bullying, classroom meetings to address bullying and other climate issues, increased monitoring of areas of the building where bullying is most likely to occur, and meetings with parents to share information across contexts. A coordinating committee is responsible for overseeing and evaluating the success of prevention efforts. Efficacy of the Olweus Bullying Prevention Program has been shown to be the greatest in Norway, where the program was developed, with somewhat less success in other European countries, and the most limited impact in the United States (Suicide Prevention Resource Center, 2011). Specifically, the Olweus program appears to be most effective at increasing awareness of bullying and its consequences, and at changing attitudes regarding the acceptability of bullying. However, especially in the United States, the Olweus program has been less successful in decreasing reports of victimization and other indications of delinquent behavior, and may not produce effects that are sustained over time without ongoing consultation and support (Melton et al., 1998).

Steps to Respect® also aims to increase adult awareness of and responsiveness to bullying, and to foster beliefs among students that encourage responsibility for intervening with bullying when it occurs. The program stresses the development of social-emotional skills that assist students in handling bullying directly, including via intervening as bystanders and reporting to adults. At the outset of the program, all staff members in the school building are trained in its implementation, which is followed up on by two in-depth trainings for administrators, mental health professionals, and teachers. Teachers go on to implement 11 skill-based lessons that take 20 – 30 minutes, and two literature based units, for which the lessons last 30 – 40 minutes. Steps to Respect® is intended for use with students ages eight to 12 years old, targeting upper elementary and early middle school students. Evaluations of the outcomes of Steps to Respect® were promising when efficacy of the program was compared via randomized trial between six schools receiving the program and six wait-listed control schools. Students reported greater responsibility as bystanders, improved perceptions of adult responsiveness, and less overall acceptability of bullying. Playground observations of bullying and bystander behavior also indicated improvements. However, self-reported bullying and teacher descriptions of social interactions did not reveal any differences over the course of intervention (Evidence-Based Program Directory). Additionally, in a one-year trial, Steps to Respect® was shown to be effective at decreasing rates of malicious playground gossip (a form of relational aggression) among elementary students who participated, an effect that was not observed in randomly assigned control groups (Low, Frey, & Brockman, 2010).

Success in Stages® is a computer-based intervention program that tailors its activities to both students' grade level and their responses to survey items about their understanding of and involvement in bullying. The program has different procedures and activities that can be used with students from nine to 18years old. Build Respect, Stop Bullying® includes two programs targeting either elementary or middle school students, while Building Respect® is specifically aimed at high school students. All the interventions involve at least three half hour computer sessions that are distributed throughout the school year. The program itself, while it asks about bullying and victimization, is based upon theories of how people proceed through change, and different stages of participation in change. Students receive feedback and additional instruction regarding their bullying behaviors based upon where their survey answers indicate that they fall on the continuum of change. Supportive materials are also included for school personnel and others who may have direct contact with students engaged in or affected by bullying (Evers, Prochaska, Van Marter, Johnson, & Prochaska, 2007). Evaluation of the outcomes of Success in Stages® was done primarily on the computer-generated self-reports of middle and high school student participants, and the percentages of students who reported no longer being a bully, victim, or passive bystander were compared across intervention and control groups. The intervention group members reported significantly less bullying, victimization, and being a passive bystander from the control group once the intervention was implemented. Often, participants in the intervention groups began to report lower participation in bullying following the second lesson in the intervention series (Evers et al., 2007).

IDENTIFYING RISK FACTORS FOR INVOLVEMENT IN BULLYING

If intervention programs are to be effective at decreasing the extent to which children and adolescents are involved in bullying and cyberbullying, intervention providers must be knowledgeable of and able to recognize factors that make a student or group of students more likely to be at risk of involvement in bullying or cyberbullying. Recent research into some of the situational and historical factors that may affect adolescents' involvement in bullying and cyberbullying provides new insight into the mechanisms through which bullying occurs and might be intervened upon. Two recent studies in which such issues were examined shed light on when and how specific students may benefit from targeted interventions designed to reduce involvement in acts of bullying and vulnerability to victimization, in both traditional and electronic forms. Study 1 focuses on age and gender differences related to cyberbullying, and examines the use of pictures and videos in cyberbullying. Study 2 examined how context variables, such as family environment and parenting style, affect adolescents' participation in bullying and cyberbullying.

Study 1

Study one examined age and gender differences related to cyberbullying, as well as how access to technology, specifically frequency of technology use, impacts the likelihood of engaging in cyberbullying or cybervictimization. Additional analyses were conducted to determine how those variables may be related to image cyberbullying and cybervictimization, which is specific to posting or sending embarrassing pictures of someone, and/or video of someone being assaulted in some way (e.g., hit or beat up) in order to hurt or embarrass them. Before the onset of the study, approval was obtained through the appropriate Institutional

Review Board. Participants for this study included 286 junior high and 87 high school students from three areas: schools in the northwestern suburbs of Chicago, schools in a small town in rural central Illinois, and schools in suburban southern Illinois. Also, 110 college-aged students were recruited from undergraduate psychology courses at a mid-western university. College-aged participants received class credit for participation. Overall, there were slightly more female participants than male participants. Over half (58.8%) of the participants were in junior high school. Before collecting data, informed consent forms were sent home to obtain parental permission to participate in the study for participants under the age of 18. Those students under the age of 18 who returned the completed informed consent were allowed to participate in the study. Students 18-years-old and older were allowed to sign their own informed consent;assent was provided by participants who were under 18-years-old. The homeroom or study hall teacher passed out both the assent forms and the surveys. After obtaining informed consent and/or assent, all participants were asked to complete the *Demographic Information and Access to Technology Survey* and the *Cyberbullying Survey*. The participants took approximately 5 minutes to complete the study. For college-aged students, data were collected in the same manner except that they all were able to sign their own informed consent.

Students at the middle school, high school, and college levels were surveyed, and asked to reflect upon a variety of behaviors, including frequency of electronic communication, frequency of cyberbullying, cybervictimization, image cyberbullying, and image cybervictimization over the course of the past year, as well as demographic information including age, ethnicity, sex, and grade. Frequency of electronic communication was assessed with questions about how often students used an instant messaging program per day, the number of text messages sent per day, and the number of hours per day spent online. Cybervictimization and cyberbullying were assessed using the *Cyberbullying Survey*, which was adapted and simplified from Bilyeu's *Traditional Bully and Cyber-bully Questionnaire* (2007). The *Cyberbullying* Survey is made up of Cyberbully, Image Cyberbully, Cybervictim, and Image Cybervictim subscales The Cyberbully and Cybervictim subscales each contain ten questions that related to cyberbullying behaviors. Questions asked about spreading gossip or rumors, threatening or insulting someone, giving out private information, using deception, and socially excluding others via electronic methods of communication. Questions regarding cyberbullying began with the phrase, "In the past year, *I have* used the internet or a cell phone to…" while questions about victimization began, "In the past year, *someone else* used the internet or a cell phone to…" Each question was answered using a 5-point Likert scale on which 0 = Never, 1 = Rarely, 2 = Once a month, 3 = Once a week, 4 = Once a day, and 5 = Several times a day. Cronbach's alphas were $\alpha=.85$ for each subscale. The Image Cyberbully and Image Cybervictim subscales each contained three questions; Cronbach's alphas for those subscales were $\alpha= .83$ and $\alpha=.72$, respectively. Responses ranged from 0 - 50 for the Cyberbully and Cybervictim Subscales; and from 0 - 15 on the Image Cyberbully and Image Cybervictim subscales. Relatively few participants reported experience with cybervictimization and cyberbullying, and even fewer reported cybervictimization or bullying through use of an image. Means and standard deviations for each subscale are reported in Table 1. Age, gender, frequency of using an instant messaging program, frequency of texting, and time spent online were all significantly correlated with being a cyberbully. In the case of cybervictimization, only frequency of using an instant messaging program and frequency of texting revealed significant correlations. Age, gender, and frequency of text messaging were associated with using an image to cyberbully someone; frequency of texting and time spent online were significantly correlated to being a victim of cyberbullying via an image. Frequency of text messaging was a significant correlate of overall involvement in both forms of cyberbullying and cybervictimization. Correlation coefficients are presented in Table 2.

Table 1. Means and standard deviations observed across subscales of the *Cyberbullying Survey*

Subscale	Mean	Standard Deviation	Potential Range
Cyberbully	2.81	4.40	0 - 50
Cybervictim	3.85	4.93	0 - 50
Image Cyberbully	.33	1.23	0 - 15
Image Cybervictim	.25	.95	0 - 15

Table 2. Correlations between demographic information, access to technology, and *Cyberbully Survey* subscale scores

Variable	Cyberbully	Cybervictim	Image Cyberbully	Image Cybervictim
Age	.17**	.06	.08**	.02
Gender	-.13**	-.03	-.12**	-.05
Instant Messaging	.11*	.18**	-.02	.05
Text Messaging	.26**	.30**	.14**	.08**
Time spent online	.09*	.07	.02	.11**

Note: * = $p < .05$; ** = $p < .01$. Male = 1. Female = 2.

Four simultaneous multiple regression equations were calculated to determine the influence of gender, frequency of instant messaging, frequency of texting, and amount of time spent online on cyberbullying and cybervictimization. A simultaneous regression was chosen because no theory of which predictors have the greatest or least influence on either of the criterion variables (cyberbullying or cybervictimization) has emerged. Gender, frequency of instant messaging, frequency of texting, and time spent online were predictors. Results of regression analyses are presented in Table 3. Gender, frequency of instant messaging, frequency of text messaging, and time spent online were entered as predictors into a simultaneous regression equation to determine their influence upon cyberbullying, cybervictimization, image cyberbullying, and image cybervictimization. Results indicated that being male, texting more frequently, and spending more time online were related to increased cyberbullying behaviors, while frequency of using an instant message program was not a significant predictor of cyberbullying. With regard to image cyberbullying, being male and texting more frequently were related to increased image cyberbullying behaviors, while frequency of using an instant message program and time spent online were not significant predictors. In the area of victimization, more frequent instant messaging and texting predicted cybervictimization; time spent online and being male were not predictors. Finally, with regard to image cybervictimization, time spent online and frequency of texting were predictors, while gender and instant messaging frequency were not.

Table 3. Simultaneous multiple regression analyses examining impact of gender and access to technology variables on cyberbullying, image cyberbullying, cybervictimization, and image cybervictimization

Variable	Cyberbully Subscale Score				Image Cyberbully Subscale Score				Cybervictim Subscale Score				Image Cybervictim Subscale Score			
	B	SE B	β	T	B	SE B	β	T	B	SE B	β	T	B	SE B	β	T
Gender	-1.74	.40	-.20	-4.39**	-.41	.11	-.16	-3.59**	-.83	.45	-.08	-1.86	-.14	.09	-.07	-1.52
Frequency of instant messaging	-.01	.12	-.01	-.12	-.05	.05	-.08	-1.51	.27	.14	.10	1.99*	.01	.03	.01	.22
Frequency of texting	.75	.11	.31	6.57**	.13	.03	.19	4.02**	.79	.13	.29	6.20**	.05	.03	.09	1.88
Time spent online	.37	.18	.09	2.02*	.05	.05	.05	1.02	.15	.21	.04	.75	.09	.04	.11	2.27*
R^2		.11				.05				.11				.02		
Adjusted R^2		.11				.04				.10				.02		
F		15.07***				6.16***				14.13***				2.87*		

Note: * = p < .05; ** = p < .01; *** = p < .001. Male = 1. Female = 2.

Table 4. Results of ANOVA analyses examining the effects of age on cyberbullying, image cyberbullying, cybervictimization, and image cybervictimization

	Cyberbully	Cybervictim	Image Cyberbully	Image Cybervictim
F	37.28	4.65	14.47	.23
P	<.001	<.01	<.001	=.77
η^2	.14	.02	.06	.001

Table 5. Means and standard deviations observed across subscales of the *Cyberbullying Survey* and the *Traditional Bullying and Victimization Survey*

Subscale	Mean	Standard Deviation	Potential Range	Observed Range
Cyberbully	1.22	2.47	0 - 50	0 – 14
Cybervictim	3.27	5.04	0 - 50	0 – 27
Traditional Bully	2.44	3.50	0 - 45	0 – 17
Traditional Victim	5.57	6.16	0 - 45	0 – 31

An examination of the means of the different age groups (e.g., middle school, high school, and college) revealed a curvilinear relationship between age and scores on the *Cyberbullying Survey*. Since age could not be entered into the simultaneous multiple regression, an ANOVA was also used to determine the influence of age on each dependent variable. Results of the ANOVA with respect to the effect of age are presented in Table 4.

ANOVA comparisons indicated that there is an overall effect of age on both cyberbullying and image cyberbullying. With regard to cyberbullying, posthoc t-tests showed that high school students cyberbullied significantly more than both middle school students and college-aged students, and that college-aged student cyberbullied significantly more than middle school students. Specific to image cyberbullying, posthoc t-tests revealed that high school student cyberbullied using an image significantly more than middle and college-aged students. No differences were observed between college and middle school students.

In the area of cybervictimization, a significant effect of age was observed upon overall cybervictimization, but not with regard to image cybervictimization. Posthoc t-tests indicated that high school students reported cybervictimization significantly more than middle school students and college-aged students, who did not differ from each other.

Study 2

Study two aimed to identify contextual variables that may be related to increased likelihood to perpetrate or be victimized by bullying and cyberbullying. Before the onset of the study, approval was obtained through the appropriate Institutional Review Board. Middle school students were asked to report on various family context variables, experiences with bullying, and experiences with cyberbullying. Two hundred twenty three students in the 6th, 7th, and 8th grades, ranging in ages from 11 to 14 years, participated via survey. The sample population was obtained from rural and suburban schools in in the Midwest. According to self-report classifications, 52% of student respondents were Caucasian, 22% were African American, 5% were Hispanic, 4.5% were Asian, and 12.5% reported another ethnicity. The responding population consisted of slightly more females than is typical of the population in general, 59.6% of respondents were female. Prior to the study, a consent form was completed by the participant's guardian, informing them of the purpose of this study. Additionally, participants were rewarded with Tootsie Rolls when completed consent forms were returned.

Survey packets were completed either during students' first hour class or during study hall. The first page of the survey packet was an assent form for the participants to read and sign. Directly following the assent form was the *Demographic Information and Access to Technology Survey,* then the *Cyber Bullying and Victimization Surveys,* and finally the *Family Assessment Survey.*

Upon distribution of the survey packets, participants were instructed to read and follow all instructions carefully, take as much time as necessary, and complete the measures in their entirety. Participants were asked to report demographic information, which consisted of their gender, ethnicity, grade, and age. In addition, they reported on how often they used an instant messaging program, how many text messages they typically sent in a day, and how many hours they spent online.

The *Cyberbullying Survey* was used to assess experiences with cyberbullying as in Study 1, with the exception that items about image cyberbullying and cybervictimization were not included. Cronbach's alpha within this study was in the good range at $\alpha=.82$ for the Cyberbullying Subscale and at $\alpha=.88$ for the Cybervictimization Subscale.

A similar tool assessing traditional forms of bullying, the *Traditional Bullying and Victimization Survey,* was developed for this study. Each subscale contained nine items that were designed to assess the participants' experience with traditional bullying. The Traditional Bullying Subscale asked about participants' experience as perpetrators of bullying with the Traditional Victimization Subscale asked about experiences being victimized. For example, one item on the Victimization Subscale asked participants, "In the past year I have been beaten up (hit, kicked, and/or pushed) by someone." Each question was answered using a 5-point Likert scale on which 0 = Never, 1 = Rarely, 2 = Once a month, 3 = Once a week, 4 = Once a day, and 5 = Several times a day. Cronbach's alphas reflected internal consistency of the Bullying Subscale at $\alpha=.77$, and $\alpha=.87$ for the Victimization Subscale.

The *Family Assessment System* (Jewell & Stark, n.d.) is comprised of 60 questions designed to measure 12 areas of family life. For the purposes of this study, 30 questions were used and the following areas were examined relative to bullying: family cohesion, authoritarian parenting style, and family conflict. Participants answered each question with "Never true," "A little true," "Sometimes true," "Mostly true," and "Always true." Sample questions included "There is a feeling of togetherness in my family," "The punishment for breaking rules in my family is too strict," and "We fight in our family." The *Family Assessment System* also asks for information regarding which parental figures participants have lived with for the past five years.

Eight-four percent of participants reported living with more than one parental figure, while 15% reported living with only one parental figure. According to interpretive guidelines provided by George and Mallery (2003), Cronbach's alphas for the various scales were in the good range $\alpha=.84$ for the cohesion scale, and in the questionable range for the authoritarian and conflict scales $\alpha=.62$ and $\alpha=.66$, respectively).

Few participants reported experience with cybervictimization and even fewer reported experience with cyberbullying; overall means for cyberbullying in this study appear to be lower than was observed in Study 1. Means and standard deviations for each subscale are reported in Table 5. A strong correlation was observed between cyberbullying and cybervictimization and moderate correlations were observed between all other subscales. Intercorrelations between subscales are reported in Table 6.

Correlations between *Family Assessment System* variables (cohesion, authoritarian parenting style, and conflict) and survey responses regarding experiences with cyber and traditional bullying and victimization are presented in Table 7. Overall, family conflict had a significant positive relationship at the moderate level with both forms of bullying and both forms of victimization. Authoritarian parenting style had a significant positive relationship at the moderate level with reported levels of cyberbullying.

To understand which *Family Assessment System* variable best predicts traditional and cyberbullying and victimization, the exclusive relationships between each family variable and bullying and victimization behaviors were examined via simultaneous multiple regression. Number of family members living in the household was also entered to determine whether having one or two parents was related to bullying or victimization. Simultaneous regression was selected because there was not prior theoretical support for one predictor having more influence than another.

Table 6. Correlations observed between responses on *Cyberbullying* and *Traditional* subscales

Variable	Cyberbully	Cybervictim	Traditional Bully	Traditional Victim
Cyberbully	-	.70**	.59*	.47*
Cybervictim	-	-	.56**	.62**
Traditional Bully	-	-	-	.61**
Traditional Victim	-	-	-	-

Note: * = $p < .05$; ** = $p < .01$.

Table 7. Correlations between *Family Assessment System* Subscale Total Scores and bullying and victimization subscale total scores

Variable	Cyberbully	Cybervictim	Traditional Bully	Traditional Victim
Parental Figures	-.10	-.05	-.05	.004
Cohesion	-.29**	-.27**	-.28**	-.29**
Authoritarianism	.35**	-	.29**	
Conflict	.32**	.31**	.33**	.39**

Note: * = $p < .05$; ** = $p < .01$. Correlations with a dash were not included in the hypotheses and, therefore, were not correlated.

Table 8. Simultaneous multiple regression analyses examining impact of *Family Assessment System* variables on Cyberbullying, Cybervictimization, Traditional Bullying, and Traditional Victimization subscale total scores

Variable	*Cyberbully* Subscale Score				*Cybervictim* Subscale Score				*Traditional Bully* Subscale Score				*Traditional Victim* Subscale Score			
	B	SE B	β	T	B	SE B	β	T	B	SE B	β	T	B	SE B	β	T
Parental Figures	-.42	.44	-.06	-.95	-.24	.94	-.02	-.25	.04	.67	.004	.06	1.19	1.11	.07	1.07
Cohesion	-.001	.06	-.002	-.02	-.04	.12	-.03	-.36	.004	.09	.005	.05	.01	.14	.01	.07
Authoritarianism	.16	.05	.25	3.16**	-	-	-	-	.17	.07	.19	2.31**	-	-	-	-
Conflict	.04	.03	.11	1.11	.24	.08	.21	3.05***	.08	.05	.17	1.60	.33	.08	.39	4.33**
R^2		.22				.20				.18				.02		
Adjusted R^2		.20				.18				.16						
F		9.07***				12.45***				7.15**				2.87*		

Note: * = p <.05; ** = p <.01; *** = p <.001. Results with a dash were not included in the hypotheses and, therefore, were not examined.

Conclusion

Summary

Results of Study 1 suggest that most middle, high school, and college students are communicating via electronic means on a daily basis. Instant messaging is likely less popular than it once was, but remains one method through which students interact socially. Others include other online forms of communication (e.g., social networking) and sending text messages. In this study, nearly 85% of respondents indicated sending one or more text messages per day, while over 90% of students spent some time online every day.

The majority of participants in both studies reported very low scores on the *Cyberbullying Survey* and *Traditional Bullying and Victimization Survey*. In Study 2, very few participants reported engaging in cyberbullying; similar levels of cybervictimization were observed across both studies. Results of Study 1 indicate that image cyberbullying and cybervictimization are occurring so infrequently that it is difficult to predict. However, there were several predictors of importance observed in these studies. Age, gender, frequency of text messaging, and time spent online were all predictive of cyberbullying in Study 1. Study 2 provided additional insight into the phenomenon of cyberbullying with the finding that authoritarian parenting style predicts both traditional and cyberbullying. Thus, the avenues through which cyberbullying becomes manifest may be similar to those through which students become traditional bullies. Indeed, the high intercorrelations between all forms of bullying and victimization observed in Study 2 suggest that not only are students often bully-victims, but those same students who are bullying and being victimized in the "physical" world are engaging in the same "digital behaviors."

Additionally, Study 1 provided important insight into the age at which students are most likely to engage in cyberbullying. High school students reported the most cyberbullying, followed by college-age students, who reported cyberbullying others more than middle school students did. This finding is similar to that observed by Smith, Mahdavi, Carvalho, Fisher, Russell, & Tippett (2008), who looked at middle school and high school students. They found that older students reported engaging in significantly more cyberbullying. Study 1 supplemented Smith et al.'s (2008) findings by demonstrating a drop in cyberbullying behaviors after high school. Additionally, the finding that males reported cyberbullying others more than females is in agreement with the findings of Dehue, Bolman, & Vollink (2008) and Li (2007). Like general cyberbullying, high school students reported engaging in more image cyberbullying than middle school or college students, but there were no significant differences between middle school and college students' reporting. Also similar to general cyberbullying, males and those who send text messages more frequently were more likely to engage in image cyberbullying.

The family context variables that were examined in Study 2 provide important insight into the background characteristics that may incline a student to engage in bullying and/or be victimized by bullying, in both electronic and traditional formats. Overall family conflict demonstrated a significant positive correlation with both forms of bullying, while cohesion demonstrated a negative relationship with both cyber and traditional bullying. However, when analyzed via multiple regression, parenting style (authoritarian) was the most influential variable predicting bullying behavior. These findings are consistent with previous research concluding that adolescents are more likely to engage in traditional bullying if they experience excessive punishment and/or frequent discipline (Oliver, Oaks, & Hoover, 1994; Ybarra & Mitchell, 2004).

In the area of victimization, high school students were more likely to be victims of cyberbullying than middle school or college students, with no differences observed between middle school and college students. This finding seems a natural reflection of the finding that high school students are more likely to engage in cyberbullying, as bullying typically occurs between same-age/grade peers. While time spent online was not a predictor of cybervictimization in Study 1, time spent texting and instant messaging were predictors, indicating that increased use of electronic communication is associated with increased risk of victimization. Unlike previous research indicating that females are more likely to be cybervictims than males (Dehue et al., 2008; Li, 2007), Study 1 did not reveal any differences in likelihood of cybervictimization due to sex. However, Beran and Li conducted a study in 2005 that also did not reveal an effect of sex on cybervictimization. Thus, the results of research to date on gender differences with respect to cybervictimization are mixed. Further work is needed to identify other variables that may mediate the link between sex and cybervictimization.

Overall, text messaging was the strongest predictor of both cyberbullying and cybervictimization in Study 1. Study 2 revealed that the strongest predictor of bullying behavior via both cyber and traditional formats was authoritarian parenting, which was a stronger effect than conflict or the potentially ameliorating effects of family cohesion. Victimization, however, was most strongly predicted by family conflict in Study 2.

Implications and Future Directions

The findings of both studies provide important implications for practitioners looking to appropriately target bullying and cyberbullying intervention and prevention programs. Specifically, despite the emergence of bullying behavior in early adolescence, cyberbullying in particular is most likely to occur during the high school years. Given the preponderance of bullying prevention programs targeting late elementary and middle school students in recent years, it is likely that at least some of the participants in this study had previously been exposed to instruction in bullying and how to respond to it. However, since more high school age students than any other age group report engaging in and being victims of bullying, intervention programs should continue to focus on preventing and intervening with bullying at the high school level. Among the evidence-based programs reviewed earlier in the chapter, only the Success in Stages® program includes materials targeting bullying behavior at the high school level. Given the rate of maturation and change during the adolescent years, it is perhaps unsurprising that high school students may easily forget or stop using the strategies they may have learned earlier on in adolescence to prevent or stop bullying and cyberbullying. Furthermore, if the majority of interventions themselves only teach strategies that are appropriate for older children and early adolescents, then high school students may find themselves ill-equipped to handle increasingly complex and sometimes confusing social relationships that involve bullying. Addressing this need will require intervention procedures that are adept at helping high school students to recognize bullying when it is occurring, proactively attempt to stop it, and resolve resulting conflicts or disruptions in social relationships that may follow instances of bullying.

Evidence regarding the predictors of bullying and cyberbullying should be used to identify and target students who are at the greatest risk of engaging in bullying or being victimized by bullying. While it appears that more high school students may benefit from bullying intervention efforts than may be currently receiving those programs, students who are male, engage in frequent electronic communication, and come from family backgrounds characterized by authoritarian parenting are even more likely to be perpetrators of bullying. Schools that administer questionnaires to ask about bullying could use this information to survey these factors as well. Given the variability in frequencies with which students sometimes report engaging in bullying, information regarding other risk factors may help school personnel to identify students who are in need of the most help. For example, a male student who reports engaging in cyberbullying, describes his parents as authoritarian, and who sends several dozen text messages a day may engage in more severe or chronic forms of cyberbullying than a male student who reports engaging in cyberbullying, but also describes his family as cohesive and sends text messages less than 20 times a day. Small group interventions may be more salient for the former student than the latter, and when resources are limited, focusing intervention efforts on the most severe offenders may result in the greatest impact for overall school climate. Conversely, knowledge of behaviors that predispose students for bullying and/or victimization, such as texting often or spending a lot of time online, may help service providers to target prevention efforts at younger students or those who do not yet report high levels of bullying or victimization.

The implications of these findings for work with family members are also important. While authoritarian parenting has been linked to many negative outcomes for youth for quite some time (e.g. Jewell, Krohn, Scott, Carlton, & Meinz, 2008), its link to bullying behavior is relatively new (Ybarra & Mitchell, 2004). Practitioners inside and outside of schools should attend to the impact of family environment on adolescents' behavior – this finding is probably particularly salient for community-based practitioners who have the opportunity to assess and target familial interactions. It may be that parents who are able to set firm limits but also to compromise when their child's well-being demands it are teaching and modeling important skills in self-regulation, seeking out social support, and maintaining positivity. Future avenues of research should examine whether learning those skills provides additional benefit in reducing bullying behaviors, which would further strengthen the link between skills gained via appropriate parenting and engagement in bullying. Meanwhile, practitioners who have the opportunity to directly address parenting style may wish to examine whether adolescents with authoritarian parents are engaging in bullying and, if so, provide additional skill instruction to both adolescents and their parents in the areas of effective communication and compromise in interpersonal relationships.

Family context also has important implications for victimization, especially in the area of conflict. Family conflict predicted victimization via both traditional and cyber routes in Study 2, suggesting that the experience of frequently witnessing conflict in the home environment may result in adolescents who are either more tolerant of receiving aggression from others and/or less skillful in effectively refuting and discouraging aggression from peers. Clearly, more research is needed to specify the exact pathways through which family conflict makes adolescents more vulnerable to bullying and cyberbullying. In light of other findings regarding age group and the protective effects of cohesion, high school students from homes with high conflict are particularly likely to be bullied traditionally and via cyber mechanisms. Additionally, practitioners should attend to the amount of conflict present in a student's family when considering whether to involve a student in a targeted intervention group or when working individually with such an adolescent. Such youth may require additional skill instruction and opportunities to rehearse proactively responding to conflict and/or aggression in a way that de-escalates the aggressor and communicates a lack of tolerance for aggressive and/or disparaging comments and actions.

In addition to the directions mentioned above, future researchers should re-examine the findings of this study to determine that the links observed between sex, age, access to technology, and family context variables are meaningfully linked to traditional, cyber, and image-based cyber bullying and victimization with a variety of adolescent populations. Of particular interest in bullying research is the extent to which self-report measures of bullying and victimization accurately reflect adolescents' actual experiences at school and in digital communication. While research examining the efficacy of bullying prevention measures has attempted in vivo observations of actual school-based behavior (e.g., Low et al., 2010), research into prevalence and factors related to bullying typically relies on self-report questionnaires to measure the extent of bullying and/or cyberbullying within a population. Expanding upon the research base by conducting observations of adolescent behavior, in particular, is likely to provide researchers and practitioners with more meaningful methods of identifying and evaluating bullying within a particular context, such as a school. Additionally, with the appropriate consent, qualitative examination of the content of adolescents' messages to and from each other in digital realms could provide meaningful insight into the types of messages and forms of bullying that are most damaging to adolescents, and could be examined in terms of the factors described above.

Just as aggression and concerns about aggression dominate discussions of human behavior from preschool through adulthood, bullying and its related forms will likely continue to be an issue requiring attention and resources for years to come. However, the extent to which social aggression is normative should always be considered in light of the potentially devastating effects that bullying can have on adolescents' lives. Understanding the conditions through which bullying is more likely to occur and the variables that may predispose an adolescent to be victimized will help practitioners and researchers alike to identify, target, and implement effective interventions to ameliorate and minimize the extent to which bullying negative impacts students of all ages.

REFERENCES

Beran, T., & Li, Q. (2005). Cyber-harassment: A study of a new method from an old behavior. *Journal of Educational Computing Research, 32*, 265 – 277.

Bilyeu, M. (2007). *The relationship of behaviors associated with childhood bullying, cyberbullying, and victimization, with adult self-esteem and anxiety.* (Unpublished master's thesis). Southern Illinois University Edwardsville, Edwardsville, Illinois.

Dehue, F., Bolman, C., & Vollink, T. (2008). Cyberbullying: Youngsters' experiences and parental perception. *CyberPsychology & Behavior, 11*, 217 – 223.

Dinkes, R., Cataldi, E. F., & Lin-Kelly, W. (2007). *Indicators of school crime and safety: 2007* (NCES 2008-021/NCJ 219553). Washington, DC: National Center for Education Statistics, Institute of Education Sciences, U.S. Department of Education and Bureau of Justice Statistics, Office of Justice Programs, U.S. Department of Justice.

Due, P., Holstein, B. E., Lynch, J., Diderichsen, F., Nic Gabhain, S., Scheidt, P., et al. (2005). Bullying and symptoms among school-aged children: International comparative cross-sectional study in 28 countries. *European Journal of Public Health, 15,* 128 – 132. doi: 10.1093/eurpub/cki105.

Espelage, D. L., Basile, K. C., & Hamburger, M. E. (2012). Bullying perpetration and subsequent sexual violence perpetration among middle school students. *Journal of Adolescent Health, 50,* 60 – 65. doi: 10.1016/j. jadohealth.2011.07.015.

Evers, K. E., Prochaska, J. O., Van Marter, D. F., Johnson, J. L., & Prochaska, J. M. (2007).Transtheoretical-based bullying prevention effectiveness trials in middle schools and high schools. *Educational Research, 49,* 397 - 414.

Evidence-Based Program Directory: Bullying. Retrieved from http://www.find youthinfo.gov/index.shtml.

George, D., & Mallery, P. (2003). *SPSS for Windows step by step: A simple guide and reference. 11.0 update* (4th ed.). Boston: Allyn & Bacon.

Hinduja, S., & Patchin, J. W. (2010). Bullying, cyberbullying, and suicide. *Archives of Suicide Research, 14,* 206 – 221. doi: 10.1080/13811118. 2010.494133.

Jewell, J., D., Krohn, E. J., Scott, V. K., Carlton, M., & Meinz, E. (2008). The differential impact of mothers' and fathers' discipline on preschool children's home and classroom behavior. *North American Journal of Psychology, 10,* 173 – 188.

Li, Q. (2005). Cyberbullying in schools: A research of gender differences. *School Psychology International, 27,* 157 – 170. doi: 10.1177/0143034306 064547.

Li, Q. (2010). An analysis of multiple factors of cyberbullying among junior high school students in Taiwan. *Computers in Human Behavior, 26,* 1581 – 1590. doi: 10.1016/j.chb.2010.06.005.

Low, S., Frey, K. S., & Brockman, C. J. (2010). Gossip on the playground: Changes associated with universal intervention, retaliation beliefs, and supportive friends. *School Psychology Review, 39,* 536 – 551.

McKenna, M., Hawk, E., Mullen, J., & Hertz, M. F. (2011). Bullying among middle school and high school students - Massachusetts, 2009. *Centers for Disease Control and Prevention: Morbidity and Mortality Weekly Report, 60,* 465 – 471.

Melton, G. B., Limber, S. P., Flerx, V., Nation, M., Osgood, W., Chambers, J. et al. (1998). Violence among rural youth: Final report to the Office of Juvenile Justice and Delinquency Prevention. Washington, DC: U.S. Department of Justice, Office of Justice Programs, Office of Juvenile Justice and Delinquency Prevention.

Oliver, R., Oaks, In. N., & Hoover, J. H. (1994). Family issues and interventions in bully and victim relationships. *School Counselor, 41,* 199 – 202.

Smith, P. K., Mahdavi, J., Carvalho, M., Fisher, S., Russell, S., & Tippett, N. (2008). Cyberbullying: Its nature and impact in secondary school pupils. *Journal of Child Psychology and Psychiatry, 49,* 376 – 385.

van der Wal, M. F., de Wit, C. A. M., & Hirasing, R. A. (2003). Psychosocial health among young victims and offenders of direct and indirect bullying. *Pediatrics, 111,* 1312 – 1317.

Wang, J., Nansel, T. R., & Iannotti, R. J. (2010). Cyber and traditional bullying: Differential association with depression. *Journal of Adolescent Health, 48,* 415 – 417. doi: 10.1016/j.jadohealth.2010.07.012.

Ybarra, M. L., & Mitchell, K. J. (2004). Youth engaging in online harassment: Associations with caregiver-child relationships, internet use, and personal characteristics. *Journal of Adolescence, 27,* 319 – 336.

In: Youth: Practices, Perspectives and Challenges
Editor: Elizabeth Trejos-Castillo

ISBN: 978-1-62618-067-3
© 2013 Nova Science Publishers, Inc.

Chapter 7

CANNABIS USE DISORDERS PREDISPOSE TO THE DEVELOPMENT OF SEXUALLY TRANSMITTED DISEASES AMONG YOUTH

Jack R. Cornelius[1] and Levent Kirisci
Center for Education and Drug Abuse Research (CEDAR)
University of Pittsburgh, PAARC Suite,
Pittsburgh, PA, US
Presented in part at the 17th Annual Scientific Meeting of the Society for Prevention Research (SPR), Washington, DC, US

ABSTRACT

Background: Previous cross-sectional studies involving adults suggest that substance use disorders (SUD) such as cocaine use disorders and opioid use disorders are associated with the development of sexually transmitted diseases (STD). However, it is less clear whether cannabis use disorders (CUD) are associated with the development of STDs, or whether those associations extend to adolescent populations. Longitudinal studies examining those associations are particularly scarce. The current report provides findings from a longitudinal study that examined the relationship between STD and CUD among youth transitioning to young adulthood.

Method: The subjects in this longitudinal study were initially recruited when the index sons of these fathers were 10-12 years of age, and subsequent assessments were conducted at age 12-14, 16, 19, and 22. Multivariate logistic regression and path analyses were conducted.

Results: At age 22, of the 345 subjects, 30 subjects were diagnosed with one or more STD, and 105 were diagnosed with a CUD. STDs were almost four times as common among those with a CUD as among those without a CUD, which was a significant difference. Path analyses demonstrated that peer deviance mediated the association

---

[1] Corresponding author: Jack R. Cornelius, M.D., M.P.H., 3811 O'Hara Street, Pittsburgh PA 15213, Telephone: 412-246-5186. E-mail: corneliusjr@upmc.edu, Address reprint requests to: Jack R. Cornelius, M.D., M.P.H., Department of Psychiatry, University of Pittsburgh School of Medicine, 3811 O'Hara Street, PAARC Suite, Pittsburgh, PA 15213, Running head: STD Associated with CUD.

between a measure of risk for SUD knows as the TLI and CUD, and that peer deviance mediated the association between TLI and STD. Risky sexual behaviors were common.

Conclusions: These finding suggest that cannabis use disorders (CUD) predispose to the development of sexually transmitted disorders (STD) among youth. These findings also suggest that peer deviance mediates the development of STD and of CUD among teenagers making the transition to young adulthood.

1. INTRODUCTION

Persons with a variety of substance use disorders have been shown to be at high risk for sexually transmitted diseases (STD) because of unsafe sexual practices associated with substance use (Lally et al., 2002). Previously, it had been shown that substance use disorders (SUD) involving "hard" drugs such as heroin and cocaine are associated with the development of STDs, but studies involving the association of cannabis use disorders (CUD) and STDs had been lacking. For example, persons with cocaine use disorders (Hser et al., 1999) and persons with heroin dependence (Kelly et al., 2000) have been shown to be at elevated risk for STDs. However, very little information is available regarding whether cannabis use disorders are associated with STDs (Nadeau et al., 2000). Recently, one cross-sectional study involving African-American girls demonstrated that those who used cannabis had a significantly higher incidence of STDs than those who were non-marijuana users (DiClemente et al., 2008) and also engaged in more unsafe sexual practices. However, it is unclear whether those findings concerning cannabis and STDs extend to populations of persons with CUD who are not female and African-American, or whether an association of CUD and STDs would be noted in a longitudinal study.

The current report provides findings from a longitudinal study that examined the relationship between CUD and STD among teenagers transitioning to young adulthood. We hypothesized that CUD would be associated with the development of STDs in that population. We also hypothesized that peer deviance would mediate the development of STD and of CUD, based on our recent findings (Cornelius et al., 2007; Kirisci et al., 2009).

2. MATERIAL AND METHODS

The subjects in this study were part of a longitudinal research study known as the Center for Education and Drug Abuse Research, or CEDAR, whose primary purpose is to examine the etiology of SUD. The children were recruited through their biological fathers, and were initially assessed in late childhood at ages 10 through 12 years of age. The recruitment procedure was designed to yield a group of children at high average risk (HAR) for SUD, identified by having fathers with a lifetime history of drug use disorders (abuse or dependence involving illicit substances) and a comparison group at low average risk (LAR), identified by having fathers without SUD or other major mental disorders. Fathers were considered to have a SUD if they ever met DSM criteria for abuse or dependence involving substances other than nicotine, caffeine, or alcohol. Diagnoses were made according to DSM-III-R, the most recent DSM edition when the study was initiated.

Multiple recruitment sources were used to minimize bias that could potentially occur if all of the subjects were recruited from one source. Approximately 89% of the families were recruited from the community through public service announcements and advertisements a well as by direct telephone contact conducted by a market research firm, and 11% were recruited from clinical sources (Cornelius et al, 2007; Cornelius et al., 2008). Psychosis, mental retardation, and neurological injury were exclusionary criteria for participation of the family. Prior to participation in the study, written informed consent was obtained from husbands and wives, and assent was obtained from minor children. The children were the focus of the current study. The study was approved by the University of Pittsburgh Institutional Review Board. The subjects were recruited at age 10-12, and follow-up evaluations were conducted at ages 12-14, 16, 19, and 22, which covered the peak years for initiation of CUD.

Assessments were comprehensive in scope, and included reports on alcohol and other substance use history, mental disorders, personality assessments, and measures of family, cognitive, and psychosocial functioning (Clark et al., 2001; Vanyukov et al., 2009). Diagnostic evaluation was conducted with an expanded version of the Structured Clinical Interview for DSM-III-R (SCID)(Spitzer et al., 1987), which was the most recent DSM edition when the study was initiated. Offspring psychopathology was assessed with the Schedule for Affective Disorders and Schizophrenia for School-Age Children-Epidemiologic Version (K-SADS-E) (Orvaschel et al., 1982). The onset date of each diagnosis was determined to the nearest month. Each family member was individually administered the research protocol in a private room by a different clinical associate. The diagnostic interviews were documented by a staff of experienced clinical associates. Training the clinical associates involved observation of several interviews and conducting joint interviews in the presence of an experienced interviewer. The training procedures were found to produce inter-rater reliabilities exceeding 0.80 for all major diagnostic categories. Diagnoses were determined in a consensus conference using the best estimate diagnostic procedure (Clark et al, 2001). The diagnostic data, in conjunction with all available pertinent medical records and social and legal history, were reviewed in a clinical case conference chaired by a board-certified psychiatrist and another psychiatrist or psychologist and the clinical associates who conducted the interviews.

Another variable included in these analyses included an index created at CEDAR known as the Transmissible Liability Index, also known as the TLI, (Vanyukov, et al., 2009; Kirisci, Tarter, et al, 2009) assessing the risk of developing SUD based on evaluations drawn from self reports, mother reports, and teacher reports. The TLI reportedly has 80% heritability, and in a family study predicted SUD outcome by age 19 with 68% accuracy (Vanyukov et al, 2009). Each standard deviation increment on the mean TLI score of the sample was associated with an increase of 70% probability that CUD would be manifest during the ensuing year. TLI has been shown to be a significant predictor of CUD (Kirisci et al., 2009). Also included was a measure of affiliation with deviant peers at age 16, which has been shown to be associated with the development of CUD and other SUD (Cornelius et al., 2007), as well as demographic information including SES of parental household when the child entered the study, race, and gender.

Logistic regression analyses (Hosmer and Lemeshow, 2000; Kirisci et al., 2009) were conducted to determine the extent to which CUD contributed to the development of STDs after allowing for the effects of deviant peers, the TLI, and demographic factors. A path analysis was conducted to assess mediational effects. Mediated paths were tested using the method described by Sobel (1982).

3. RESULTS

A total of 345 subjects were included in this study, including 30 subjects with lifetime STDs and 105 persons with lifetime CUD. The 30 subjects with STDs included 15 male participants (50.0%) and 15 female participants (50.0%), of whom 13 were Caucasian (43.3%) and 17 were African American (56.7%). The 110 subjects who met diagnostic criteria for a CUD included 83 male participants and 22 female participants, including 64 Caucasian participants and 41 participants of other races. STDs were almost four times as common among those with a cannabis use disorder as compared to those with no history of a CUD, which was a significant difference. Specifically, STDs were reported in 4.7% of those with no history of a lifetime CUD, while 17.3% of those with a history of a lifetime CUD reported a history of at least one STD (Chi-square=15.0, df=1, p<0.001). The most common STD in the sample was clamydia (n=17, 53.3%), followed by genital warts (n=7, 23.3%), gonorrhea (n=4, 13.3%), trichomoniasis (n=4, 13.3%), other STD (n=4, 13.3%), herpes (n=3, 10.0%), and pelvic inflammatory disease (n=1, 3.3%). No cases of syphilis or HIV infection were noted.

Logistic regression demonstrated that CUD were associated with STD (OR=4.71, Wald=9.51, p=0.002), deviance of peers (OR=2.27, Wald=27.39, p≤=0.001), the TLI of the offspring (OR=1.56, Wald=9.11, p=0.003), and Caucasian race (OR=2.46, Wald=8.24, p=0.00). In addition, as shown in Figure 1, path analysis confirmed the results of logistic regression analysis: TLI predicted deviance of peers (beta=.13, z=3.75, p<.001) and CUD (beta=.16, z=4.10, p<.001), deviance of peers predicted STD (beta=.11, z=3.34, p<.001) and CUD (beta=.32, z=9.00, p<.001), and finally, CUD and STD were correlated (beta=.20, z=3.88, p<.001). Peer deviance mediated the association between TLI and CUD (beta=.04, z=3.39, p=.001), and peer deviance mediated the association between TLI and STD (beta=.01, z=2.35, p=.019). Risky sexual behaviors were common. For example, 29.4% of females and 22.7% of males reported a history of vaginal intercourse without a condom while under the influence of alcohol or other drugs.

4. DISCUSSION

The findings of this longitudinal study suggest that CUD are associated with the development of STDs. Specifically, STDs were almost four times as common among those with a cannabis use disorder as compared to those with no history of a CUD, which was a clinically significant and statistically significant difference. These findings confirm and extend the findings of DiClemente and colleagues (2008), who had conducted a cross-sectional study involving a population of African-American girls. Previously it had been shown that other substance use disorders involving "hard" drugs such as heroin and cocaine (Hser et al., 1999; Kelly et al., 2000) are associated with STDs, but studies involving the association of CUD and STDs had been lacking. Our current findings also suggest that peer deviance mediates the development of STD and of CUD among youth making the transition to young adulthood. Thus, the study hypotheses were confirmed by the findings of the study.

There are limitations to our research design that should be noted when interpreting our findings. First, the sample was not a random sample from across the United States, so the results may not generalize to the United States as a whole. Also, the study sample was primarily male, so the results of the study may not generalize to women. In addition, the number of study subjects was limited. However, this study had the methodological advantage of being a longitudinal study, while most studies assessing STDs in persons with SUD have been cross-sectional studies. Future studies are warranted to further clarify the association between CUD and STDs and to clarify optimal prevention strategies for prevention of STDs among young persons with CUD (Lally et al., 2002; Cornelius et al, 2007).

ACKNOWLEDGMENTS

This research was supported in part by grants from the National Institute on Drug Abuse (P50 DA05605, R01 DA019142, R01 DA14635, K02 DA017822, and the NIDA Clinical Trials Network); from the National Institute on Alcohol Abuse and Alcoholism (R01 AA013370, R01 AA015173, R01 AA14357, R01 AA13397, K24 AA15320, and K02 AA000291), and a Veterans Affairs MIRECC grant to VISN 4.

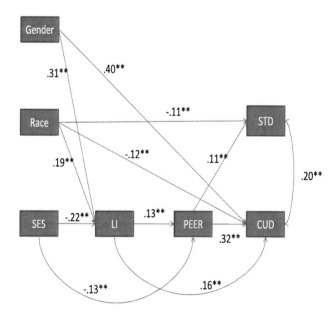

Figure 1. Mediation analyses. Chi-square=5.54, df=3, p=.14, RMSEA=.033 *:p<.05, **:p<.01.

REFERENCES

Clark, D.B., Cornelius, M.S., Kirisci, L., and Tarter, R.E. (2005). Childhood risk categories for adolescent substance involvement: a general liability typology. *Drug and Alcohol Dependence, 77*, 13-21.

Clark, D.B., Pollock, N.K., Mezzich, A., Cornelius, J., Martin, C. (2001). Diachronic assessment and the emergence of substance use disorders. *Journal of Child and Adolescent Substance Abuse, 10*:13-22.

Cornelius, J.R., Clark, D.B., Reynolds, M., Kirisci, L., and Tarter, R. (2007). Early age of first sexual intercourse and affiliation with deviant peers predict development of SUD: A prospective longitudinal study. *Addictive Behaviors, 32;*850-854.

Cornelius, J.R., Reynolds, M., Martz, B.M., Clark, D.B., Kirisci, L., and Tarter, R. (2008). Premature mortality among males with substance use disorders. *Addictive Behaviors, 33*:156-160.

DiClemente, R.J., Wingood G.M., Crosby, R.A., Salazar, L.F., Rose, E., Sales, J.M., Caliendo, A.M. (2008). Prevalence, correlates, and efficacy of selective avoidance as a sexually transmitted disease prevention strategy among African-American adolescent females. *Archives of Pediatric Adolescent Medicine, 83*:223-7.

Hosmer, D.W., and Lemeshow, S. (2000). Applied Logistic Regression, Second Edition. John Wiley and Sons, New York.

Hser, Y.I., Chou, C.P., Hoffman, V., Anglin, M.D. (1999). Cocaine use and high-risk sexual behavior among STD clinic patients. *Sexually Transmitted Diseases, 26*:82-86.

Kelly, P.J., Blair, R.M., Baillargeon, J., German, V. (2000). Risk behaviors and the prevalence of Chlamydia in a juvenile detention facility. *Clinical Pediatrics, 39*:521-527.

Kirisci, L, Tarter, R., Mezzich, A., Ridenour, T., Reynolds, M., and Vanyukov, M. (2009). Prediction of cannabis use disorder between boyhood and young adulthood: clarifying the phenotype and environtype. *The American Journal on Addictions, 18*:36-47.

Lally, M.A., Alvarez, S., Macnevin, R., Cenedella, C., Dispigno, M., Harwell, J.I., Pugatch, D., Flanigan, T.P. (2002). *Sexually Transmitted Diseases, 29*:752-755.

Nadeau, L., Truchon, M., Biron, C. (2000) High-risk sexual behaviors in a context of substance abuse: A focus group approach. *Journal of Substance Abuse Treatment,* 19:319-328.

Orvaschel, H., Puig-Antich, J., Chambers, W.J., Tabrizi, M.A., Johnson, R. (1982). Retrospective assessment of prepubertal major depression with the Kiddie-SADS-E. *Journal of the American Academy of Child Psychiatry, 21*:392-397.

Sobell, M.D. (1982). Asymptotic confidence intervals for indirect effects in structural equation models. In Sociological Methodology Leinhardt, S., ed. Washington, DDS: *American Sociological Association*, p. 290-312.

Vanyukov M.M., Kirisci, L., Moss, L., Tarter, R.E., Reynolds, M.D., Maher, B.S., Kirillova, G.P., Ridenour, T., Clark, D.B. (2009). Measurement of the risk for substance use disorders: Phenotypic and genetic analysis of an index of common liability. *Behavior Genetics, 39*:233-244.

In: Youth: Practices, Perspectives and Challenges
Editor: Elizabeth Trejos-Castillo
ISBN: 978-1-62618-067-3
© 2013 Nova Science Publishers, Inc.

Chapter 8

BEYOND SCHOOL AND FAMILY: THE BASIS AND THE STRUCTURE OF THE TERTIARY SOCIALISATION FIELD AND THE "YOUTH-AFFAIRS" AS AN AUTONOMOUS AREA

Adam Nagy[*] *and Levente Székely*[†]
Excenter Research Centre, Hungary

ABSTRACT

Many models have been made during the study of the chronology and areas of the socialisation process[1] and thus the extrafamilial and extracurricular platforms have often been in focus. A new area deserves thorough analysis with a focus on theoretical background since models of leisure environments outside the family and the school. The current study deals with the extra familiar and curricular environment, setting up the theoretical background of youth work and try to answer the following questions: Is there any homogenious socialization field beyond the school and the family?, What are its characteristics?, What does the youth work field involve? It reviews theories of socialisation environments and venues, provides a grouping of them. It must be stressed that the present study does not deal with the repertory of socialisation themes, such as gender socialisation, moral socialisation, political socialisation and others, but merely those environments where these take place. It is our objective to create a sound

---

[*] nagyadam@excenter.eu.
[†] szekelylevente@excenter.eu.
[1] In the present case socialisation is defined as the process of acquiring knowledge and skills enabling the individual to become a member of society. During this process the individual acquires knowledge of himself and his society, acquires the rules of living together as well as the possible and expected behavioural patterns (Bagdy, 1994). Education is aimed at influencing this process, while socialisation can be an unconscious process. Therefore, in our definition socialisation is a broad category: it is not restricted to a closely delineable process but rather a wide range of phenomena (from formal socialisation agencies to non-formal actors) (Vajda-Kósa, 2005), where the socialisation process is not only the result of conscious learning but can occur via hidden mechanisms (Pecheron, quoted in Murányi, 2006). Socialisation, one of the notions shared by psychology and sociology, and in this sense is not identical with social development, part of which is the formation of the individual with a distinct emotional world and individual behaviour.

theoretical framework without the empirical evidence; our model will become vital after some theoretical tests have been conducted.

We were devoted to justifying the existence of the tertiary socialisation environment (Nagy, 2011) and the role it plays in the youth field. Because the tertiary socialization field is not the main focus of other professions related activities require knowledge whichother professions do not fully cover. That is why we can outline, the mission of the youth workers: working with young people (people and communities) in the tertiary socialization field (in resocialization situation even all of the fields).

At the same time, we do not how to approach youth activities (primarily those carried out in the tertiary socialisation environment) and what distinct characteristics they have based on which they can be divided into specific areas. The following is an attempt at raising a discussion about our proposed model of youth activities.

I. THEORIES OF SOCIALISATION ENVIRONMENTS

The term agencies of socialization coined by Giddens (Giddens, 2006) refers to groups or social contexts in which socialisation processes and cultural learning take place[2].He asserts that certain stages of an individual's socialisation might be realised through several agencies, which can be structured groups or environments where the key socialisation processes take place. Giddens introduces four agencies of socialisation: the family, peer groups, schools/the workplace and mass communication devices, but also adds that in fact there are as many agencies of socialisation as groups or social situations in which an individual spends a considerable period of his life[3].

Other models differentiate only two environments of socialisation. The first one is the family, generally referred to as early socialisation or the primary or early environment of socialisation. The family as a small, informal group is the first source of patterns, the scene of the first "we-experience" where the individual's habits and behaviours[4] are formed. The second one is the school, where late, or secondary (chronologically and not in order of importance) socialisation takes place.

Socialisation in the school can be examined from the following perspectives: that of child peers, the class as a social environment, and that of the teachers. Parson also distinguishes between primary socialisation in the early years when the basic structure of personality forms and secondary socialisation when social patterns are acquired in an institutionalised system (Parsons, 1955). According to another theory derived from this one, the most important environments of secondary socialisation are the school, peer groups and the media. (Bodonyi-Busi-Hegedűs-Magyar-Vizely, 2006).

---

[2] Although the socialisation agencies and social mobility share many characteristics, in the present study these agencies are not defined as areas of mobility (about social mobility, see: Sorokin's studies).

[3] These agencies of course do not trigger mechanic responses but rather urge the individual to participate in a particular framework in his social practice (Giddens, 2006).

[4] We first see the relations between roles, symmetrical and asymmetrical relationships here, and we learn the status value of different roles, the hierarchy of statuses and the principle of mutuality in the family. The socialisation functions of the family: care and protection (learning love as the primary social emotion), providing interaction space – providing models and learning roles, acquiring the fundamentals of the I, the I system, and inner control functions (formation of systems of stimulating and inhibiting action, delaying, frustration tolerance and the ability to control oneself in receiving reward and punishment) and the foundations of the order of communication (verbal and non-verbal communication and their harmony).

Yet other theories propose a tripartite system with the family being the scene of primary socialisation, the kindergarten and school those of secondary socialisation and the workplace that of tertiary socialisation: "secondary socialisation refers to learning processes in groups of the same rank and takes place during childhood[5]... tertiary socialisation is linked to adulthood, the period after school studies are completed, or more precisely to the years of active working life" (Kiss, 2002; Szabó, www). During the study of the chronological order of socialisation environments in which he was examining whether there is a recession in the use of obscene language after childhood, Czeglédi (Czeglédi, manuscript) defines secondary socialisation as overlapping with childhood and regards tertiary socialisation as the period of employment and active work[6]. In further classifications the family is the environment of primary socialisation, obligatory (elementary) schools are that of secondary socialisation, while colleges and universities are the scenes of tertiary socialisation when the individual is preparing for a chosen career. Csaba Dupcsik (Dupcsik, www) agrees that tertiary socialisation involves training for a vocation or a profession.

Some research outlines a structure of four socialisation environments: the family is defined as the scene of primary socialisation, when basic norms and rules are acquired; the kindergarten and the school as scenes of secondary socialisation; career socialisation is defined as tertiary (secondary and teriary education, and training for work); and the workplace is the environment of quaternary socialisation. Trencsényi (Trencsényi, 2006) classifies the socialisation environments according to the organisation that carries out the task of teaching and thus differentiates natural communities and learning environments (family, relatives, neighbours), state institutions (children's surgery, nursery, kindergarten, boarding school, advisory centre for education, centre for child well-being, children's home, crisis care home, youth detention centre, youth prison, foster home, art school, cultural centre – institution with multiple purposes, cultural house, cinema, library, theatre, museum, concert hall, dance house, stadium), as well as service providers (childcare, youth entertainment facilities – arcades – disco, extracurricular courses, training courses (language school, driving school, dance school), swimming pool, sports centre-gym) and civil initiative (churches, organisations for children and adolescents, sports associations, cultural associations, art associations). The introduction of educational media (children's magazines, children's books, radio, TV, the Internet) is an advanced element in Trencsényi's four-partite division[7]. He calls into doubt the generally highlighted and exclusive role in secondary socialisation of "traditional" educational institutions that are historically not so old since they developed at the time of social modernisation (Trencsényi, 2009).

---

[5] These groups of various sizes (school classes, gangs, associations, clubs, etc.) contain individuals with shared interests and represent typical social patterns, themes as well as a relatively homogenous language and style.

[6] Musgrave (Musgrave, 1979) explores the areas of work and professions. In his view, the first stage of career socialisation is determined by learning the occupational roles linked to the system of careers and after every decision the repertory of roles decreases since the range of available opportunities is narrowing down. Musgrave discusses professional socialisation in detail, the developmental stages of which include, firstly, the (concealed) learning of the roles of preliminary professional socialisation (attainment of career knowledge), followed by entering a professional field, stepping onto a career path, career expectations and reality, and, finally, real professional socialisation begins when the individual's final role behaviour and meeting the requirements of the given career is formed. For Musgrave tertiary socialisation emerges when an individual changes his career or activity, but since this is only a coincidental overlap of terms, we will not deal with this area in detail.

[7] In this division Trencsényi only includes conscious actors (not denying the existence of "spontaneous" socialisation effect).

Another division defines seven categories: childhood family, adult family, school, peer groups, mass communication, workplace, and other socialisation environments (e.g. church and civil communities) (Vukovich, in Nagy 2006). Kozma (Kozma, 1984) also reviews socialisation environments and discusses each segment in detail; however, he does not apply a unified approach to the examination of the extrafamilial and – curricular domains. He claims that the school is the environment of formal education, while the family, the neighbours, the workplace, the army, politics, religion and the media are those of non-formal and informal (sic!) education.

Some other theories interpret socialisation environments in relation to special groups and not general life situations. Csanád Bodó studies the issue from the perspective of minorities, who learn Hungarian during secondary or tertiary socialisation. "Adult speakers also use Hungarian during the tertiary linguistic socialisation of teenagers, since young people at this stage are seen by the community as adults, individuals being initiated in the world of work, with whom the linguistic code characteristically used in typical community activities, i.e. the local Hungarian dialect, is regarded as adequate." (Bodó, www). Edina Szabó (Szabó, www) applies the terms secondary and tertiary linguistic socialisation to penal institutions.

A shared feature of the above theories is that the family (relatives) is defined as the primary environment of socialisation, where private relationship patterns and communication skills develop, identity is defined, and basic behavioural (e.g. health behavioural) habits are formed. Learning takes place through personal experience: the persons involved in this environment cannot be substituted and the fundamentals of the individual's interpretation of the world are created at this stage (these are very difficult to alter later on). The most important scene of secondary socialisation are the kindergarten and school the aim of which is for children to acquire all the information, skills and values regarded by society as important (sense of duty, reliability, accuracy, etc.). Secondary socialisation occurs at a later stage of development, when new interpretations of the world appear, showing new sections of society and introduces new hierarchies. In this environment – in contrast to the family, where mostly everything worked at a "subjective" level – individuals are primarily assessed based on their characteristics, and expectations and norms are becoming increasingly abstracted from concrete persons. Cooperation with others must be learnt, expectations of others must be met and new rules of behaviour are needed (sharing, competing).

With regard to their framework of interpretation, some of the theories (e.g. Giddens, Kozma) focus on a given stage of life and examines the related places, life situations and social time as its imprints, while others analyse and describe environments and main socialisation stages of the individual's development (eg. Parsons, Kiss, Szabó, Dupcsik, Czeglédi). However, there are differences between schools based on developmental stages and also between those analysing a given social time (differences often occur within one particular school), with regard to their terminology (using words such as environment, scene, domain, group, etc.) and the number of environments (two, three, four) they define. Even similar schools differ in what these environments are – if there are more than two – and what their main drivers and postulations are. Thus, not all of these theories include a teriary socialisation environment, and even those that do differ in defining it (most of them refer to career socialisation and preparing for work, but there are a number of exceptions) and in establishing if tertiary socialisation has additional elements. The basis, conceptual background, reason and explanation found in literature are predominantly mainly based on conjecture and declarations (what is more, the same term is often used to denote different notions) instead of deduction and inference.

With regard to socialisation beyond the family and the school, it is of key importance whether prior to adulthood the environment beyond the school and the family can be treated as a homogenous entity. It must also be established if the areas involved have any shared characteristics, and, if they do, what characteristics are distinct to all of these areas and at the same time distinguish them from primary and secondary environments[8]. Another question is if peer groups play a synthesising role and if they can be defined as an environment or only as an additional group (in order to avoid the confusion of concepts, a qualitatively new socialisation interface will from now on be referred to as an environment or a (macro)domain, and those that are only new in regard to their content – e.g. if we enter a new workplace or group – will be called a scene or a group.). An interesting proposition is if relationships, friends, peers, loves differ in their essence to relationships in the family and the school.

II. TERTIARY SOCIALISATION ENVIRONMENT

Simply defined, free time is the period of an individual's day when he does what he wants. Two general approaches exist: free time can be understood as the time left over after work is finished and everyday needs (meals, daily errands, workplace- and school-related activities) are satisfied (left-over time approach) or the time (and use of time) when an individual can engage in free time activities (activity approach). A distinction can also be made between objective and subjective free time: objectively speaking, e.g. Sunday can be seen as free time, however, if someone feels it their duty to do work around the garden, it is not free time in a subjective sense (Gábor, 2000; Gábor, www, Azzopardi-Furlong-Stadler, 2003). Fundamentally, only subjective time is real free time, i.e. when the individual feels that he is in control and free of any external obligation.

This means that free time is not defined by time and activity but by the individual. That is, free time is a personal commitment rather than an opportunity presented by circumstances. Free time is the scene related to private life, belonging to a group and consumption[9].

---

[8] The delineation of this environment is necessitated by theoretical (does extrafamilial and –curricular socialisation have shared motives, elements and a foundation that link them into a distinct category with shared characteristics) and practical reasons (establishing the basic statements of the youth professions).

[9] Free time for youth is also a trial of adulthood: it is a time of autonomy, self-management and self-realisation where multiidentity manifests itself the most visibly. Due to the cyclical nature of a year, the following types of free time activities can be examined:
 a) free time on weekdays (typically afternoons)
 b) free time at week-ends
 c) free time during holidays (especially in summer).

Free time during weekdays, week-ends and holidays can be described based on the results of free time and youth research (Demetrovics-Paksi-Dúll, 2010; Szapu, 2002; Szabó-Bauer, 2009, 2006, 2001; Gábor, 2000; Gábor, www; Azzopardi-Furlong-Stadler, 2003; Nagy, 1991 etc.):
 a) free time during weekdays: watching TV, listening to music, "hanging about", going out to places of entertainment, shopping (consumption), going to shopping centres, entertainment in general, going to the cinema, studying and home work, computer and internet games, time spent together with friends or peers in a community or organisation (sport, cultural or art, student body, local government body, church, civil/youth organisation), reading, doing sport or dancing, raising children, non-computer games, cultural programmes: theatre, concert, exhibition, restaurant, café, pub, other activities.
 b) free time at weekends: same as during the weekdays, plus going to a disco, house party, trips, other activities.

Since the strength of socialisation is determined by the time and intensity of participation (Vukovich, in Nagy 2006), we can only apply the term environment when the individual spends sufficient time (and intensely enough) – without these a scene can certainly not be called a socialisation environment (just socialization elements, of which we can find dozens or hundreds).

There are at least three places where a young person spends sufficient time, which can be divided into at least three impact groups in the present context: the family, the school (work) and the free time (see also research on social time: Demetrovics-Paksi-Dúll, 2010; Szapu, 2002; Szabó-Bauer, 2009, 2006, 2001; Gábor, 2000; Gábor, www; Azzopardi-Furlong-Stalder, 2003; Nagy, 1991, etc). Thus, today a third one can be added to the primary and secondary socialisation environments[10]: "a new socialisation group agency, the peer group, can be added to the family, first complementing it, and later providing a counter-pattern" (Csepeli, 2006). While the impact of traditional institutions of socialisation (family, school) are weakening (Mátóné, in Bábosik, 2009), the peer group[11] as a platform of interaction increases in importance (Váriné, in Somlai, 1975). The activities in peer groups share many characteristics with those in the family and the school, but also differ from these in many respects. "The peer group is the single social scene where a young person can reckon on relationships based on equality and where, he does not experience one-sided dependence from another individual, such as a parent or teacher" (Csepeli, 2006, 406). While in the family the prescribed norms are obedience and authoritarian love, the peer group operates on the basis of cooperation and mutual agreement (Piaget 1970, 40). The essence in the peer group phenomenon is not the seemingly deviant content but the process in which the individual takes voluntary action which is also determined by the community, and in conforming to the group steps outside the scope of individual interests. Informal groups are quintessential to the individual (Csepeli, 2006). The table below (see: Table 1) is an attempt to sum up those similarities and differences between the three environments that outline a unified tertiary socialisation environment. It can be seen that some of the characteristics of the proposed tertiary environment are shared by the other two, while there are some distinct characteristics that set it apart from them. From now on we will call this area tertiary socialisation (free time) environment, within which we will differentiate between generally applicable scenes of socialisation: neighbours, etc, and special scenes applicable only to certain individuals or groups: church, army. However, these scenes will not be analysed in depth in the current paper. The literature on socialisation environments (see previously) does not say on what basis an environment can be defined as a socialisation environment and therefore which environments do not qualify as such; nevertheless it suggests that the intensity of the socialisation environment and the autonomy that results from it depend on the following three factors:

---

c) free time during holidays: same as free time at weekends, plus going on holiday with friends, with family, with partner, alone, other activities.

In these periods of time the activities can be divided into two main groups based on the intensity of the activity: there is a strong distinction between functional, physically, intellectually and emotionally demanding free time activities (shopping, meals) and non-functional, passive reception (hanging about). (About the shopping centre as social space, and about functional and non-functional free time activities, see: Demetrovics-Paksi-Dúll, 2010).

[10] Peer groups, without a predetermined hierarchy of people with equal rank, the world of shopping centres, the Internet, the media and small community interaction, etc. Large institutional systems of education (work) and family affairs are unable to substitute the predominantly voluntary and self-organised third socialisation environment, and it is not their task either.

[11] About peer groups and more about globalisation, see: Hervainé in Bábosik 2009.

Table 1. Similarities and differences in the socialisation environments

Characteristics	Family	School	Extrafamilial- and curricular (mainly free-time) activities
Main characteristics, organisational principles	• Main characteristic: a "given" • Organisational principle: unconditional	• Main characteristic: obligatory • Organisational principle: conditional	• Main characteristic: voluntary (particular elements can be used voluntarily, joining can be voluntary) • Organisational principle: optional (independent, free use of time)
Changeability	Cannot be changed in regard to the people or the framework	Changes over time	Relationships can be freely ended and started[14]
Mutuality	None	None	yes[15]
Presence of authority	There is predetermined authority in the form of a natural hierarchy (parents); accepting discipline and rules is not voluntary.	There is predetermined authority in the form of an artificial hierarchy (teachers); accepting discipline and rules is not voluntary.[16]	There is no predetermined authority, nor predetermined hierarchy[17]; accepting discipline and rules is voluntary[18].
Appearance of environment	From birth (0--)	From school (kindergarten) years (3-6---)	The need for its elements arises approx. At the same time (8-12---)
Level of institutionalisation	More institutionalised	Institutionalised	Less institutionalised[19]
Relations	Given	Obligatory	Optional
Time spent (ages 14-16)	Approx. 2-6h	Approx. 5-7h	Approx. 3-9h

---

[14] Csepeli, 2006.
[15] "If we examine the world of youth ... interaction, we must see that the principle of mutuality cannot be practised in any other context." (Csepeli, 2006, 406)
[16] There are attempts (e.g.: Nahalka, 2003) to introduce extracurricular developmental activities into the classroom, however, these do not go beyond the traditional approach to roles, with the teacher playing the key role, and do not provide the opportunity for real community roles to be formed. The tertiary socialisation environment is different from school exactly because the roles develop in relation to the forming community.
[17] For more about authority in the family and the school, see: Vajda-Kósa, 2005, about peer groups Csepeli, 2006, Piaget, 1970.
[18] Csepeli, 2006.
[19] Cf. disco dance floor vs. shooting association. The peer group falls outside the institutionalised social network (in our case institutionalised constitutes an objective existence independent of the will of the group members). Adopting an extreme approach we could say that formal groups play an essential role by carrying out activities directly beneficial to society (e.g. work), while informal groups play a similarly essential role by engaging in activities directly beneficial to the individuals (e.g. games, leisure time, entertainment) (Csepeli, 2006), although the borders between these two groups are becoming less and less defined. The institutions of a consolidated society try to "tame" initiatives organised outside the official institutions with varying degrees of success (Trencsényi, 2006).

Table 2. The impact of socialisation environments on the individual, in relation to age

Socialisation environments	0	1	2	3	4	5	6	7	8	9	10	11	12	13	14	15	16	17	18	19	20	21	22	23	24	25	26	27	28	29	30
Primary (family-relatives)																															
Secondary (kindergarten-school)																															
Extra-curricular and familiar activities																															

- The time spent in the socialisation environment: most obviously, the individual spends a considerable amount of time in the family and the school, while it can also be ascertained that the time he spends outside these two socialisation environments will reach and then supercede (even many times over) this level as he progresses in age (see: Table 1).
- The intensity of the time spent in the socialisation environment: in our case this intensity refers to the involvement of the individual in the given socialisation environment, the depth of his participation and the strength of his ties to this environment. In the family and the school this intensity is by definition very high, with manyfold and deep ties. Authors who have written on the environment outside the family and the school maintain that the aforementioned relationship of the individual is of a similar intensity in the third socialisation environment.
- A socialisation environment must have its own system of rules and its own principles of participation: as can be seen from the table (Table 1), the set of rules governing the extrafamilial- and –curricular environment fundamentally differs from the rules and principles of the socialisation environments of the family and the school.

Based on the above it can be stated that there *is* a distinctly delineable socialisation environment outside the family and the school. Furthermore, with regard to the chronological emergence of this socialisation environment in the life of the individual, we propose that it be called the tertiary socialisation environment.

This tertiary socialisation environment does not form the basis of any profession, since it is not regarded by any one of them as their main focus, especially not with the youth age groups at its centre. The activities related to this environment require knowledge that is not covered by other professions; thus, the mission of the youth profession can gradually be outlined: to render unsubstitutable support to the members of the youth age groups in becoming citizens responsible for their own actions and their communities primarily in the tertiary socialisation area but in (re)socialisation emergency situations in all the socialisation fields.

Although extracurricular and extrafamilial environment not only includes free time but other obligatory activities –e.g. official affairs, medical check-ups – the amount of time spent on these is not significant, and, broadly speaking, they can be linked to the tertiary as well as to other environments (medical check-ups at the workplace, medical test for employment, or annual screenings, applying for a birth certificate, certificate of good character required for university admission, or various affairs at public utility works, etc.). Vajda (Vajda, 2006) claims that research into socialisation mainly focus on families, schools and peers (and less on broader spheres of interaction, primarily on mass communication), although Vajda includes the Internet in mass communication it can be disputed in many respects (activity-passivity, individual-mass etc.). In the present context it is not so essential to establish whether mass communication can be regarded as an autonomous environment (cf.: cultural identity is now not formed in classrooms but in TV studios (György, in Buckingham, 2002). The situation is somewhat similar to the differences between theories pertaining to the sectoral division of society, where the three-sectoral (state, market, non-profit) approach clashes with the four-sectoral theory (state, market, non-profit, household), although the existence of the non-profit sector is not debated by either. Here we have a similar case: the existence or non-existence of a quaternary environment does not affect the existence (or non-existence) of the tertiary environment. What is more, we can toy around with the idea that the "official world" (offices, healthcare, etc.) can be proposed as a quinary socialisation environment in regard to its impact, although not in regard to temporality. The impact of this environment cannot be underestimated (see the public conditions in Hungary), and indeed: this element appears to come after the other four, as the fifth one.

III. YOUTH WORK, THE YOUTH PROFESSION[20]

In the following part of the study a model will be presented to systematise youth support activities. The model is based on the direct (concrete) orindirect (abstract) nature of activities involvingindividuals/communities. In the focus of the model is the individual (or the community he belongs to) carrying out the youth activity (in this study youth activity comprises activities outside the educational system, conducted on a voluntary basis in one's free time to help youth groups). The innermost layer of the structure is formed by activities carried out directly by individuals (communities). The middle layer contains activities that are only indirectly connected with the individuals (communities) and "merely" provide an organisational structure creating synthesising theories for them. The outermost layer represents a horizontal youth approach and contains borderline areas, professions linked with youth work.

   a) Youth work is defined as the sum of activities realised through interaction between youth groups and actors directly in contact with them. It is social, community and personal development and empowering work aimed at solving the problems specific to the examined age groups and facilitating their social inclusion partly based on their active participation and partly on the special tools of the youth profession. The key words of youth work are: exploration of self-image, self-knowledge, self-activity, community dialogue, group socialisation, dealing with challenges, free time activities, informal learning. Youth work is predominantly linked with factors directed at development (personality, community, group, regional, settlement development...) inherent in which are the positive signs, promise and potential of support, modernisation and renewal, which are also indicated by key words such as empowering, encouraging, and inclusion. Youth work entails notions like solidarity, the active ability and skill to accept differences (and within that empathy). The range of its services differs from those offered by businesses in that they are (theoretically) generally available, low-threshold services without financial or other requirements.
   b) Youth profession: the middle section of youth activities which, through their content and methodology, can facilitate indirect youth work. It is a sum of activities at higher levels of abstraction aimed at providing the "background" for youth work.
   c) outh field: any activity associated with youth groups, primarily within the activities of other sectors (education, social work, culture, economy, etc.), and aimed at the

---

[20] The youth paradigm is tossed about like Charon's boat: although it can be primarily regarded as an autonomous pedagogical discipline, it can form part of sociology, can be seen as a politological entity, youth work, partly social work and partly a pedagogical activity. It being an autonomous entity is supported by the very fact that it does not fully form part of any one science or profession.

development of areas ranging from the development of family planning competences, support schemes, labour market and entrepreneurial competences, through child benefit schemes and learning, to youth media and culture (representing a horizontal approach).

It has been obvious that the tertiary socialisation environment is not a highlighted aspect of any profession, since it is not regarded by any of them as being specific to its profile, especially not in regard to youth groups. Activities related to youth require knowledge that is not available in any other profession; thus, the task of the youth profession can be outlined: to render support – that cannot be substituted by any other – in regard to the process of young people becoming citizens responsible for themselves and their communities, primarily achieved through the development of the tertiary socialisation environment and, in a (re)socialisation emergency[21], of all socialisation environments.

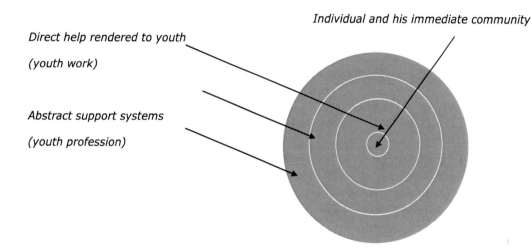

Figure 1. Structure of youth activities.

Youth work is a collective term aimed in part and whole at helping young people in the process of growing up. Two important aspects must be focussed on in regard to youth work targeting these age groups: the participants and the areas. Direct and indirect youth work will be examined from both these aspects, since the overall standard of youth work depends on how successfully the various activities and groups of activities strengthen one another and thus facilitate the process of growing up. Numerous synonyms are known in everyday communication for the terms and expressions (e.g. youth profession, youth work) used in the youth field.

The phrase 'youth work' offers a wide range of interpretations, regardless of the fact whether the given uses are linked to one another; however, to some extent each one concerns young people growing up. Therefore, the term must be properly defined first. Many people

---

[21] More about the decomposition of the primary socialisation environment, see e.g.: Alpár, 2009, the problems within the secondary environment, and primarily about behavioural issues and learning difficulties, see: Kósáné, 1989, Kósáné – Münnich, 1985 (although only in relation to its solution within the school).

associate youth work with some concrete job done by a young person, as if at a workplace (youth work agencies target this area). Moreover, in an everyday sense, youth work is done by the official working for a local government if he deals with tasks related to youth age groups. In the commonly used meaning of the term doctors, teachers, training officers, youth workers, swimming coaches also do youth work. There are a lot of people in the field engaged in a lot of activities, working in many areas, with entirely different qualifications and ideas, as well as fundamentally different methods and objectives. Indeed, young people who come into contact with them can also completely differ from each other, in regard to age, life situation, level of maturity, etc. People in the youth field only have two things in common: the role they play in the lives of young generations is in some way connected to growing up, and their work is characterised by activity and concrete actions. Strange as it may sound, only these can link a grandmother reading a bedtime story to his grandchild and a children's dentist...

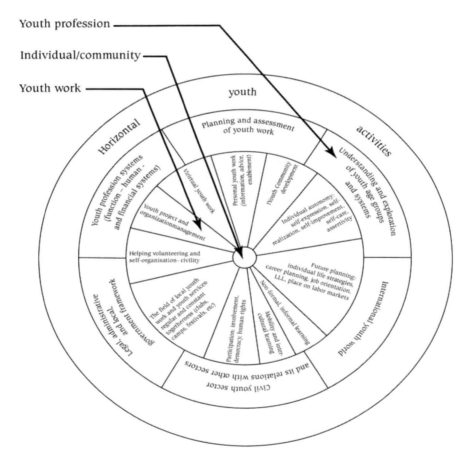

The definition previously used in the section about the youth profession can be made more accurate by establishing which three groups youth activity is related to:
- directly to the youth age groups – youth work;
- to the community of youth professionals and the youth sector of the state (government, local government, etc.) – youth profession; and

- to the borderline areas of youth activities that do not form part of the youth profession but are affiliated with it; horizontal approach to youth – youth field (i.e. in our model youth culture, health, inhabitance, allowances, education, family, employment, etc. all belong to the horizontal youth area).

Regarding the areas of youth work, focus will be placed on those areas in which activities are directly aimed at the young generation and their members. As regards the youth profession, it contains those segments in which work carried out for young people is more abstracted than the previously mentioned direct work, i.e. it is at a higher level of abstraction.

IV. AREAS OF YOUTH WORK

Informal Learning and Youth Activities

In the triangle of formal, non-formal and informal learning methods, the latter one appears the most characteristically in the youth area. Informal learning is a kind of learning in which the learning process as such is lost in other types of activities and contents, that is it is not planned and assessed. Among others, edutainment (learning through entertainment) belongs to this category, but knowledge acquired through experience is also a form of informal learning. There is a close connection between informal learning and indirect (bottom-up) learning, in which tasks are the sources of impact, conditions are like relations and interrelations between pupils, and interactions are the primary means and mediators of behaviour patterns (e.g. mutual check, mutual help, etc.). Besides informal methods, the youth field applies non-formal and, in our case, formal pedagogical methods. (Accordingly, e.g. organising leisure programmes can only be regarded as youth work if it fits into a pedagogical process.) This segment is a special transition between the group-oriented approach of community development and the individual approach of youth assistance, since the activities are conducted in groups but are aimed at the development of the individual.

Local Youth Work-Institutionalised Youth Services

Youth services are generally, although not exclusively, (rendered to the) public services aimed at catering to the needs and other manifestations of different age groups of the generations growing up and expected to fulfil specific professional requirements (e.g. legal, labour market, psychological, drug-related, etc.). In addition, they must be relevant to the youth, i.e. the services not only have to meet the professional criteria of a given area but also include developmental tasks, or elements of socialisation (preparing young people for adulthood).

Thus, youth services must effectively satisfy both demands. This area involves everything that facilitates the understanding of social processes through services (and not directly) and encourages the active participation of youth age groups in these, empowering them to become active shapers of their life. Youth clubs, playgroups, adolescent centres, youth offices, youth information centres, festivals, camps, etc. are all regarded as youth services.

Personal Youth Work

Acquiring basic self-knowledge and peer knowledge and its development are quintessential to any assistance activity. The methodology of youth advisory activity has person to person relationships at its focal point – providing information, advice and assistance – determining assistance models, conflicts, conflict management, etc. Youth work is mainly built on communication, factors that facilitate or hinder it, and personality development methods. Although in general help is provided for and comes to fruition in a community, the emphasis in this area is still on person-to-person interaction[22].

Youth Community Development

Living in society we all partake in various organisations, groups, associations and – if lucky – communities that represent quality. It is generally accepted that youth work can be done efficiently and effectively mainly in communities. One of the reasons why youth work is built on communities is that, besides its multifariousness, one of its main objectives is to ensure and develop the passing on of social and cultural values.

The area deals with the youth elements of this, which includes peer assistance and other methodologies. In dealing with youth groups, their establishment and development, special

---

[22] It is not age (or age difference) that plays the main role in the counselling interview but that the helper should not have any selfish motives in his relationship with the one helped during the period of the helping relationship. (Here anything that did not form part of the personality of the helped person at the outset, or anything that was initially and remained the monopoly of the helper can be regarded as selfish, even the most positive manipulation by a priest, doctor, psychologist, teacher, etc. in the counselling interview is forbidden. This requirement constitutes a problem because even today the experts working in the area of the so-called helping professions unquestionably regard themselves as the knowers in the counselling interview, thus establishing an asymmetrical relationship of roles and excluding the chance for a symmetrical interpersonal relationship. Helpers only have the right to bring to the surface the inner "powers" of the person they are helping and let these powers move into action. Helpers must also be fully aware of the limitations of their own competence.) Moreover, it is important that helpers know exactly up to which point an interview is successful and effective but does not overstep the limit by interfering in the others' life (keeping a symmetrical relationship, and staying within the familiar stranger status). Situations requiring medical treatment and help rendered to people in a psychologically critical condition do not fall within the parameters of helping relationships, only those who need temporary help in a given situation and under given circumstances, e.g.: if those helped need information and, facts or applicable procedures they do not know about; they need help to be able to face their real situation, knowledge, competences, and opportunities; they need to be "released" from the various consequences of pangs of conscience or need help to let the accumulated excess emotions and anger be "purged" from their system; need help to recognise their values and powers, achieve a positive self-evaluation, confirmation and support; or they need help with (psychological) cramps resulting from misconceptions, false beliefs, and misunderstandings. The helping relationship is always based on a request, is always individual and unique. (In an ideal case, the request is formulated, but often the potential helper has to decide if the communication conducted with him contained the element of a request.) Taking on the role of a helper is also always a matter of the free, personal decision of the potential helper. The helping relationship occurs within the framework of a kind of contract concluded for the duration and aimed at the concrete subject of the relationship even if this contract is unspoken.

emphasis is placed on the inner mechanisms of youth communities and their development, as well as community development procedures implementable among the youth[23].

Youth Project and Organisation Management

This area involves project activity specifically for youth communities. The segment is aimed at handling the youth aspects of stakeholder management, project cycle management and project area management (project focus, integration, time, cost, human resource, quality, communication and risk management).

In another approach, it is the management of youth projects to the benefit of youth age groups, the initiation, planning, organisation, implementation and direction of programmes organised for youth (various events, festivals, camps, training courses, publications, etc.) as well as checking their realisation and closing them.

Mobility and Intercultural Learning

The balance of a given society largely depends on the relationship between the majority and minority cultures and the personal aptitude of the representatives of given groups. Key elements of mobility and intercultural learning are the assumable and real presence of diversity and pluralism, their acceptance by the wider and smaller communities involved, as well as the existence and necessity of learning openness and acceptance.

Intercultural learning means more than cultural, national, ethnic and religious sensitisation but also the acceptance of "everyday othernesses" such as disabilities, sexual differences and identities, ideological differences, as well as age and generational or even geographical differences that define the given stage of life of the individual.

---

[23] The more communities the members of the youth age groups actively participate in, the more they strengthen the local and ultimately the entire society, especially if they do not forget the patterns learnt as young people when they enter adulthood. Key words of the area: community, community development, guided conversation, voluntariness, animation. This activity providing help for the youth is development aimed at the social environment and the (human) community which young people need to learnt to accommodate to and in which they have to be able to find their way, role, self-expression, self-validation, self-representation and the representation of others, as well as assuming responsibility and bearing consequences, i.e. they have to learn decision-making. Self-expression is not the only focus in community development, but the exploitation of the potential and resources inherent in communities enabling them to achieve things they individually could not. Thus, the other focal point in community development is locality, i.e. action and development at local, municipal or regional levels. Community development primarily constitutes the development of the skills of initiative and action, in which citizens play a key role, along with communities and their networks, as well as – depending on the local tasks – community developers, whose encouraging, stimulating, informing, and networking work is often invaluable. Community development has the potential of exploring, complementing and strengthening the resources of a community. Youth community development is also realised at least in two spheres: in an informal world (street workers) and in formalised youth organisations, and in neither of these two areas do the participants have to possess simple attributes linked to a teacher role. Moreover, community development can be studied in a further dimension: there are activities carried out by young people, and those by experts that started working in the field in their youth.

Voluntariness

Voluntariness is the self-activity of citizens based on the solidarity between the members of society: it is action freely rendered to persons (not relatives), their communities or others, without expecting compensation. Cooperation with youth groups and organisations forms part of youth work. In certain cases it facilitates youth public life from the individual initiative all the way to the establishment of an organised entity. It is, therefore, important to mention altruism, youth cooperation, assistance to youth self-organisation and the nature of voluntariness.

Virtual Youth Work

The opportunities provided by the information society fundamentally transform the notions of social environment, youth community space, youth social networking, etc. Virtual youth work addresses the following issue: in what regard can youth age groups be regarded as occupying a special position in virtual space (primarily but not exclusively on the Internet) (Tapscott, 2008; Tapscott-Williams, 2006). The area also deals with the changes of youth culture and youth communities (and their characteristics) organised in virtual space.

Participation: Involvement, Democracy, Human Rights

This means all the activities carried out by youth commnunities and organisations to involve young people in the lives of the local communities; for example, to promote youth participation in the lives of settlements/regions etc. (organisation and operation of local youth governments, youth representation), activities carried out by formal youth organisations and non-formal youth communities, assistance rendered to youth by other organisations and professionals, as well as other activities aimed at the better interiorisation of democracy and its institutions, and activities promoting the education, practice and reception of human rights etc.

Future Planning (Life Strategies, Career Planning, LLL)

This involves everything that concerns "not the present but the future": life strategies, personal and vocational planning, learning competences necessary for employment, career planning, etc.

Individual Autonomy: Self-expression, Self-realization, Self-improvement, Self-care, Assertivity

This area is mainly concerned with the individual and identity: how responses should be expressed, how to respond to impulses, how to organise, express and develop one's self, body, mind and spirit. Self-expression and assisting others in their development can be the most effectively done while people are still young.

V. AREAS OF THE YOUTH PROFESSION

Legal Framework of Youth Activities

This area primarily covers youth legislation (specifically applicable to the youth field and adopting a youth approach across its entire volume) and justice, its examination and implementation. It defines child rights (limitation of autonomy, assertion of legal capacity), youth rights (operation of special support systems), youth law (one of the principal arguments for the autonomy of the youth field is the need for a separate legal framework). The legal framework of youth activities examines the position of youth in law: regulations pertaining to youth must pervade the entire legal system. It deals with the theoretical (constitutional) starting points of the legal approach taken to children, i.e. the fundamental characteristics of legal relations, the consideration of age-specific characteristics of individuals otherwise having the same legal capacity, the restriction of exercising rights and enhanced legal protection as well as with the rights and obligations of those working with children (youth workers). The legal framework for youth activities raises awareness regarding the state's obligations in connection to children's rights which are stipulated by the constitution and international agreements and relevant laws. The area also addresses issues that have not been defined and settled legally (e.g. what happens, what is the legal assessment in the case of adolescents taking on public roles; is the youth worker regarded as a person of public authority, i.e. if someone confides in him that he smoked a joint, what is his legal duty, is he obliged to report the case?). The problem of the youth act also forms part of this area, and although there is no legal obligation to draw up such an act, its existence would indicate the state's commitment and systematic approach to the situation of the youth. Borderline areas that are not specifically part of the youth field but play a significant role regarding the legal regulation of the area (organisations, legal regulation of civil framework, procedures, etc.) also fall within the legal framework of youth activities.

Study and Research of Youth Age Groups

This area essentially examines the social layers of youth, stratification, the local cross-sections of youth, as well as small and big groups organised along specific values, model patterns, free-time and work. Important disciplines that form part of the study and research of youth age groups include cultural anthropology, ethnography and political sciences. This area reviews the various youth research activities from the preparatory work required by projects, the collection and processing of data, through their interpretation and to their systematic study-level presentation and publication. This segment also reviews the methodology of youth research, which, in addition to its sociological foundation, applied, already at the very beginning, various psychological approaches and some of their tools, the approach and study methods of social psychology, combining the research methods used in sociology, management theory and pedagogy. The development of applied methods determined by the objectives of concrete projects also belong here, as do comparative analyses.

Planning and Assessment of Youth Work

This area covers the forming of youth strategy and the related action plan, as well as their monitoring. Youth strategy is the long-term (10-20-year-long) arrangement of the actions of a given community, society or large social group in regard to youth, according to specific objective(s), as well as the designation of resources for its implementation. The content of the area pertains to youth age groups, although truly "usable" strategies and action plans cannot disregard the adult population. Action plans elaborate the actions to be implemented in the short term (2-4 years), as inferred from the strategy, and designate the sources and people in charge. Monitoring examines the rationale behind the implemented measures and compares them with the plans. However, strategies and action plans are not only "youth" because they focus on youth but also because youth generations, communities and organisations actively participate in their formulation and implementation.

Youth Systems

This area deals with the definition and operation of the public tasks of the youth, determines their indicators and evaluates them. The area also deals with the financial systems (from the tender system to the governmental development activity) and human systems (training system, youth networks, etc.).

International Youth Activity

This area analyses the supranational cooperation in regard to youth activities. Youth organisations, government structures, and research processes have grown beyond their initial frameworks and have introduced services, opportunities and challenges that can only be realised through broad-based cooperation extending beyond national borders. The area deals with the objectives, content, methods and forms (e.g. networks, cross-border cooperation) of international youth activity, the framework institutions, organisations, their operation, interdependence, structure, important documents, support programmes, primarily – but not exclusively – in a European dimension.

Civil Youth Sector and its Relations with other Sectors

The most important element of the non-profit sector is that in regard to its fundamental attributes it differs from the state and economic organisations (in addition to the traditional division of state and economic, the third one is the so-called non-profit sector). The non-profit sector is distinct from the state (it has no functions of public authority) and the economy (it is not driven by making a profit), and it most often comprises civil organisations, i.e.

organisations established by volunteers and operated on a self-active basis. The area focuses on the rules and phenomena of the youth segment of the civil sector, and the youth work conducted in the segment.

This area involves the strategies and techniques regarding the representation of the members of a given community, organisation, government or local government organisation, etc. and the assertion of the interests of youth age groups (or a part of them), as well as the communication of these strategies and techniques and its special characteristics in the youth segment also. Youth representation involves the analysis, discussion and communication of situations, problems, action plans and consequences carried out by the members and representatives of youth age groups in order to impact decisions affecting the youth and influence decision-makers – both individuals and institutions – to the benefit of the youth. The members and representatives of youth age groups can be local non-formal communities and their leaders, local or higher level – regional, county, nationwide, international – formal organisations and their leaders, as well as forums of cooperation affiliated with certain institutions (e.g. student government of public educational institutions, youth divisions of company trade unions). The area of youth representation also includes institutions and actors with a leading role in the youth field and the authority to impact it, and entails cooperation with decision-making bodies, youth dialogues, preparatory work carried out before decision-making, the role of control, as well as lobbying for youth interests in the profit or non-profit sector alike.

VI. HORIZONTAL YOUTH ACTIVITY

We did not divide the so-called horizontal youth activities into parts, since different social systems, countries, and approaches require different divisions they deem sensible and compliant with their own social philosophy (since horizontal youth activities concern the relationship between the youth sector and other sectors). The following division has started to take shape in Hungary:

- youth and formal education,
- youth and family,
- youth and culture, consumption and media,
- youth and the world of health,
- youth and the world of work,
- youth and politics,
- youth and deviance crime,
- youth and poverty, segregation, marginalisation,
- youth and those living with disabilities,
- youth and liveable environments,
- youth and europeanness,
- youth and national identity.

Summary

Many sociologists and pedagogues deal with those scenes, periods of life and phases in which socialisation occurs. However, up until now, no comprehensive study approached the extrafamilial and -curricular scenes of socialisation based on their shared characteristics. The present study was aimed at describing the tertiary socialisation environment in regard to the social time of young people and the groups of impacts affecting them.

The tertiary socialization field is not the main focus of other professions, and related activities require knowledge whichother professionsdo not fully cover . That is why we can outline the mission of the youth workers: to work with young people (people and communities) in the tertiary socialization field (in resocialization situations even all of the fields).

We made an attempt to classify youth activities in the tertiary socialisation environment from the perspective of the individual (community), applying this approach to youth work, the youth profession and horizontal youth activities. We divided youth work into eleven and the youth profession into six areas, while we did not divide horizontal youth activities. We propose to start a discussion that will establish the foundations for the youth areas.

References

Alpár Zsuzsa – Lux Elvira - Pál Mária - Popper Péter: *Legfeljebb elválunk- az élet dolgai*, 2009, Saxum, Budapest.

Bagdy Emőke: *A csoport specifikus hatótényezői: a csoportdinamikai történések. In: Konfliktuspedagógiai szöveggyűjtemény,* Veszprérni Egyetemi Kiadó, 1994, Veszprém.

Bodó Csanád: *Nyelvi szocializáció és nyelvi tervezés a moldvai magyar–román kétnyelvű beszélőközösségekben. adatbank.transindex.ro/html/cim_pdf436.pdf,* downloaded: 2010.03.01.

Bodonyi Edit-Busi Etelka-Hegedűs Judit-Magyar Erzsébet-Vizely Ágnes: *A gyakorlati pedagógia néhány alapkérdése,* Család, Gyerek, Társadalom, Bölcsész Konzorcium, 2006, Budapest.

Buckingham David: *A gyerekkor halála után - Felnőni az elektronikus média világában.* 2002, Helikon, Budapest.

Czeglédi Sándor: *Az ifjúsági nyelv szóhasználati jellegzetességei egy veszprémi felmérés tükrében,* Veszprémi Egyetem Angol Tanszék, kézirat.

Csepeli György: *Szociálpszichológia,* 2006, Osiris Kiadó, Budapest.

Demetrovics Zsolt - Paksi Borbála - Dúll Andrea (ed.): *Pláza, ifjúság, életmód – egészséglélektani vizsgálatok a fiatalok körében,* 2010, L'Harmattan Kiadó, Budapest.

Dupcsik Csaba: *Magyar Virtuális Enciklopédia* Szocializáció cikkszó, *www.enc.hu/ 1enciklopedia/fogalmi/szoc/szocializacio.htm,* downloaded: 2010.03.01.

Furlong, A., Stalder, B., and Azzopardi A.: *Vulnerable Youth: perspectives on vulnerability in education, employment and leisure,* Council of Europe, Strasbourg, 2000.

Gábor Kálmán (ed.): *Társadalmi átalakulás és ifjúság.* Belvedere Kiadó, 2000, Szeged.

Gábor Kálmán: *Az ifjúsági kultúra és a fiatalok társadalmi orientációs mintái* in. Civilizációs korszakváltás és ifjúság, 1992, Miniszterelnöki Hivatal Ifjúsági Koordinációs Titkárság, Budapest.

Gábor Kálmán: *Társadalmi egyenlőtlenségek,* www.*ifjusagsegito.hu/belvedere/ tarsadalmi_egyenlotlensegek.pdf,* downloaded: 2010.03.01.

Giddens Anthony: *Sociology,* Polity, 2006.

Hervainé Szabó Gyöngyvér: *A globalizáció és az ifjúsági bandák kapcsolata,* in Bábosik István - Torgyik Judit(ed.): az iskola szocializációs funkciói, 2009, Eötvös Kiadó, Budapest.

Kiss Jenő: Társadalom és nyelvhasználat. *Szociolingvisztikai alapfogalmak,* Nemzeti Tankönyvkiadó, 2002 Budapest.

Kósáné Ormai Vera: *Szocializációs zavarok és az iskola,* in Gáti Ferenc-Horányi Annabella-Kósáné Ormai Vera (ed.): Szemelvények a hazai gyermek- és ifjúságvédelem irodalmából, 1989, Tankönyvkiadó, Budapest.

Kozma Tamás: *Bevezetés a nevelésszociológiába,* A nevelésszociológia alapjai Tankönyvkiadó, 1999, Budapest.

Mátóné Szabó Csilla: *Az ifjúsági szubkultúrák szocializációs hatásainak iskolai kezelése,* in Bábosik István - Torgyik Judit (ed.): Az iskola szocializációs funkciói, 2009, Eötvös Kiadó, Budapest.

Murányi István: *Identitás és előítélet,* 2006, Új mandátum Kiadó, Budapest.

Musgrave P. W. *The Sociology of Education,* 1979, 3rd edition, Routledge.

Nagy Ádám: *Beyond school and family – the theoretical foundations of the tertiary socialisation environment and the youth profession as an autonomous field,* manuscript.

Nagy Attila: *Keresik életük értelmét?* Olvasás-könyvtár-szocializáció, 1991, OSzK KMK, Budapest .

Nahalka István: *Túl a falakon: az iskolán kívüli nevelés módszerei,* Elte Btk, Neveléstudományi Intézet 2003, Gondolat Kiadói Kör, Budapest .

Parsons T. - Bales R.F: *Family, socialization and interaction process,* 1995, Free Press, Glencoe.

Piaget Jean: *Sociological Studies.* London, Routledge, 1995.

Somlai Péter (ed.) : Álláspontok a *szocializációról,* Szociológiai füzetek, 1975, Oktatási Minisztérium Budapest.

Szabó Edina: *„Nagyobb lesz az ember, ha kicsit dumásabb" A börtönszleng használók véleménye nyelvváltozatukról,* Magyar Nyelvjárások, Debreceni Egyetem Magyar Nyelvtudományi Tanszék évkönyve, Debrecen, 2003 http://mnytud.arts.klte.hu/ szleng/tanulmanyok/73szaboe.doc, downloaded: 2010.03.01.

Szabó Andrea - Bauer Béla - Laki László: *Ifjúság 2000* Tanulmányok, 2002, Nemzeti Ifjúságkutató Intézet, Budapest.

Szabó Andrea-Bauer Béla: *Ifjúság 2004 Gyorsjelentés,* 2005, Mobilitás Ifjúságkutatási Iroda, Budapest.

Szabó Andrea-Bauer Béla: *Ifjúság 2008 gyorsjelentés,* 2009 Szociálpolitikai es Munkaügyi Intézet Budapest.

Szapu Magda: *A zűrkorszak gyermekei: mai ifjúsági csoportkultúrák,* 2002, Századvég, Budapest.

Székely Levente: *Virtuális ifjúsági munka,* In Földi-Nagy (ed.): Ifjúságügy – ifjúsági szakma, ifjúsági munka, Módszertani kézikönyv, 2010, Mobilitás-ISzT-ÚMK, Budapest .

Székely Levente–Rab Árpád–Nagy Ádám: *Virtuális ifjúsági munka*, In Nagy (ed.): Ifjúságügy - Ifjúsági szakma, ifjúsági munka, 2008, Palócvilág – Új Mandátum, Budapest.

Tapscott Don: *Growing up digital*, McGraw-Hill, New York,2008.

Tapscott Don –Williams Anthony D.: *Wikinomics*, Tantor Media, 2006.

Trencsényi László: *Az iskola funkcióiról a nevelési intézmények történeti rendszertanában*. In: Kiss Éva (szerk.): Pedagógián innen és túl. Pécs–Veszprém 2006.

Trencsényi László: *Nagy Ádám Ifjúságügye*, in. Új Pedagógiai Szemle 2009/2.

Vajda Zsuzsaanna - Kósa Éva: *Neveléslélektan*, 2005, Osiris, Budapest.

Vukovich Gabriella: *Szocializáció*, in Nagy Katalin (ed.): Szociológia, 2006, Typotex, Budapest.

In: Youth: Practices, Perspectives and Challenges
Editor: Elizabeth Trejos-Castillo

ISBN: 978-1-62618-067-3
© 2013 Nova Science Publishers, Inc.

Chapter 9

HISPANIC ADOLESCENT CHALLENGES IN THE SCHOOL ENVIRONMENT

Fernando Valle and Francisco B. Debaran
Texas Tech University, Texas, US

ABSTRACT

The world of adolescence challenges students to find their optimal place in and out of school environments. Hispanic students are currently the fastest growing adolescent population in the United States. As a group they continue to face the storms and stress of adolescence and are relentlessly impacted by the socio-political challenges placed on their identities through stereotypes, low expectations, language barriers and questioning the value of their culture. This chapter utilizes the person environment fit theory as a framework to examine existing structures in the pipeline of Hispanic adolescent education. It calls for the re-examination of obstacles faced by Hispanic students during adolescent development to fit into U.S. school environments. Finally, the authors argue for conclusions and recommendations which encourage policy makers and educational leaders to scrutinize Hispanic adolescent realities and create inclusive spaces for educational opportunities.

As Hispanic adolescents navigate American public schools, a cascade of labels continue to define their educational opportunities and shape their lives. With adolescents in this country, labels can easily serve as factors that impact their success in the educational pipeline. Adolescence is a time characterized by change—hormonally, physically, and mentally (Blakemore and Frith, 2005).

The idea of adolescence being a period of 'storm and stress' is a perspective introduced by Hall (1904), supported by the psychoanalytic tradition of Freud (1958) and congruent with Erikson's (1968) definition of adolescence as a time of identity crisis (Op de Beeck, 2009). Such characterizations of adolescence reflect the negative consequences that youth experience, from changes in their interpersonal relationships to being confronted with social expectations about their roles in the world. For young Hispanics, adolescence is a particularly difficult period of 'storm and stress,' as they must navigate labels of identity such as ethnicity, physical appearance, social and economic status, poverty, race, and intelligence. Hispanic students must not only steer through the minefield of adolescence but must overcome challenges inherent in the policies and practices of American public schools. Tracking, stereotypes, cultural disengagement and perceptions of low expectations are a few persistent factors that contribute to academic achievement gaps. Such challenges function as at-risk school factors that promote the generalization of student abilities based on ethnicities, creating the ongoing exclusion and push out of this growing American population.

Our schools are often run by -- and therefore reflect -- the dominant white culture, which determines how minorities are treated in schools (Ogbu, 1988). Those students who "conform" will be nurtured and helped to succeed while those who look or act differently will be tolerated, ignored, or even discarded (George and Aronson, 2003). This chapter addresses the unique intersection of Hispanic adolescents in the school environment, the challenges they continue to face and the progress made as research, publications, scholars, schools, states and the 2010 Census continue to document Hispanic numbers across the country.

As the Hispanic population across the country increases, adolescents are becoming a greater part of the fabric of many states and communities. Their documented obstacles, struggles and progress in empirical studies and qualitative work is proof of the labor Hispanic families must endure to navigate public education as they seek local schools in their communities and the educational environment for "goodness of fit". We use the person-environment fit theory as a framework to guide the critical discourse on the diverse perspectives, cultural competencies and broader training needed to advance the practice in schools serving Hispanic adolescent students; moving away from deficit thinking and exclusion to a more strengths based and inclusive environment. A national shift within institutional and educator mindset is long overdue; one from exclusionary practices and limited belief of academic success to inclusion by providing culturally responsive opportunities in public education. The aim of this chapter is to provide constructive information on the Hispanic adolescent, highlight current school challenges and give voice to their unique passage through the American educational pipeline.

[*]A note in terminology, the terms "Hispanic" and "Latino" will be cited as found in the literature and used interchangeably in this chapter.

PERSON-ENVIRONMENT FIT THEORY

Students have the knowledge and ability to achieve, and schools provide opportunities for educational growth; however, Hispanic students are more likely to find that educational environments do not promote the use of their strengths and makes them susceptible to risks linked to underachievement. According to the person-environment fit theory, individual characteristics and the educational environment interact to account for student behavior (Hunt, 1975).

The interaction that occurs accesses characteristics of the student thus creating a behavioral, motivational, and/or emotional susceptibility towards positive or negative learning outcomes. Some educational psychologists emphasize the person component of the theory by taking a developmental stages approach (Eccles and Midgley, 1989). Psychosocial and cognitive changes then become important factors to consider when determining a student's developmental stage. Hispanic students are less likely to find adults in school, where they share a sense of belonging and who can identify and meet their psychological and interpersonal needs.

In this fashion, the teacher-student relationship as well as classroom climate plays an important role in the educational environment. If a teacher-student relationship does not foster a student's academic self-concept, nor if the academic work does not lead to student investment in learning outcomes, then a student's academic motivation can decrease (Eccles and Roeser, 1999). Educators and practitioners in the field have researched, documented and pondered interventions for the downward academic and affective-spiral affecting students moving from elementary to middle school environments. Therefore, in addition to the person's culture, language, achievement and poverty factors, we include developmental stages as another factor relevant to the learning environment and susceptible of learning outcomes. We borrow Jacquelynne Eccles view of optimal development, viewing it as a momentary event "that takes place when there is a good stage-environment fit between the needs of developing individuals and the opportunities afforded them by their social environments (Eccles, et al., 1993, p. 98)". We identify elements in the environment that should be considered not only in theory but in actual professional development and practice when meeting the needs of Hispanic students, and discuss sociopolitical factors as environmental forces that make these students susceptible to further exclusion in school settings. With respect to the person, adolescence for Hispanics is unlike that of non-Hispanic Whites in that ethnicity becomes a salient characteristic in the form of a self-representation. Similarly, unlike African Americans and Asians, Hispanics must contend with the unique combination of obstacles like stereotypes of low academic competence, poor English mastery, and questions about their immigrant status. Understanding the person-environment fit can reveal deficit thinking, subtractive schooling practices and forces that have historically impeded the establishment of optimal development for Hispanic success in U.S. school settings.

SCHOOLING CONCERNS AND AREAS FOR OPPORTUNITY

Population Growth of the Hispanic Adolescent

The Hispanic population makes up 16% of the U.S. population with 50 million plus U.S. Hispanics (DeNavas-Walt, Proctor, and Smith, 2011)). According to the Pew Research Center (2008) the vast majority of Hispanic public school students (84%), were born in the United States and are one in five of the student population.

Most Hispanic students are of Mexican origin (69%), followed by Puerto Rican (9%), Dominican (3%), Salvadoran (3%) and Cuban (2%) (Fry and Gonzales, 2008).

The Hispanic population is the fastest-growing ethnic group in the U.S. (U.S. Census Bureau, 2005). At a median age of 27.2 years, with 34% under the age of 18 years, Hispanics also constitute the youngest single ethnic group. The U.S. Census Bureau (2009) School Enrollment Below Post Secondary table reports more than 11,165,000 Hispanic students enrolled in K-12 schools. Yet, current statistics as well as past trends of persons 25 years or older indicate Hispanics, and in particular those of Mexican heritage, have the lowest high school and college graduation rates (U.S. Census Bureau, 2008).

These low rates suggest, as a group, Hispanics are the least likely to experience academic achievement or attain developmental benefits derived from continued participation in a school setting (Lerner and Lerner, 2006). Indeed, "study after study has indicated that people with bachelor's degrees have better health, more rewarding employment, more financial security, and greater satisfaction with their lives than do people who never achieve the degree" (Kegley and Kennedy, 2002, p. 2). If the attainment of a post-secondary education continues to be a marker of psychosocial development and societal success, we must look not only to post secondary environments for retention of Hispanic students but scrutinize the gate keeping practices which target and impact Hispanic adolescents along the educational pipeline. The U.S. educational pipeline by race and ethnicity (Hurtado, Cervantez, and Eccleston, 2010) synthesizes graduation rates for five major subpopulations found in American public Schools. The number of Latinos completing high school, post secondary educations, and professional degrees in this chart are dismal at best. From high school to professional schools, the disparities are another cold reality of the small number of Hispanic students nationally that find an environment conducive to their academic and developmental success in American schools.

A visual reminder of the flow of knowledge and skills our academic institutions -- especially public schools -- facilitate and stream to selected student populations is presented in figure 1.

The leaks in the Latino education pipeline are serious at all levels. This figure serves as a reminder of the unequal public, post secondary and graduate school conditions and educational efforts Latinos face in the academic pipeline.

Identifying practices, factors, and programming that improves the transition of Hispanic adolescents in public schools and their graduation rates requires a culturally informed framework of Hispanic academic achievement. The sections which follow provide a brief overview of the continued educational challenges forming deficit mindsets and impacting the progress and achievement of Hispanic adolescents.

Reprinted from the *pg. 249.*

Poverty, The Hispanic Adolescent and The Public Education Pipeline- As an illustration of environmental factors fostering individual susceptibility to underachievement, Steven A. Carbone's (2010) study on the Trends in International Mathematics and Science (TIMS) reports that American schools with the most wealth possessed the highest test scores. Carbone presents statistical data concerning the math and science achievements by American fourth- and eighth-graders broken down by the percentage of incidence of poverty in each population group, a U.S. average and international averages are then presented. The pattern in findings for this international study is clear: 75% or more of the American schools with the greatest levels of poverty achieved the lowest grades on math and science tests, falling below average in comparison to American and international scores in both subjects and grades (Carbone, 2010). TIMS data has been collected in 1995, 1999, 2003 and 2007 and in 2011 it will have more than 20,000 students in over 1,000 schools across the United States added as part of the fourth-through-eighth-grade data set. The relationships are clearly established in this longitudinal study between the poverty levels and academic achievement of certain populations. Berliner (2006) goes on to emphasize that the lowest scoring students come from schools where at least 75% of the student population are eligible for free or reduced lunch programs, a marker of extreme poverty.

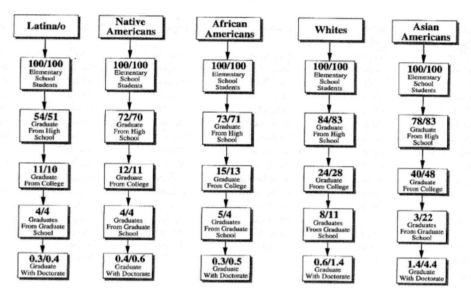

Figure 1. The U.S. educational pipeline by race/ethnicity and gender, 2000. From Hurtado, Cervantez, and Eccleston, 2010.

Hodgkinson (2008) reports that in addition to test scores, international studies document another alarming statistic; among industrialized nations, international studies since 1995 have shown the United States to be No. 1 in the number of children living below the poverty line. These comparisons of poverty and academic achievement play an especially important role in the nature of the educational environment as they freeze school and district ability to provide proper intervention and support. In addition to facing educational issues similar to those of other minority groups, Hispanic adolescents and their families must also contend with issues of learning the English Language, equity in school funding, quality of schooling, stereotyping and some of the highest number of children living in poverty than any other racial or ethnic group. Indeed, data from the U.S. Census Bureau reveals that 37.3% of poor children were Latino, 30.5% were white and 26.6% were black (Lopez and Velasco, 2011). Children in concentrated-poverty schools (i.e. schools with high proportions of students in poverty) face enormous challenges. In such schools, students' peers are generally less prepared, have lower aspirations and graduation rates and have greater mobility and absences; parents are less involved, with less political and financial clout; and teachers tend to be less experienced and more commonly teach outside their fields of concentration (Aud et al., 2010; Kahlenberg, 2001; McArdle, Osypuk, and Acevedo-Garcia, 2010). The association between poverty trends and achievement described above suggests that Hispanic students are likely to be placed in environments that do not provide the motivational and behavioral opportunities to achieve comparable to more affluent environments.

Schools are a key environment, influencing child and student development. Research has documented the negative effects of concentrated-poverty schools as well as the advantages of racially/ethnically diverse learning environments. McArdle, Osypuk and Acevedo-Garcia (2010) report on segregation and poverty, they point out minority children continue to attend high-poverty, high-minority schools, separate from the vast majority of white children. Even as the racial and ethnic composition of urban, suburban, and rural communities continue to change, the documented increase in Hispanic populations in the last census is generating further racial and ethnic segregation in many schools and communities. Research at the national level has found increasing segregation for blacks and Latinos since 1988 (McArdle et al., 2010). The authors further note, in that year, the average black student was in a school that was one-third white and just one-third of black students were in intensely segregated schools (i.e., those with 90-100 percent minority students.) Hispanic student also attended schools with average enrollments that were one-third white, while only one-third of Hispanics were in intensely segregated schools. By 2006, both minority groups were in schools that were almost three-fourths minority on average, and about 40% were in intensely segregated schools. For Hispanics, community and school enrollment increases are associated with the quick growing numbers, causing a rise in housing and neighborhood segregation. McArdle and colleagues further document high levels of neighborhood segregation fueled by high levels of primary school segregation, as the vast majority of children attend neighborhood schools, based on geographic proximity. The report further clarifies most children do not attend schools that reflect the racial/ethnic composition or the poverty composition of their metro areas. White students attend schools with disproportionate shares of white, non-poor classmates, while racial/ethnic minority students attend schools with disproportionate shares of minority, poor classmates.

As evidenced by these poverty trends, Hispanic students are likely to find themselves in schools with poor physical environments and be placed in classrooms where the average learning outcomes are inadequate. Schools in low-income areas are more likely to suffer from being inadequately maintained and overcrowded facilities (Evans, 2004). With overcrowding, classroom instructional tools and access to books and computers becomes increasingly scarce. Students at low-income schools are more likely to be characterized by low efficacy for academic achievement and less connection to one's school than students in affluent communities. A pattern of increasing segregation in low-income schools suggests that, for Hispanic students, the characteristics linked to achievement will continue to be subdued by the inherent disadvantages posed by economic obstacles and the deleterious effects on segregated public schools.

The English Language Learner- According to census data, approximately 80 percent of all English Language Learners (ELLs) in the U.S. are Hispanic. Most of these students were born in the U.S. and approximately 2.5 percent of teachers who instruct ELL students possess a degree in ESL or bilingual education (NCES, 1997). In fact, it has been found that as many as 20% of all high school and 12% of all middle school ELLs have missed two or more years of formal education since the age of six (Ruiz de-Velasco and Fix, 2000). With the culmination of language, poverty, academic achievement gaps and stereotypes looming over the Hispanic ethnic identity it is clearer how policies and sparsely embedded inclusive practices can push students out of school. For example, although states vary in their definition of a dropout, the National Center for Educational Statistics (NCES) reported that the percentage of dropouts in the non-native born Hispanic youth population between the ages of 16 and 24 years old is 43.4% (Kaufman and Alt, 2004). Further, while some high-poverty schools have attained high academic achievement, a study of more than 60,000 schools found that low-poverty schools were 22 times more likely to reach consistently high academic achievement compared with high-poverty schools (McArdle et al., 2010).

In response to the theories surrounding the correlation between poor socio-economic class and low academic achievement, Berliner (2006) asserts that an increase in the incomes of our poorest citizens might spur an increase in student achievement scores. Hodgkinson (2008) adds that solutions to the achievement gap in economically challenged populations would be most successfully remedied by a long-term commitment by educational, government and business leaders to invest in the communities surrounding low performing schools. Similarly, In Kozol's (2005) examination of per pupil spending in six metropolitan areas throughout the 2002-2003 school year, the author reveals a clear disparity in spending with the predominantly Caucasian schools holding the greatest per pupil spending and predominantly African American and Latino schools having the lowest.

Teachers have a powerful role in educating children. The power extends beyond the effective delivery of academic content (Stevens, Hamman, Olivarez, 2007). Particularly in early adolescences when academic motivation dramatically decreases, teacher assistance and instruction can prevent a student from falling to far behind. Students who are learning the English language are in need of educators who have English Language Learner training. Communities with emerging Hispanic populations face the absence of ELL programs and trained teachers. The school environment can function as an obstacle for Hispanic adolescents by farming them out to other programs and schools and by neglecting to promote English language development. The persistent use of first language can leave students more susceptible to heightened feelings of being lost, unprepared and show a greater dependence on the teacher.

During the middle school years, when children reach early adolescence, cognitive changes result in the sense that others' thoughts are directed at the adolescent, which makes the role of social interactions salient (Elkind, 1967). For Hispanic adolescent students, academic disconnect, minimal student-teacher engagement and a marginalized environment gives way to boredom, academic disidentification and discipline issues. By not addressing the language needs of English language learners, public schools continue to funnel immigrant and non-immigrant Hispanic students alike into academically unprepared territory, pushing them through the cracks and leaks of public education.

Hispanic Adolescent and the School To Prison Pipeline- The environment factors that can interact with student characteristics go beyond the direct effects of schools and include policies at the state and national level. The efforts made in public education to reform both middle and high school schools have been noted by the quest of accountability, the scope of testing, school turn around initiatives and meeting requirements of The No Child Left Behind Act of 2001 (NCLB). The use of high-stakes standardized testing to determine school success has produced marginalized education avenues for Hispanic adolescents and increased the pursuit to find alternative routes to completing a secondary education. In her work on urban youth and schools, *Eve Tuck (2012)* unearths the unintentional cost of ever-increasing accountability policies on secondary school completion by focusing specifically on the use and over-use of the General Education Diploma (GED) credential. Tuck (2012) discovered accountability tacitly and explicitly pushes under-performing students out of the system. The curriculum and school opportunities providing meaningful routes to graduation are missing for the under-performing. This ongoing practice of pushing out underperforming students from U.S. schools illustrates the humiliating ironies and the dangerous dignity of American schooling for the marginalized.

The National Council for La Raza (NCLR) argues the enforcement of zero-tolerance policies has further contributed to the marginalization of students of color and has resulted in racial and ethnic disparities with school systems nationwide. In their *Models for Change* fact sheet, Latino students are 1.5 times more likely to be suspended and twice as likely to be expelled as their White peers (Advancement Project, 2010). Every seven seconds during the school year, a Latino public school student is suspended (Children's Defense Fund, 2011). School suspension is the top predictor of contact with the justice system for students who become incarcerated by ninth grade (Balfanz, Spirikakis, Neild, and Legters, 2003).

The focus on middle school and the Hispanic adolescent is in concert with the importance of a student's middle school experience in determining future academic success (Losen and Skiba, 2010). The author's further report suspension in middle school may have significant long-term repercussions. Balfanz, Spirikakis, Neild, and Legters (2003) provide a comprehensive look at incarcerated youth and connect the dots between youths that experience difficulty in school and those wind up in prison. Balfanz and colleagues chronicle the educational paths of more than 400 incarcerated ninth- graders and found that the youths most at risk of incarceration were clearly identifiable by middle school, and that nearly all had "struggled profoundly" in school. According to their finding, the typical ninth-grader who went to prison had previously attended school only 58% of the time, and two-thirds had been suspended at least once in eighth grade, failed at least one quarter of their classes, and read at a sixth grade level at the end of eighth grade. In their sample, 80% were black, and 85% came from neighborhood non-selective schools.

The NAACP Legal Defense and Education Fund School to Prison Pipeline report (2011) further noted historical inequalities in the education system—segregated education, concentrated poverty, and longstanding stereotypes—influence how school officials and law enforcement both label children and treat students who present challenging behavior. Studies show that students of color receive harsher punishments for engaging in the same conduct as white students and racially isolated schools that primarily educate students of color are more likely to be among the nation's "dropout factories" and among those utilizing the harshest, most exclusionary means of discipline (NAACP Legal Defense and Education Fund, 2011). Given the importance of the instructional time in predicting achievement outcomes (Greenwood, Horton, and Utley, 2002;Wang, Haertel, and Walberg, 1997), one might argue that concerns about high suspension rates should be treated with the same level of concern often expressed for low test scores, poor attendance, and high dropout rates (Losen and Skiba, 2010).

The Civil Rights Project at UCLA and the Southern Poverty Law Center along with other national partners advocated the 2010 report in which authors Losen and Skiba further document longitudinal studies showing students suspended in sixth grade are *more* likely to receive office referrals or suspensions by eighth grade, prompting researchers to conclude that suspension may act more as a *reinforcer* than a punisher for inappropriate behavior (Tobin, Sugai, and Colvin, 1998). In the long term, school suspension has been found to be a moderate-to-strong predictor of school dropout (Balfanz et al., 2003), and may in some cases be used as a tool to "cleanse" the school of students who are perceived by school administrators as troublemakers (Bowditch, 1993). National suspension rates show 17%, or 1 out of every 6 Black school children and 1 in 14 Latinos (7%) enrolled in K-12 were susupended at least once, compared to 1 in 20 (5%) Whites (Losen & Gillespie, 2012). Emerging data indicates that schools with higher rates of school suspension and expulsion have poorer outcomes on standardized achievement tests, regardless of the economic level or demographics of their students (Losen and Skiba, 2010).

The criminalization of certain kinds of school misconduct has created what is often referred to as the "school-to-prison pipeline" (Wald and Losen, 2003). The pressure for educators to ensure all adolescents fit into the evolving blueprint of secondary education is passed on to students. According to the U.S. Department of Education Office for Civil Rights (OCR), nearly three million students are suspended at least once each year and more than 100,000 students are expelled. In 2007, nearly 70% of our nation's public school student's ages 12 through 18 reported that police officers or security guards patrol their hallways (Thurau, 2009). Secondary school environments continue to face high number of classroom and school removals to alternative school campuses. The additional need for school discipline, expulsion, and zero-tolerance policies—especially in middle and high schools criminalizes school behaviors. Losen and Gillespie (2012) through their work at the UCLA Civil Rights Project assert it is critically important to keep students, especially those facing inquality in other parts of their lives, enrolled in school. Hispanic students are suspect to face the discipline side of schooling in disproportionately higher numbers and systematically being pushed out of school. In essence, they are provided with fewer and fewer safe spaces in public schools.

BEYOND STEREOTYPES AND LOW EXPECTATIONS

Building Cultural Coherence- The hardest culture to examine is often our own, because it shapes our actions in ways that seem second nature, like the air we breathe, permeating all we do (Rothstein-Fisch, 2003). Teachers and educators also bring their culture into the classroom and the school. A students' sense of school belonging, which refers to psychological membership in a supportive school community (Patrick, Anderman, and Ryan, 2002), becomes an especially important social variable to consider with Hispanic students during their middle school years (Stevens et al., 2007). Fewer than 13% of current public school teachers come from underrepresented groups, which reflect the lowest representation in decades (American Association of Colleges for Teacher Education, 1999). Addressing this disparity will be difficult, as only 5% of students enrolled in teacher education programs described themselves as Hispanic as recently as 1995 (American Association of Colleges for Teacher Education, 1999).

Schools are capable of taking advantage of multicultural environments, including and embracing families, students and communities or maintain a culture of tolerance distributing knowledge, opportunity and cultural resources to select student populations—further separating and segregating minority students. The victims of this hidden curriculum are the traditionally underserved students who struggle every day to overcome cultural bias and racial stereotypes that set them apart from their white peers (George and Aronson, 2003). Gandara (1999) suggests African-American, Latino, and Native-American students often have different learning opportunities because of their ethnic and socioeconomic backgrounds – opportunities dictated by the predominant cultural beliefs of our society, which, in turn, translate into teacher expectations. Teacher expectations, educational opportunities and the culture of the school and local community must be aligned, congruent and a process of learning for all parties involved that is continuous (George and Aronson, 2003).

Spradlin and Parsons (2008) point out class distinctions are incredibly powerful determinants of the quality of schooling an individual receives as well as how that individual might interact with peers and society as a whole. Their work suggests teachers take steps to explore their own beliefs about social class and determine the influence those beliefs have on curriculum and teaching. Viewing Hispanic families and students as holders of knowledge, providing learning opportunities in the context of culture and providing diverse ways of knowing and understanding, encourages multicultural perspectives and teacher-student cultural congruency. It is the work necessary in our school to move toward culturally responsive pedagogy and teaching.

Unfortunately, the stereotypes Americans hold of specific races and ethnic groups have not disappeared (George and Aronson, 2003). The National Opinion Research Center revealed that in general, Americans evaluate minority groups more negatively than whites after respondents were asked to evaluate characteristics of Whites, Jews, African-Americans, Asian-Americans, Latinos, and southern Whites on a scale of 1 to 7 (George and Aronson, 2003). Latinos and African-Americans were ranked last or next to last on almost every characteristic measured which included intelligence, laziness, and motivation to be self-sufficient (Association of American Colleges and Universities, 1998).

Good and Brophy (2003) echo this in a more tangible manner and point out those interactions between teacher and students may well be impacted by race. Teachers might feel a sense of hostility or rejection of minority students, or even rate those students less favorably than their classmates (Carbone, 2010; Good and Brophy, 2003). Teachers must be sensitive to the diversity found in the classroom and foster a learning environment that incorporates that diversity (Carbone, 2010). Developing a consciousness for differences amongst adolescent students as well as differences between teachers and students is the practice and development of cultural competencies. Such competencies create the coherence needed to meet the accountability, demographic and assessment demands currently placed in our schools. Genuine efforts by teachers and school leaders to embrace facets of multicultural environments are important educational tasks which build social justice foundations, foster equity in schools and move the work toward academic justice forward.

An additional cultural framework aimed at recognizing the educational needs of the Hispanic adolescent is that of the individual versus the collective present in curriculum and American public school culture. Our U.S. schools and classrooms have taught students to be exceptional and distinctive individuals—empowered by individual thinking for independence and personal achievement. A collective culture, representative of many immigrant cultures, adheres to family norms, maintains respect for authority and elders, embraces a social context for learning and is associated with shared and group learning.

For educators working with Hispanic students, finding ways to bridge cultural differences has a profound influence on learning (Rothstein-Fisch, 2003). This practical framework for understanding cultural differences describes two contrasting value systems: individualism vs. collectivism. The individualism approach fosters independence and success of the individual and a collectivism approach fosters interdependence and success of the group (Greenfield,

1994). A profound challenge of students from collectivistic backgrounds is the separation of "social experience" from the school assessments of "content knowledge" (Quiroz, Greenfield, and Altchech, 1999). The table below provides salient features prevailing in U.S. cultures compared with those of many immigrant cultures.

Table 1. Salient Features of Individualism and Collectivism

Individualism (Representative of prevailing U.S. culture)	Collectivism (Representative of many immigrant cultures)
1. Fostering independence and individual achievement	1. Fostering interdependence and group success
2. Promoting self-expression, individual thinking, and personal choice?	2. Promoting adherence to norms, respect for authority/ elders, group consensus
3. Associated with egalitarian relationships and flexibility in roles (e.g., upward mobility)	3. Associated with stable, hierarchical roles (dependent on gender, family background, age)?
4. Understanding the physical world as knowable apart from its meaning for human life	4. Understanding the physical world in the context of its meaning for human life
5. Associated with private property, individual ownership	5. Associated with shared property, group ownership

Protective Factors- Hispanic adolescents maintain the greatest dropout rates of any ethnic group in the country. School assessments and accountability factors presents a catch-22 for Hispanic youth who are expected to achieve similarly to that of non-Hispanic Whites but are more likely than them to miss out on instruction due to discipline placements, poverty, school suspensions, language barriers and subsequent placement in alternative education settings which providing minimal curricular and academic support. Hispanic students facing suspension and discipline issues have traditionally been pushed out of their schools under the auspices of obtaining an alternative education or a General Education Development (GED). Educators across the nation are facing pressures to educate *all* students. However, to truly engage in transformative work for schools, educators must create an inclusive environment where goodness of fit and achievement and student outcomes are new molds of school success. Indeed, grants and programs which include parental support, academic interventions, college readiness and community engagement and outreach have provided spaces for adolescent Hispanics to develop protective factors—extracurricular activities, spaces where bonding occurs, academic and tutoring support, development of transferrable skills and being surrounded by people who have positive beliefs and standards toward education.

Communities and educators serving Hispanic adolescents must move from viewing their status as purely at-risk to conversations which include family, school and community protective factors to support and shape adolescents. Schools policies can lag behind with outdated and deficit practices that do not meet the cultural needs of students. Hispanic parents and students are still targets for the continued disconnect between communities and schools. The shaping of school belonging not only refers to how students perceive the social context of schooling but how they view their place in the school structure (Anderman, 2003). Shaking up the status quo and elitist's logic suggesting not all students deserve high engaging curriculum and only a few students are college material, will be important to the economic development and global standing of this country in the next decade. Therefore, the closed mindset of past decades, which concluded American public schools were only capable of serving certain types of students—those who fit into the traditional mold of schooling—requires a cultural shift to meet the needs of the Unites State's 21st century learners.

Coping and Hoping Skills- Research suggests that participation in extracurricular activities may increase students' sense of engagement or attachment to their school, and thereby decrease the likelihood of school failure and dropping out (Lamborn, Brown, Mounts, and Steinberg, 1992; Finn, 1993). Research on high schools continues to demonstrate the correlation between extracurricular activity participation, which requires student and often parent involvement and social support to support the successful school experiences. Davalos, Chavez, and Guardiola (1999) studied the effects of participation in extracurricular activities on Mexican American students and found that those involved in such activities were more likely to stay in school than their uninvolved peers. Such findings, which counter the Hispanic high school dropout rate, has expanded the attention and focus on the complex factors that contribute to Hispanics' academic success.

Ortiz and Gonzalez, (2000) illustrate that joint organizational efforts between a high school principal, university president, institutional units responsible for student preparation, students, and their parents can create social relationships and pathways to raise Latino students' eligibility for college admission. These efforts coupled with individual initiative were found to counteract social structures inhibiting Latino students' pursuit of higher education (Ortiz and Gonzalez, 2000). In contrast, Jonathan Kozol (2005) identified hopelessness among students interviewed in several New York City high schools. Through his narratives, it is clear that students' plans for the future following high school are uncertain as only one out the seven students interviewed indicated plans to go to college. Other students articulated frustration and anger through obscenities and sarcasm. Given current bleak public school achievement conditions, it is often uncertain how a student could strive to succeed academically if they have no hope of a positive future (Carbone, 2010).

Challenging this notion of hopelessness among Latinas, Ceja (2004) examined the parental support and resilience of Latina students. Ceja's definitions of resiliency suggest that individuals develop a certain consciousness or mental outlook that allows them to form a critical perspective of their surroundings and lived experiences. This perspective in turn functions as a coping mechanism which allows them to survive in deleterious school conditions and in many cases thrive within those realities. The concept of resiliency in Ceja's study allows us to further understand how Latina students are able to find strength and empowerment from their often marginalized social conditions. Solorzano and Villalpando (1998) remind us of the hope and resilience required for Latino students to endure, "Marginality is a complex and contentious location and process whereby students of color are subordinated because of their race, gender, and class" (p. 301).

Countering the culture of marginalization in their school environment, Hispanics are the majority population in many communities yet still the majority of alienated individuals. Tan and Pope (2007) state students who participate in extracurricular activities develop more positive academic identities and have higher retention and higher graduation rates. However, for many Hispanic adolescent students, the option to participate in extracurricular activities is not always present. Many factors exist that prevent Hispanic students from experiencing a well-rounded school experience: family commitments, financial obligations, working during school, being the oldest in the home, contributing to the family income. With such factors weighing on the needed coping skills in secondary education, Hispanic students can easily become disconnected from a successful path of middle to high school, and on to college completion. To help Hispanic students persist, we advocate a framework that emphasizes the person by identifying values, principles, and practices that we believe are essential for increasing the goodness of fit to environmental factors such as educators, parents, schools and training institutions. Only when the person-environment interaction is considered can public schools in the U.S. be responsive to the needs and preferences of students of Latino background. The Education Development Center, Inc. (2002) challenges educators and families to address the following area of values, principles, and practices:

Familia/Family: Forming alliances with the family network. Redefining partnerships with parents as teacher involvement includes the whole community surrounding the student/adolescent.

Pertenencia/Belonging: Creating a sense of family. Building a student/adolescent environment that echoes the positive relationships and bonds within families, where children form identity, feel part of something greater than themselves, and feel supported.

Educación/Education: Learning together. Discussing, developing, and generating life-long skills that go beyond building knowledge to building capacity to act and solve problems collectively.

Compromiso/Commitment: Reaching beyond boundaries. The role of the responsive teacher and school extends to action and initiative within the grade level, within school programs, within the field, and within the community in order to serve the student/adolescent and families.

POSITIVE ACTION AND CONCLUSION: DEBUNKING THE HISPANIC ADOLESCENT MYTH

Implications for policy makers- Hispanic students along with other students of color have been at the mercy of deficit thinking systems in schools. The use of models and theories created for majority students is well intentioned, yet it may not be appropriate (Torres, 2006). Valencia (2001) explains deficit thinking as an "endogenous theory of school failure, [which] 'blames the victim' rather than examining how schools and the political economy are structured to prevent students from learning optimally" (p. 83). Before definitions of social justice surfaced, scholars like Freire (1970), described social injustices in detail as strategies that dehumanized people and maintained the status quo of elitist groups. Consistent with Reyes and Valencia (1993) we suggest policy makers and *administrator preparation programs* embrace school policies that are embedded in multiculturalism *to provide new and different perspectives in tune with the diversity which currently exists in schools.* We assert that policy makers and agencies *outside* of education continue to influence and institute agendas (i.e, No Child Left Behind, Equity of School Finance, Immigration Issues, Language Programs, etc...) into the practice of schools and classrooms that do not fit the needs of the growing Hispanic student population.

Implications for Public Schools Leaders: The assumptions that students are homogenous is argued and debunked by Reyes and Valencia (1993) as it creates barriers in comprehending and appreciating Latino student diversity. The authors of this chapter concur with scholars who believe schools are racialized spaces (Barajas and Ronnkvist, 2007), and our practice as educators is not divorced from who we are (Calderón, 2008; Contreras and Lee, 1990; Rousseau and Tate, 2003). In other words, school leaders enter the profession with core beliefs, dispositions and motivations which can contribute to student susceptibility to underachievement. School leaders must understand *who* they are translates into *what* they do. In fact educational leaders play a central role in constructing the achievement environment for students. These roles include the importance of school leaders' as moral and ethical stewards, as distributive and transformational and culturally conscious community builders (Murphy, 2002; Northouse, 2012).

Yosso (2005) similarly stressed the importance of building on community cultural wealth (i.e., aspirational, linguistic, familial, social, navigational) to challenge traditional interpretations of social and cultural capital which elevates and values the dominant culture over others. We affirm school leaders are the creators and guardians of successful environments for students. Specifically for Hispanics, school leaders must be reflective and acknowledge that their own experiences may be incongruent with the identity needs of the students they serve. To achieve congruencies, school leaders must view languages other than English as mechanisms for success. Efforts to access the cultural wealth of Hispanic communities through direct interaction can lead to greater understanding of Hispanic student ethnic identity and serve as a gauge of school connectedness.

Programs for Success A report by the Education Commission of the States (Ruppert, 2003) revealed that, among those of eligible age, only 15% of the Hispanic population earns a postsecondary degree, and an astounding 48% have less than a high school credential. Whatever the particular contexts and reasons for Hispanic dropouts, the condition is intolerable. One sound approach is primary prevention, providing students with high quality elementary and middle experiences to deal with the precursors to drop out: low achievement; retention in grade, and dislike of school (Fashola, Slavin, Calderón, and Duran, 1996).

Fashola and Slavin (1998) researched programs designed to reduce dropout rates and increase college attendance among at-risk students in middle and high schools. Programs such as these provide at-risk student groups with the college preparation skills and knowledge needed to enter and succeed in college (Perna and Swail, 2001). These authors discovered programs such as Upward Bound, SCORE, Advancement Via Individual Determination (AVID), and Graduation Really Achieves Dreams improved school to college pipeline rates for Hispanics (Fashola and Slavin, 1998). These academic programs demonstrated a strong impact in reducing dropout rates by creating meaningful bonds between students and teachers, connecting students to an attainable future, giving students opportunities to work while in school, providing academic assistance, and giving students high-status roles in the school.

Recommendations and Final Thoughts

Hispanic student population growth across campuses in the U.S. has not translated into academic gains and graduation rates relative to their African American and European American peers. Hispanic students continue to attend schools classified as dropout factories (Balfanz and Letgers, 2004). Hispanic students struggle to form a sense of belonging to the educational and interpersonal environments they encounter in U.S. schools. In addition media messages provide mixed acceptance of the defining characteristics of Hispanic students' ethnic identity. Schools are still the key environments where college readiness is transferred to all students. Student placements in advanced courses or classes that offer college credit often do not reflect the proportion of Hispanic students enrolled in the school. Hispanic students are still over-represented in school discipline cases, vocational tracks, and are found participating in less advanced or average level courses. Such disproportion and unequity can also be found in clubs and other forms extracurricular activities. School-sponsored student organizations often require large financial out of pocket expenses and a faculty member to serve as an advisor, and yet many schools do not employ faculty who share knowledge of student's ethnic and cultural backgrounds. Attempts to form a school sponsored organization which reflects a culturally imbued mission will fail if students do not have access to faculty who share their passion and interest.

Few books on the shelves in school libraries and book stores identify American born Hispanics who have made significant contributions to this country. Curriculum discourse on the positive contributions of Hispanics is also rare. Adolescence is a time when role models inspire and motivate students to pursue goals in emerging adulthood. If school policies and curriculum do not provide opportunities for students to identify with parts of American history that connect with their Hispanic heritage then an opportunity to reverse school disengagement and drop out trends is lost.

Hispanic students also struggle to achieve belonging at the interpersonal level when ethnic heritage and culturally grounded beliefs are aspects of cultural wealth that is not valued by peers and adults. Peer-to-peer discrimination and the presence of stereotypes are both forms of hostile interpersonal environments. When Hispanic students experience such interpersonal environments, they may either reject such beliefs or may begin to believe there is some truth behind stereotypes. The effects of stereotypes are most toxic when Hispanic students address hostile interpersonal environments. The complex interaction of educational and interpersonal environments on the developing adolescent can help account for negative learning outcomes and failure to graduate.

Given the growing youthful presence of Hispanics in the U.S., we recommend secondary public schools emphasize college readiness for Hispanic students who are increasingly targeted as prospective applicants by colleges and universities. The current cultural and demographic shift in the U.S. provides our country with an opportunity to include Hispanics in the race to meet demands of globalization. The goal of producing a workforce viable in a global market should be a platform for educators and policy makers to embrace diversity and reduce the marginalization of ethnic minority students. The history of the Hispanic adolescent is currently being written. It is our responsibility as educators, leaders and policy makers to provide environments which are inclusive to the needs of Hispanic students, making them feel connected, academically and part of a good fit in schools.

Recommended Readings

Freire, P. (1970). *Pedagogy of the oppressed.* New York: Continuum Publishing.
Gonzalez, N., Moll, L.C., & Amanti, C. (2005). *Funds of Knowledge: Theorizing practices in households, communities and classrooms.* New Jersey: Laurence Erlbaum Associates.
Kozol, J. (2005). *The shame of the nation.* New York: Three Rivers Press.
Kozol, J. (2003). *Savage inequalities.* New York: Harper Perennial.
Murillo, E.G., Villenas, S. A., Trinidad Galvan, R., Sanchez Munoz, J., Martinez, C., & Machado-Casas, M. (2009). *Handbook of Latinos and education: Theory, research and practice.* New York: Routledge.
Reyes, P., Scribner, J.D., & Scribner, A. P. (1999). *Lessons from high performing Hispanic schools: Creating learning communities.* New York: Teachers College Press.
Tilman, L.C. & Scheurich, J.J. (2013). *Hanbook of research on educational leadership for equity and diversity.* New York: Routledge.
Valencia, R. (1997). *The evolution of deficit thinking.* New York: Routledge.
Valencia, R. (2010). *Dismantling contemporary deficit thinking.* New York: Routledge.
Valenzuela, A. (1999). *Subtractive schooling.* New York: State University of New York Press.
Villarreal, F. A., Carlo, G., Grau, J.M, Azmitia, M., Cabrera, N. J., & Chahin, T. J. (2009). *Handbook of U.S. Latino psychology: Developmental and community-based practices.* Los Angeles: Sage Publications.
Yosso, T. J. (2005). Whose culture has capital? A critical race theory discussion of community and cultural wealth. *Race Ethnicity and Education*, 8(1), 69-91.

REFERENCES

Anderman, L. H. (2003). Academic and social perceptions as predictors of change in middle school students' sense of school belonging. *Journal of Experimental Education*, 72, 5–22.
American Association of Colleges for Teacher Education. (1999). *Teacher education pipeline IV: Schools, colleges, and departments of education enrollments by race, ethnicity, and gender.* Retrieved from http://www.eric.ed.gov/PDFS/ED432571.pdf.
Advancement Project, (2010). *Test, punish, and push out: How "zero tolerance" and high-stakes testing funnel youth into the school-to-prison pipeline.* Retrieved from http://www.advancementproject.org/sites/default/files/publications/rev_fin.pdf.
Association of American Colleges and Universities. (1998, Winter). *How do Americans view one another? The persistence of racial/ethnic stereotypes.* Retrieved from http://www.diversityweb.org/Digest/W98/research2.html.
Aud, S., Hussar, W., Planty, M., Snyder, T., Bianco, K., Fox. M.,... & Drake, L. (2010). *The condition of education 2010 (NCES 2010–028).* Retrieved from the National Center for Education Statistics website: http://nces.ed.gov/pubs2010/2010028.pdf.
Balfanz, R., Spiridakis, K., Neild, R. C., & Legters, N. (2003). *High poverty secondary schools and the juvenile justice system: How neither helps the other and how that could*

change. In J. Wald and D. J. Losen (Eds.), Deconstructing the school-to-prison pipeline, 71–79. San Francisco: Jossey-Bass.

Berliner, D. (2006). Our impoverished view of educational research. *Teachers College Record, 108*(6), 949-995. Retrieved 5 February 2012 from http://www.education anddemocracy.org/Resources/Berliner.pdf

Blakemore, S. J. & Frith, U. (2005). The learning brain: Lessons for education: a précis. *Developmental Science,* 8, 459- 471. doi: 10.1111/j.1467-7687.2005.00434.x.

Ceja, M. (2004). Chicana college aspirations and the role of parents: Developing educational resiliency. *Journal of Hispanics in Higher Education,* 3, 338-362. Retrieved from http://dx.doi.org/10.1177/1538192704268428.

Carbone II, Steven A. (2010). *Race, class, and oppression: Solutions for active learning and literacy in the classroom.* Online publication Student Pulse. Retrieved from http://www.studentpulse.com/a?id=113.

Children's Defense Fund. (2011). *Moments in America for Latino children.* Retrieved from http://www.childrensdefense.org/child-research-data-publications/moments-in-america-for-latino-children.html

Davalos, D. B., Chavez, E. L., & Guardiola, R. J. (1999). The effects of extracurricular activity, ethnic identification, and perception of school on student dropout rates. *Hispanic Journal of Behavioral Sciences,* 21, 61–78. doi: 10.1177/0739986399211005.

DeNavas-Walt, C., Proctor, B. D., & Smith, J. C. (2011). *Income, poverty, and health insurance coverage in the United States: 2010 (Current Population Reports 60–239).* Washington, DC: U.S. Government Printing Office.

Eccles, J. S., & Midgley, C. (1989). *Stage-environment fit: Developmentally appropriate classrooms for young adolescents.* In C. Ames & R. Ames (Eds.), Research on motivation in education (pp. 139–186). San Diego, CA: Academic Press.

Eccles, J. S., Midgley, C., Wigfield, A., Buchanan, C., Reuman, D., Flanagan., & MacIver, D. (1993). Development during adolescence: The impact of stage–environment fit on adolescents' experiences in schools and families. *American Psychologist,* 48, 90–101. doi: 10.1037/0003-066X.48.2.90.

Eccles, J. S., & Roeser. R. W. (2005). *School and community influences on human development.* In M. H. Bornstein and M. E. Lamb (Eds.), Developmental science: An advanced textbook (pp. 513–556). Mahwah, NJ: Erlbaum.

Elkind, D. (1967) Egocentrism in adolescence. *Child Development,* 38 (4), 1025–1034.

Erikson, E. H. (1968). *Identity, youth and crisis.* New York: Norton.

Finn, J. D. (1993). *School engagement and students at risk.* Washington, DC: National Center for Education Statistics..

Freud, A. (1958). Psychoanalytic study of the child. *Adolescence,* 15, 255–278.

Fry, R., & Gonzalez, F. (2008). *One-in-five and growing fast: A profile of Hispanic public school students.* Retrieved from Pew Hispanic Center website: http://www.pewhispanic.org/files/reports/92.pdf.

Gandara, P. (1999). *Paving the way to higher education: K-12 intervention programs for underrepresented youth.* Washington, DC: National Postsecondary Education Cooperative.

George, P. & Aronson, R. (2003). *How do educators' cultural belief systems affect underserved students' pursuit of Postsecondary education? A white paper sponsored by*

NASSP in conjunction with the Pathways to College Network. Retrieved from http://www.eric.ed.gov/PDFS/ED475881.pdf

Good, T., & Brophy, J. (2003). *Looking in classrooms* (9th ed.). Boston: Pearson Education, Inc.

Greenfield, P. M. (1994). *Independence and interdependence as developmental scripts: Implications for theory, research and practice*. In P. M. Greenfield and R. R. Cocking. (Eds.), Cross-cultural roots of minority child development (pp. 1–37). Hillsdale, NJ: Lawrence Erlbaum Associates.

Greenwood, C. R., Horton, B. T., & Utley, C. A. (2002). Academic engagement: Current perspectives on research and practice. *School Psychology Review, 31* (3),328–349.-349. Retrieved from http://www.nasponline.org/index2.html.

Hall, G. S. (1904-1905). *Adolescence: Its psychology and its relation to physiology, anthropology, sociology, sex, crime, religion, and education* (Vols. 1–2). Englewood Cliffs, NJ: Prentice-Hall.

Hodgkinson, H. (2008). *Demographic trends and the federal role in education. Center on Education Policy*, (ERIC Document Reproduction Service No. ED503865) Retrieved from the Center on Education Policy website: http://www.eric.ed.gov/PDFS/ED503865.pdf.

Hurtado, A., Cervantez, K., & Eccleston, M. (2010). *Infinite possibilities, many obstacles: Language, culture, identity, and Latino/a educational achievement*. In E. G. Murillo, Jr., S. A. Villenas, R. T. Galván, J. S. Muńoz, C. Martínez, and M. Machado-Casas (eds.), Handbook of Latinos in education: Theory, research, and practice (pp. 284–300). New York: Routledge.

Hunt, D. E. (1975). Person-environment interaction: A challenge found wanting before it was tried. *Review of Educational Research, 45*, 209–230.

Kaufman, P., & Alt, M. N. (2004). *Dropout rates in the United States: 2001* (NCES 2005–046). Washington, DC: U.S. Government Printing Office.

Kahlenberg, R. D., (2001). *All together now: Creating middle-class schools through public school choice*. Washington, DC: Brookings Institution Press.

Kegley, J., & Kennedy, L. (2002). *Facilitating student success in achieving the baccalaureate degree: Report of the California State University task force on facilitating graduation*. Retrieved from http://www.calstate.edu/acadaff/facilitatinggraduation.pdf.

Kozol, J. (2005). *The shame of the nation*. New York: Three Rivers Press.

Lamborn, S. D., Brown, B. B., Mounts, N. S., & Steinberg, L. (1992). *Putting school in perspective: The influence of family, peers, extracurricular participation, and part-time work on academic engagement*. In F. M. Newman (Ed.), Student engagement and achievement in American secondary schools (pp. 153 – 181). New York: Teachers College Press.

Lerner, R. M., & Lerner, J. V. (2006). *Toward a new vision and vocabulary about adolescence: Theoretical, empirical, and applied bases of a "positive youth development" perspective*. In L. Balter and C. S. Tamis-LeMonda (Eds.), Child psychology: A handbook of contemporary issues (2nd ed., pp. 445–469). New York: Psychology Press.

Lopez, M. H., & Velasco, G. (2011). *The toll of the great recession: Childhood poverty among Hispanic sets record, leads nation*. Retrieved from Pew Hispanic Center website: http://www.pewhispanic.org/files/2011/10/147.pdf.

Losen, D.J. & Gillespie, J. (2012). *Opportunities suspended: The disparate impact of disciplinary exclusion from school.* The Civil Rights Project: UCLA. Retrieved from: http://civilrightsproject.ucla.edu/resources/projects/center-for-civil-rights-remedies/school-to-prison-folder/federal-reports/upcoming-ccrr-research.

McArdle, H., Osypuk, T., & Acevedo-Garcia, D. (2010). *Segregation and exposure to high-poverty schools in large metropolitan areas: 2008-09.* Retrieved from diversitydata.org website: http://diversitydata.sph.harvard.edu/Publications/school_segregation_report.pdf.

Ogbu, J. U. (1988). *Diversity and equity in public education: Community forces and minority school adjustment and performance.* In R. Haskins and D. MacRae (Eds.), Policies for America's public schools: Teachers, equity, and indicators (pp. 127–170). Norwood, NJ: Ablex.

Ortiz, F. I., & Gonzalez, R. (2000). Latino high school students' pursuit of higher education. *Aztlan: A Journal of Chicano Studies*, 25 (1), 67–107. Retrieved from http://aztlanjournal.metapress.com/media/h83kwkmuqmdbfqqyhnr2/contributions/b/6/8/4/b684j4l20772th86.pdf.

Op de Beeck, H. (2009). *Adolescent times of storm and stress revised.* Retrieved from http://www.jeugdonderzoeksplatform.be/publicaties/Paper_Adolescent_times_of_storm_and_stress_revised.pdf.

Patrick, H., Anderman, L. H., & Ryan, A. M. (2002). *Social motivation in the classroom social environment.* In C. Midgley (Ed.), Goal, goal structures, and patterns of adaptive learning (pp. 85–108). Mahwah, NJ: Lawrence Erlbaum Associates, Inc.

Quiroz, B., Greenfield, P. M., & Altchech, M. (1999). Bridging cultures with a parent-teacher conference. *Educational Leadership,* 56 (7), 68–70.

Rothstein-Fisch, C. (2003). *Readings for bridging cultures: Teacher education module.* New Jersey: Lawrence Erlbaum Associates.

Ruiz-de- Velasco, J., Fix, M., & Clewell, B. C. (2000). *Overlooked and underserved: Immigrant students in U.S. schools.* Washington, DC: The Urban Institute Press.

Stevens, T., Hamman, D., & Olivarez, A. (2007). Hispanic students' perception of White teachers' mastery goal orientation influences sense of school belonging. *Journal of Latinos and Education*, 6, 55–70. doi: 10.1207/s1532771xjle0601_4.

Solorzano, D. G., & Villalpando, O. (1998). *Critical race theory, marginality, and the experience of students of color in higher education.* In C. A. Torres and T. R. Mitchell (Eds.), Sociology of education: Emerging perspectives (pp. 211-224). Albany, NY: State University of New York Press.

Spradlin, L. K., & Parsons, R. D. (2008). *Diversity matters: Understanding diversity in schools.* Belmont, CA: Thomson Wadsworth.

Tan, D. L., & Pope, M. L. (2007). Participation in co-curricular activities: Nontraditional student perspectives. *College and University*, 83, 2-9. Retrieved from http://www.aacrao.org/publications/college_and_university_journal.aspx.

Thurau, L., (2009). Rethinking how we police youth: Incorporating knowledge of adolescence into policing teens. *Children's Legal Rights Journal,* 29(3), 30-48. Retrieved from http://www.nlg-npap.org/html/documents/RethinkingPolicingYouthLT.pdf.

Tuck, E. (2012). *Urban youth and school pushout: Gateways, getaways, and the GED.* New York: Routledge.

U.S. Census Bureau (2005). *Race and Hispanic origin in 2005.* Retrieved from http://www.census.gov/population/pop-profile/dynamic/RACEHO.pdf.

U.S. Census Bureau (2008). *Section 4: Education.* Retrieved from http://www.census.gov/prod/2007pubs/08abstract/educ.pdf.

U.S. Census Bureau. (2009). *School enrollment below postsecondary-summary by sex, race, and Hispanic origin.* Retrieved from http://www.census.gov/compendia/statab/2012/tables/12s0253.pdf.

Wald, J. and Losen, D. J. (2003). Defining and redirecting a school-to-prison pipeline. *New Directions for Youth Development,* 99, 9–15. Retrieved from http://www3.interscience.wiley.com/journal/117944414/grouphome

Wang, M. C., Haertel, G. D., and Walberg, H. J. (1997). *Learning influences.* In H. J. Walberg and G. D. Haertel (Eds.), Psychology and educational practice (pp. 199-211). Berkeley: McCutchan.

Yosso, T. J. (2005). Whose culture has capital? A critical race theory discussion of community and cultural wealth. *Race Ethnicity and Education,* 8(1), 69-91.

Section 3. Treatment and Intervention Issues

In: Youth: Practices, Perspectives and Challenges
Editor: Elizabeth Trejos-Castillo
ISBN: 978-1-62618-067-3
© 2013 Nova Science Publishers, Inc.

Chapter 10

AGGRESSION REPLACEMENT TRAINING FOR DISRUPTIVE ADOLESCENTS: EFFICACY, EFFECTIVENESS, AND NEW DIRECTIONS INVOLVING FAMILIES

Robert Weis and Ellen R. Pucke*
Denison University, Granville, OH, US

ABSTRACT

Aggression Replacement Training (ART) is a multimodal treatment designed for adolescents who show disruptive, aggressive, and antisocial behavior. It consists of structured, cognitive-behavioral activities designed to increase youths' social, emotion-regulation, and moral-reasoning skills. Research conducted in juvenile justice facilities, residential treatment centers, clinics, schools, and communities indicates that ART is associated with improvements in adolescents' behavioral and socioemotional functioning and may lead to reduced recidivism.

In this chapter, we describe ART and review the research literature regarding its efficacy and effectiveness. We then present a new development in ART research, specifically, the practice of including parents and other caregivers in ART sessions. Finally, we evaluate a new program, Adolescent and Family Anger Management, which administers the components of ART to adolescents and parents together.

Our findings provide experimental data supporting the effectiveness of social skills, anger management, and moral reasoning training for disruptive adolescents and their families.

Keywords: Aggression replacement training, aggression, delinquency, treatment, adolescents, families

---

* Correspondence should be addressed to Robert Weis, Department of Psychology, Denison University, Granville, OH 43023. Email: weisr@denison.edu.

WHAT IS AGGRESSION REPLACEMENT TRAINING?

Aggression Replacement Training (ART) is a multimodal treatment designed for adolescents with histories of disruptive, aggressive, and antisocial behavior (Glick and Gibbs, 2011; Reddy and Goldstein, 2001). ART is founded on the premise that adolescents who engage in antisocial acts lack the behavioral, affective, and cognitive skills that underlie prosocial actions. Instead, these adolescents show delays in social skills, social problem-solving, emotion regulation, and moral reasoning that interfere with their ability to engage in compliant, constructive behaviors. Furthermore, disruptive and aggressive behavior is sometimes modeled and reinforced by other people in these adolescents' lives, especially family members and peers (Goldstein, 2002).

In ART, adolescents engage in structured group activities designed to teach behavioral, emotional, and cognitive skills (Glick, 2006; Goldstein and Martens, 2000; Hollin, 2004). These skills are systematically taught using a system of modeling, behavioral rehearsal, and social reinforcement. Specifically, ART consists of three components: skillstreaming, anger control training, and moral reasoning training.

The goal of skillstreaming, the behavioral component of ART, is to enhance prosocial skills that help adolescents avoid arguments and aggressive displays and promote social competence (Goldstein, 1997). These skills are taught in small groups through a combination of modeling, roleplay, reinforcement and feedback, and transfer to other settings. Skills fall into six categories: beginning social skills (e.g., listening), advanced social skills (e.g., apologizing), skills for dealing with feelings (e.g., understanding the feelings of others), skill alternatives to aggression (e.g., keeping out of fights), skills for dealing with stress (e.g., dealing with group pressure), and skills related to planning (e.g., setting a goal).

Skillstreaming is a structured, psychoeducational activity. First, a skill is introduced by the facilitator and defined by the group. It is important for the group members to collectively synthesize a definition of the skill and outline the behavioral steps needed to practice it. Second, the skill is modeled by the facilitator in a fashion that clearly follows each step. The facilitator then prompts each group member to identify with whom they might utilize the skill in their everyday life.

Next, a volunteer is selected from the group to roleplay the skill. The volunteer describes a real-life situation in which he or she might practice the skill and gives details about the setting, preceding events, and feelings of everyone involved. The volunteer assumes the role of the main actor and chooses another group member to play the part of the individual with whom he or she might use the skill. The pair rehearses their roleplay outside the group setting, reviewing each step of the skill with the facilitator. While the pair rehearses, a second facilitator asks other members to carefully observe the roleplay and evaluate each step of the skill, so that they might later provide feedback to the actors. When ready, the actors return to the group and perform the roleplay. The observers, the actors, and the facilitator, in turn, provide feedback on the main actor's ability to use the skill. The roleplay and feedback process is repeated until all group members have the opportunity to practice the skill. Then, the facilitator asks each group member to practice the skill outside the group and reflect on the outcome of this practice.

Anger control training comprises the emotion-regulation component of ART (Feindler and Engel, 2011; Hollin and Bloxsom, 2007; Novaco, 1975). A primary goal of anger control training is to help adolescents understand the Angry Behavior Cycle—a model for the external triggers and internal cues that prompt adolescents' anger. The group first discusses and roleplays situations that trigger anger. Once group members have identified their triggers, the facilitator encourages them to recognize what physiological markers serve as cues that they are angry. Next, anger-reducing techniques, such as deep breathing, are presented and practiced. Members are also taught to use "reminders"--self-statements designed to decrease arousal, such as *"Take it easy, he didn't mean to bump into me on purpose."* Group members are also encouraged to identify and use skillstreaming techniques to solve social problems and avoid angry/aggressive displays. In later sessions, facilitators teach "self-evaluation," in which adolescents review their handling of a conflict, reward themselves for successfully avoiding anger, or find ways to deal with social problems more effectively in the future. Throughout anger control training, these triggers, cues, reducers, reminders, skillstreaming applications, and self-evaluation skills are practiced step-by-step via roleplay and feedback.

The final element of ART is moral reasoning training (Arbuthnot and Gordon, 1986; Gibbs, 2010; Palmer, 2007). The goal of moral reasoning training is to move group members from immature moral reasoning to more advanced Kohlbergian stages of moral development. Facilitators provide the group with a relatable story in which an adolescent encounters a moral dilemma (e.g., cheating, stealing, fighting). Group members discuss questions posed by facilitators, which highlight cognitive distortions, moral values, and the rights and feelings of others. During the course of discussion, facilitators attempt to create a state of disequilibration, or cognitive tension, among group members, prompting them to adopt more mature, less egocentric moral decision making.

EVALUATIONS OF ART

Considerable research has been directed at examining the efficacy and effectiveness of ART with aggressive children, adolescents, and young adults. ART has also been evaluated in a wide range of treatment settings (e.g., prisons, residential centers, schools) and in different cultures. Overall, results indicate associations between ART and improvements in socioemotional functioning and behavior. However, inconsistent findings and limitations in the designs of these evaluation studies suggest caution when inferring a causal relationship between ART and these beneficial outcomes (Amendola and Oliver, 2010; Glick and Gibbs, 2011; Gundersen and Scartdal, 2009).

Original Evaluations

The first evaluation of ART (Goldstein and Glick, 1987) was conducted by its developers at Annsville Youth Center, a residential facility in New York State for adolescent boys arrested for assault, burglary, theft, robbery, and similar crimes. Youths were randomly assigned to one of three conditions: (a) ART, (b) a brief instructions control group, designed to control for youths' motivation to complete posttest measures in a positive manner, or (c) a no-treatment control condition.

The evaluation yielded mostly positive results. Adolescents who participated in ART demonstrated knowledge of five of the ten social skills presented during training; furthermore, these adolescents were able to apply three out of the ten skills to new social situations. Adolescents who received treatment did not differ in moral reasoning compared to youths in the control groups. However, staff members reported less disruptiveness and impulsiveness among youths in the treatment condition compared to controls. The researchers also examined the outcomes of a nonrandom sample of 54 youths, three months after release. Youth service workers reported significantly greater adjustment in the community for youths who received ART than controls.

A second evaluation (Goldstein and Glick, 1987), conducted at the MacCormick Youth Center, was designed to replicate the first evaluation with a new sample of youths convicted of more serious felonies (e.g., murder, rape, assault). Social skill outcomes were similar to the first evaluation. Youths who received ART demonstrated knowledge of four of the ten social skills presented during training, and were able to apply three of the ten skills to new situations. Outcomes for moral reasoning and behavior problems diverged from the first evaluation. In contrast to Annsville, youths who received ART at MacCormick showed significantly higher moral reasoning scores than controls. Also in contrast to Annsville, youths who received ART at MacCormick did not show reduced disruptiveness or impulsiveness compared to controls. The authors speculate that this lack of behavioral change might be due to the fact that MacCormick was a locked facility; youths may not have had opportunities to engage in disruptive or impulsive behavior.

A third evaluation (Goldstein, Glick, Irwin, Pask-McCartney, and Rubama, 1989) was conducted with a community-based sample of 84 antisocial adolescents recently released from residential treatment. Youths were assigned to one of three conditions: (a) ART, (b) ART plus a modified ART program for parents and other family members, or (c) a no-treatment control condition. The authors reasoned that involving parents in ART might help them recognize and reinforce their adolescents' use of social and anger management skills at home. Consequently, caregivers engaged in skillstreaming and anger control exercises similar to youths.

Results showed that youths who participated in either of the two treatment conditions reported significantly greater social skills and anger management than controls. There were no differences in self-report outcomes across the treatment conditions. Six months after release from residential treatment, there were no significant differences in recidivism for youths assigned to ART (15%), ART plus caregiver sessions (30%), and controls (43%).

The final evaluation (Goldstein and Glick, 1994) was also conducted in the community. Young adult gang members ($N = 65$) were assigned to either ART or to a no-treatment control condition. Results were mixed. Therapists who administered ART reported significantly greater interpersonal skills among youths who participated in ART than controls. However, youths who received ART reported no differences in their capacity to manage anger compared to controls. Furthermore, youths in the ART group differed from comparison youths in only one of five behavioral outcomes. Specifically, youths who received ART had superior work-related outcomes; there were no differences in home and family, school, peer, and legal outcomes across conditions. Recidivism outcomes were more positive. Youths who participated in ART were less likely to be arrested (13%) than comparison youths (52%) eight months after the beginning of the study.

Peer-Reviewed Evaluations in the United States

The first evaluations of ART, conducted by its developers, provided initial evidence that it can help adolescents acquire and apply social skills and regulate their emotions. Three independent evaluation studies have also been published examining ART. These studies are noteworthy because, unlike the original studies, they were conducted by independent researchers and published in peer-reviewed journals. The first study examined 39 adolescents in residential treatment (Coleman, Pfeiffer, and Oakland, 1992). Most adolescents had histories of conduct problems. Adolescents were randomly assigned to 10 weeks of ART or to traditional residential treatment. Adolescents who participated in ART showed increased knowledge of social skills; however, adolescents in the treatment and control conditions showed similar outcomes on all other measures. Specifically, staff members reported no differences in observed social skills, anger and aggression, or overall behavior problems across groups. Furthermore, adolescents in the treatment group showed no differences in moral reasoning compared to controls.

Leeman, Gibbs, and Fuller (1993) found more tangible benefits of ART in their evaluation of 57 adolescent boys assigned to a medium security correctional facility. Most adolescents had violated parole or committed less serious felonies (e.g., breaking and entering, burglary). Youths were randomly assigned to one of three conditions: treatment, simple control, or motivational control. The treatment program, entitled EQUIP, combined ART with daily group meetings designed to foster social support and positive peer culture among residents. Youths in the simple control condition completed pre- and post-treatment measures only. Youths in the motivational control condition also completed pre- and post-treatment measures, but were told that their behavior would be assessed during treatment.

Youths in the treatment condition reported significantly greater social skills and fewer behavior problems than youths in the control conditions. Furthermore, staff members observed fewer behavior problems and unexpected school absences among youths in the treatment condition than controls. No differences in moral reasoning were observed across groups. Six months after release, youths in the treatment group showed comparable recidivism rates as youths in the control groups. However, one year after release, recidivism was significantly lower for youths in the treatment (15%) compared to the control (40.5%) conditions.

A final evaluation examined the effectiveness of ART in reducing disruptive behavior among adolescents living in a runaway shelter (Nugent, Bruley, and Allen, 1999; Nugent and Ely, 2010). The researchers used an interrupted time-series design, investigating changes in therapist-reported behavior problems among adolescents in the shelter before and after the implementation of ART. Data from 522 homeless adolescents were analyzed. A condensed version of ART was administered, consisting of social skills and anger control training only. Results varied as a function of gender. Girls showed a significant (29.4%) reduction in disruptive behavior over time; however, the reduction in boys' disruptive behavior (14%) was not significant. Regression analyses revealed that the number of other males in the shelter moderated the effects of ART on boys' outcomes. Specifically, ART significantly reduced boys' disruptive behavior only when there were fewer than nine other boys in the shelter.

Peer-Reviewed Evaluations in Europe

Several other evaluations of ART have been conducted in Europe. The first published evaluation examined the effects of ART on 39 Norwegian youths referred by teachers because of behavior problems or social skill deficits (Moynahan and Stromgren, 2005). Youths were randomly assigned to either a modified version of ART or to a no-treatment control group. Results varied as a function of age. Children who participated in ART showed a significant increase in teacher-reported social skills and decrease in teacher-reported behavior problems over time. In contrast, adolescents who participated in ART showed no change in skills or behavior. Unfortunately, analyses examining between-group differences in outcomes were not reported.

A second Norwegian study also explored the use of ART with children and young adolescents displaying behavior problems or social skill deficits (Gundersen and Svartdal, 2010). Youths ($N = 140$) were randomly assigned to either ART or to a no-treatment control condition. Results showed significant increases in parent- and teacher-reported social skills for youths in both conditions. Teachers also reported significant reductions in disruptive behavior among children in both groups. Parents reported significant reductions in disruptive behavior among youths in the ART condition only. As in the previous study, analyses examining between-group differences in outcomes were not reported.

In a third Norwegian study, Gundersen and Svartdal (2006) also examined the effects of ART on youths showing disruptive behavior or social skill deficits. However, in this study, the researchers examined outcomes both within and between groups. Youths ($N = 65$) were randomly assigned to two conditions: 24 sessions of ART or standard social and educational services. Outcomes were assessed after treatment based on parent-, teacher-, and youth-report questionnaires. Results varied as a function of outcome measure and informant. Parents of youths in the ART condition reported greater improvement in children's social skills than parents of youths in the control condition. However, no such improvements were reported by teachers or children. Similarly, the researchers were unable to detect significant treatment x time interactions for youths' disruptive behavior (as assessed by any informant) or youths' social problem-solving ability.

Recently, a Swedish study (Holmqvist, Hill, and Lang, 2009) compared ART to more traditional, supportive psychotherapy for adolescent offenders. Fifty-seven older adolescent offenders participated in either (a) ART plus token economy or (b) supportive psychotherapy that emphasized empathy with a trusted adult. Both interventions were administered in residential treatment facilities. Average duration of treatment was 14 months; consequently, youths in the ART condition participated in the program repeatedly. One and two years after release, there were no differences in overall recidivism, severity of reoffense, or frequency of reoffense across treatment groups.

Another evaluation, conducted in Great Britain, examined young adult male offenders assigned to community rehabilitation (Hatcher et al., 2008). Fifty-three offenders ordered to participate in ART were compared to 53 offenders matched according to age, offense, and number of previous convictions. Recidivism was assessed 10 months after treatment. Results showed no significant differences in recidivism for adults who were assigned to ART (39.2%) and matched controls (50.9%). Closer inspection showed that many individuals assigned to ART did not complete the program. Furthermore, outcomes varied as a function of completion status. Specifically, recidivism was lowest among adults who completed ART

(20%). Adults assigned to ART but who never began the program (36%) and adults who withdrew from ART after beginning it (61.5%) showed higher recidivism.

Finally, Dutch researchers examined the effectiveness of ART for adult offenders (Hornsveld, 2004; Hornsveld, Nijman, Hollin, and Kraaimaat, 2008). In their first study, 25 adults with histories of violent offending were examined over time. All participants received ART. Results showed no significant change in self-reported, other-reported, or observational measures of anger and disruptive behavior over time. In a second study, 38 adult offenders who received ART were compared to a matched sample of controls. All participants were inpatients at a forensic psychiatric hospital. Outcomes were based on observations of participants' behavior in the facility. Patients who received ART showed greater reduction in aggressive behavior than controls. However, no differences were seen across groups on any other outcome measure. Furthermore, participants in both groups showed a significant *decrease* in social skills over the course of treatment.

Large Community-Based Evaluations

The effectiveness of ART has also been evaluated in several large community-based interventions. The strength of these evaluations is that they involve large numbers of aggressive youths and, consequently, have sufficient power to detect beneficial treatment outcomes. The chief weaknesses of these studies are twofold. First, all are quasi-experimental or rely on within-subjects analyses to evaluate outcomes. Consequently, they suffer from threats to internal validity making causal statements regarding the merits of ART tentative. Second, none have been adequately peer reviewed.

McGuire and Clark (1994) describe the implementation of ART in England. Adult offenders ($N= 153$) who received ART were compared to a matched sample of controls. Recidivism, using government arrest records, was assessed after one year. Results suggested differences in recidivism between adults who received ART (20.4%) and controls (34.5%), although inferential statistics were not reported.

A similar study, examining 283 adolescent offenders was conducted in the United States (Hosley, 2005). Adolescents were referred to ART by probation officers or the local juvenile court. Most youths had histories of family conflict, truancy, or aggressive behavior. Youths participated in ART in residential settings, school-based treatment programs, or outpatient clinics. Three months after treatment, youths reported significant improvements in social skills and significant reductions in anger and aggression. Youths did not report significant improvement in interpersonal functioning, however. One year after treatment, 32% of adolescents who received ART had reoffended (Ramsey County Community Corrections, 2005). This percentage was higher than the overall rate of reoffending for youths on probation (21%) but comparable to the rate of reoffending for similar youths referred to other multimodal treatments (29%).

In 1997, the Washington State Legislature passed the Community Juvenile Accountability Act which initiated the adoption of several evidence-based interventions for youths with antisocial behavior (Barnoski, 2004). The most frequently adopted intervention was ART. Approximately 1200 youths were assigned by juvenile courts, on a nonrandom basis, to receive either ART or regular child and family services. Recidivism was assessed at

18 months. Results showed no significant differences between youths who received ART and controls in terms of overall recidivism, felonies, or violent felonies.

After data analysis had begun, the researchers retrospectively classified each juvenile court as either "competently" or "not competently" administering ART. Then, the researchers reevaluated outcome data, comparing only "competent" ART programs with youths in the control condition. Results of the reevaluation continued to show no significant differences in total recidivism and violent felony recidivism across "competent" ART programs and control groups. However, reevaluation did indicate that youths who received "competent" ART showed lower recidivism for nonviolent felonies (18.8%) than controls (24.8%).

A larger and more recent evaluation was conducted by the California Institute for Mental Health (Mitchell, 2010). This evaluation included approximately 4,700 youths who received ART in juvenile justice centers, residential treatment facilities, alternative schools, or the community. All youths received ART; no control group was used. Results, based largely on youths' self-reports, were positive. Youths reported significant increases in both direct and generalized social skills over time. Youths also reported increased capacity for anger control and moral reasoning. Finally, youths reported reductions in behavioral and emotional problems. In general, youths who received treatment in correctional or residential facilities reported greater improvement than youths who received ART in the community.

Most recently, Amendola and Oliver (2010) provide initial findings of their evaluation of ART at Perseus House, an agency that delivers mental health services to youths in Pennsylvania. Youths received ART during residential ($n=300$) or community-based treatment ($n=599$). Their analyses examined changes in functioning before and after treatment; no control group was used. Results suggested improvements in youths' self-reported social skills, anger control, and moral reasoning, although inferential statistics were not provided.

Unpublished Studies

At least 14 unpublished theses or dissertations address the effectiveness of ART (Table 1). The most consistent result of these studies is that ART is associated with increased social skills or prosocial behavior. In contrast, only two studies indicate that ART is associated with a significant reduction in anger or other behavior problems. None of the studies demonstrate increased moral reasoning or decreased recidivism associated with ART. The lack of random assignment and adequate control groups limit the conclusions that can be drawn from these studies.

Summary of ART Evaluations

The first evaluations of ART, conducted by its developers, were encouraging (Goldstein and Glick, 1987, 1994; Goldstein et al., 1989). Overall, youths who participated in ART showed moderate acquisition and application of social skills compared to comparison youths who did not receive ART. Furthermore, in half of the studies, youths also showed increased anger control, improved moral reasoning, and decreased recidivism.

Table 1. Unpublished Theses and Dissertations Evaluating ART

Author (Year)	Treatment/Participants	N	Design	Results
Barto (1995)	ART; adult offenders	57	3	Increased social skills; decreased moral reasoning; no change in hostility/aggression
Billings (2003)	Brief ART; adolescent offenders	21	3	Decreased parent- and youth-reported behavior problems on 50% outcomes measures
Byrne (2008)	ART + goal setting; middle school	36	2	Increased child-reported social competence
Cleare (2001)	ART; residential, aggressive girls	27	3	Increased observed positive behavior; no change in behavior problems, aggression
Currie (2010)	ART; older adolescent offenders	20	3	Increased self-reported social skills; no change in observed behavior problems
Curulla (1991)	Modified ART; adult offenders	67	3	No differences in recidivism, anger/aggression, or moral reasoning
Gonzalez (2008)	ART; gang members and families	15	3	Improved communication; increased anger/provocation (youth- and parent-report)
Jackson (1991)	Modified ART; disruptive adolescents	40	1	Decreased youth-reported anger; no differences in parent-reported physical aggression
Kennedy (1990)	ART; adult offenders	37	3	Decreased self-reported anger, criminal sentiments; no change in observed behavior
Metz (1996)	ART; adolescent offenders	54	3	No differences in problem-solving, moral reasoning, or observed behavior problems
Nodarse (1997)	ART; youths w/ emotional problems	50	3	Increase social skills, decreased aggression (teacher-reported)
Roberts (2009)	ART; adolescent offenders	511	3	No differences in self-reported attitudes toward violence and guns
Torchin (2003)	ART; adolescents on probation	21	3	No changes in social skills, anger/aggression, or recidivism
Zimmerman (1987)	ART; adolescent offenders	36	1	Increased social skills; no differences in moral reasoning, behavior control or problems

Note. Design: (1) random assignment, between-group analyses reported; (2) random assignment, within-group analyses reported; (3) quasi-experimental. Participants in Zimmerman (1987) may overlap with participants in Goldstein and Glick's (1987) evaluation at Annsville.

The results of independent, peer-reviewed evaluations of ART conducted in the United States were more mixed (Coleman et al., 1992; Leeman et al., 1993; Nugent et al., 1999; Nugent and Ely, 2010). On one hand, these studies also showed increased social skill acquisition associated with ART.

On the other hand, the effects of ART on observed behavior was inconsistent. Furthermore, none of the studies showed increased moral reasoning associated with ART.

European evaluations of ART also yielded mixed results (Gundersen and Svartdal, 2006, 2010; Hatcher et al., 2008; Holmquist et al., 2009; Hornsveld et al., 2008; Moynahan and Stromgren, 2005). The Norwegian studies provide initial evidence that ART can be administered to young children and that ART is associated with improvements in teacher- and parent-reported behavior and social competence. The effects of ART on older adolescents are less consistent, with two studies showing no significant improvement over time or no improvement relative to controls. Studies investigating the effects of ART with adult offenders also show mixed results. Whereas the Dutch studies suggest that ART is helpful in reducing aggressive behavior among adult offenders participating in residential treatment, the study conducted in Great Britain indicates no effects of ART on recidivism after release.

Finally, the results of large-scale evaluations are promising and suggest that ART is helpful in improving youths' self-reported social skills, anger control capacities, and sociomoral reasoning (Amendola and Oliver, 2010; Barnoski, 2004; Hosley, 2005; McGuire and Clark, 1994; Mitchell, 2010). The effects of ART on recidivism are less clear. Overall, community-based evaluations provide little evidence that ART affects recidivism overall; however, competently administered ART programs are associated with a reduction in non-violent felonies.

Evidence-based treatment programs can be categorized based on their research design and empirical support (Amendola and Oliver, 2010; Nathan and Gorman, 2002). Researchers, practitioners, and policymakers can have greater confidence in interventions whose support is based on studies relying on carefully controlled, reliable, and valid measurement. In general, four levels of empirical support are possible:

- Efficacious programs: These programs yield positive outcomes under carefully controlled settings. Studies are characterized by random assignment to treatment and control groups, between-group outcome analyses, and high treatment fidelity. Outcomes have also been replicated by independent researchers.
- Effective programs: These programs yield positive outcomes under usual care settings (e.g., hospitals, clinics, residential facilities). Studies are characterized by random assignment, between-group outcome analyses, and acceptable treatment fidelity. Outcomes may or may not be replicated by independent researchers.
- Model programs: These programs yield generally positive outcomes, although some outcomes can be mixed. Studies are often quasi-experimental (e.g., matched comparison groups) although they usually include between-group outcome analyses. Outcomes may not be replicated by independent researchers.
- Promising programs: These programs are believed to yield positive outcomes based on either empirical evidence or expert consensus. Empirical data come largely from quasi-experimental studies using within-group (pre- vs. post-treatment) outcome analyses.

Currently, ART is classified as a "Model Program" by the United States Office of Juvenile Justice and Delinquency Prevention and is classified as a "Promising Program" by the United States Department of Education (Glick and Gibbs, 2011). These classifications appear to be based on the multiple empirical research studies demonstrating that ART is associated with increased social skills, decreased angry and aggressive displays, and (less frequently) improved moral reasoning. At this time, ART is not yet considered "Efficacious" or "Effective."

Statements regarding ART's empirical support and clinical utility must be made cautiously. Research investigating ART is limited in several ways. First, most research evaluating ART is based on quasi-experimental research or studies without adequate control groups. Indeed, many studies evaluate outcomes using only within-subjects (pre- vs. post-treatment) analyses. Carefully controlled experimental studies, characterized by random assignment to treatment and control conditions, are needed to demonstrate causality between ART and improvements in participants' functioning.

Second, most empirical evaluations of ART are not presented in peer-reviewed publications. Rather, the majority of results are only available in book chapters, government reports, or unpublished works. Professionals typically have greater confidence in results presented in peer-reviewed journals given the independent scrutiny of these publications.

Third, ART appears to have differential effects on participants' social skills, anger control, and moral reasoning. Overall, ART is most consistently associated with significant improvements in participants' social skills. Fewer studies demonstrate associations between ART and reductions in anger, aggression, or disruptive behavior. Even fewer studies show improvements in moral reasoning associated with ART. These findings are similar to the results of several meta-analyses examining the efficacy of psychosocial treatments for youths with social deficits or behavioral problems. Overall, interventions that target social skills or overt behavior yield larger effect sizes than interventions characterized by anger management, mood regulation, or moral education (Lipsey and Wilson, 1998; McGuire, 2008; Sukhodolsky, Kassinove, and Gorman, 2004; Wilson and Lipsey, 2007). Although ART may target social skills, anger control, and moral reasoning, its effects on these targets may be unequal.

Outcomes also seem to vary as a function of informant. Although there is considerable heterogeneity in findings, ART is most often associated with positive outcomes when these outcomes are based on participants' self-reports. Although two of the earliest evaluations showed improvements in social skills, anger control, and moral reasoning based on objective tests, most of the later studies relied on self-report instruments to evaluate these constructs. Fewer studies demonstrated benefits when outcomes were assessed based on parent-report, teacher-report, observed behavior, or recidivism. Differential outcomes as a function of informant have also been reported in several meta-analyses of treatment for disruptive youths. Overall, antisocial youths tend to show better outcomes when assessed by self-report compared to parental-report, observation, or other objective measures (Quinn, Kavale, Mathur, Rutherford, and Forness, 1999; Sukhodolsky et al., 2004).

Finally, some data suggest possible iatrogenic effects of ART when administered to adult offenders. Hornsveld and colleagues (2008) found decreased social skills among incarcerated adults who participated in ART. Similarly, Barto (1995) found decreased sociomoral reasoning among adult offenders who received ART. Finally, Hatcher and colleagues (2008) found increased recidivism among adults who began ART but did not successfully complete treatment. It is possible that ART, a group-based intervention, can provide antisocial adults opportunities to model and reinforce maladaptive thoughts, feelings, and actions during the course of treatment, especially if treatment is not carried to completion. Similar iatrogenic effects of group therapy for antisocial youths have been reported in some studies (Dishion, Poulin, and Burraston, 2001; Macgowan and Wagner, 2005) but not others (Weiss et al., 2005). Clinicians should be mindful of possible deleterious outcomes, especially for adult offenders who withdraw from ART prematurely.

Taken together, the evidence supports the notion that ART is a promising, model approach to helping children and adolescents with disruptive behavior problems. Its strengths rest in its integrated interventions based on behavioral, social learning, and developmental theory; its clear objectives, strategies and tactics; and its emphasis on systematic measurement to evaluate outcomes. ART deserves attention from researchers and clinicians interested in establishing it as an effective or efficacious intervention for at-risk youths.

ADMINISTERING ART TO FAMILIES

Family ART

The developers of ART emphasized the importance of involving parents and other caregivers in therapy (Goldstein et al., 1988). Parental involvement was considered valuable because caregivers can model and reinforce skills introduced to adolescents during ART. Most recently, Glick and Gibbs (2011) restated the importance of parental involvement in the transfer of social skills, anger control strategies, and moral reasoning from treatment facility to home and community:

"Real-life reinforcement…is critically important and takes some effort on the part of group facilitators. At times, group members are encouraged to use the skill situation outside the session with individuals who will be likely to provide reinforcement and to persist if they do not get what they desire in the first instance. Persons in the group members' real-life environment can also be assisted in providing coaching and reinforcement" (p. 36).

In traditional therapy, parental involvement is typically accomplished through periodic consultations (e.g., meetings, telephone calls) and written homework assignments. However, the creators of ART began developing ways to include systematic involvement from parents and other caregivers in their treatment.

As previously described, Goldstein and colleagues (1989) piloted a family ART program for aggressive adolescents recently released from residential treatment. As in traditional ART, adolescents participated in 10 group sessions of social skill, anger management, and moral education training. In addition, parents and other family members were invited to participate in group sessions for caregivers. Each parent session included: (a) a review of the week's activities, including parents' ability to reinforce skills discussed during the previous session; (b) social skill, problem-solving, and anger control training; and (c) activities to foster group cohesiveness. The topics for parent sessions were typically generated by parents themselves. Therapists tended to emphasize the importance of recognizing and reinforcing social skills and emotion-regulation techniques used by adolescents at home. A secondary goal of parent sessions was to foster a sense of social support among caregivers.

The program was evaluated by comparing outcomes of youths who participated in ART, ART plus parent sessions, and no-treatment controls. Results showed significant improvements in interpersonal skills and anger control for youths in the two treatment groups compared to controls. However, the addition of parent sessions did not yield benefits above and beyond ART alone. Furthermore, there was only a trend toward reduced recidivism among youths who participated in ART plus parent sessions (15%), ART alone (30%), and controls (43%). It is possible that the lack of differential outcomes across the two treatment groups can be attributed to poor adherence among parents. The authors report that many parents did not attend sessions and, instead, received individual home visits or telephone calls from therapists to replace missed sessions.

Despite generally positive outcomes, very little research was directed at investigating the efficacy of family-based ART programs. One exception has been the development of "Family ART" at Batshaw Youth and Family Centres in Montreal (Calame et al., 2001; Calame and Parker, 2003; 2004). The goal of Family ART is to involve parents in adolescents' skill development to maximize the transfer of skills from therapy to home. This goal is achieved by fostering social support among parents, introducing them to many of the skills taught to adolescents, and encouraging them to model, identify, and reinforce these skills at home with their youths.

During the first three sessions of Family ART, adolescent and parent groups are separated. While adolescents practice skill acquisition, anger management, and moral reasoning, parents discuss events that prompted their adolescents' treatment referral. Later, parents discuss positive aspects of their adolescents. Next, parents are introduced to many of the same social skills that their adolescents are developing. Parents may focus on additional skills depending on their needs and interests.

For the remaining sessions, parent and adolescent groups are brought together. The focus of combined sessions is learning about and roleplaying the Angry Behavior Cycle--a model for hostile-coercive interactions in the family. Parents and adolescents identify behaviors that each member of the dyad does to make the other angry.

Then, dyads roleplay events that occur at home, showing how these behaviors trigger anger and hostility. Later, parents and adolescents practice social and anger management skills to avoid these triggers and promise to use these skills at home. Subsequent sessions are spent managing families' progress learning and applying skills outside the therapy setting.

Unfortunately, there has been little published research examining the outcomes of family-based approaches to ART (Calame and Parker, 2004; Gonzalez, 2008). Consequently, we now describe a new family-based intervention that is based on ART than might have promise for disruptive youths and their caregivers.

Adolescent and Family Anger Management

Adolescent and Family Anger Management (AFAM) is a 10-session, community-based program designed for delinquent adolescents. It is currently used by a juvenile court in central Ohio. Court-involved adolescents may be referred to AFAM by their probation officers or the juvenile court. Participation is typically compulsory.

AFAM is based on other family-based ART programs (Calame and Parker, 2004; Goldstein et al., 1989). AFAM requires the participation of at least one parent or guardian.

Parents assume the role of "coach" for their adolescent. The theoretical foundation of AFAM, like traditional ART, is that aggression is primarily a learned behavior; therefore, parents have the opportunity to influence their adolescent's aggressive tendencies by modeling and reinforcing social and anger management skills at home.

AFAM is also designed to help parents develop their own capacities for emotion regulation, problem-solving, and parenting skills which can help alleviate family discord. Considerable research indicates that many parents of aggressive youths have skill deficits that increase the likelihood that they will contribute to their children's behavior problems (Conger, Neppl, Kim, and Scaramella, 2003; Kimonis and Frick, 2010). For example, the caregivers of disruptive youths often have unrealistic expectations for their children, interpret their children's misbehavior as deliberately hostile, show rigid problem-solving strategies, engage in hostile-coercive discipline techniques, and experience high levels of parenting stress (Stern and Azar, 1998). Interventions which address these deficits in parents and children together appear to yield greater benefits than interventions designed for youths alone (Henggeler and Schaeffer, 2010; Kazdin, 2010; Lochman, Boxmeyer, Powell, Barry, and Pardini, 2010; Webster-Stratton and Reid, 2010).

There are two AFAM facilitators: one directs adolescents, the other leads parents. At the start of every session, adolescents and parents gather in a large classroom for "check-in." Each adolescent describes one positive action that his or her parent has done in the past week, and each parent shares one positive action by his or her adolescent. These reports provide an opportunity for affective sharing and permit facilitators to gauge how well skills are being implemented at home.

For the first 4-6 sessions of AFAM, parents and adolescents are separated after "check in." Each group is then introduced to the three components of AFAM which are modeled after traditional ART: social skills training, anger control training, and character trait education.

All groups learn four "core" social skills: *listening*, *negotiating*, *understanding your own feelings*, and *understanding the feelings of others*. Other skills are selected from ART skillstreaming techniques based on the needs and interests of families. Skills are first explained by a facilitator and modeled by the facilitator and a volunteer. Then group members identify situations in which they might use skills at home. Finally, in pairs, group members roleplay these situations and receive feedback from each other and the facilitator.

Parents and adolescents also learn anger control techniques. Specifically, facilitators teach adolescents and parents about external and internal triggers for anger, body cues (physical signs) of anger, reducers (techniques to decrease anger), reminders (self-statements to increase positive feelings), and thinking-ahead strategies to help individuals consider the consequences of their actions.

Each component of the anger control sequence is introduced, discussed, and roleplayed. In addition, participants learn four cognitive errors that often predispose them toward anger: *minimizing*, *self-centered thinking*, *assuming the worst*, and *blaming others*. Each error is introduced and discussed by groups. Then, facilitators teach group members how to challenge each maladaptive way of thinking and replace it with more realistic cognitions.

The character trait component of AFAM differs from the moral training component of ART. AFAM character trait education begins by asking participants to complete a "traits inventory." Specifically, participants review a list of prosocial traits and identify traits they would like to improve (e.g., patience, honesty, responsibility, gratitude). In later sessions, group members listen to and discuss stories that exemplify specific character traits. Group members are also asked to report instances in which they observed certain prosocial traits in their everyday lives. Finally, participants develop strategies to practice desired character traits and reinforce family members and peers for prosocial behaviors.

In later sessions, adolescent and parent groups meet conjointly. Many activities that occur during conjoint sessions introduce members to new social skills or provide opportunities for dyads to roleplay previously-learned skills together. Other activities focus on how dyads might model and reinforce social skills or anger control techniques at home. Still other activities focus on ways to recognize and encourage prosocial behaviors in the family. All skills and techniques are first modeled by a facilitator and volunteer. Then, adolescent-parent pairs rehearse scenarios in which they might utilize each skill. Finally, family teams present and receive feedback from the entire group on their skill development.

EVALUATION OF AFAM

Involving parents in ART may improve the outcomes of youths who participate in this program. A family-based ART program may not only help generalize skills acquired in the clinic to the home and community, but also educate and support parents as they work to manage their adolescents' disruptive behavior. Unfortunately, besides an early pilot study of family-based ART (Goldstein et al., 1989), little empirical research has investigated the efficacy of providing skillstreaming, anger management training, and moral education to adolescents and parents together.

The purpose of our study was to investigate the effectiveness of AFAM as a means to reduce behavior problems, improve social skills, and decrease recidivism among court-involved adolescents. We conducted an experimental study comparing disruptive youths assigned to AFAM with youths assigned to traditional individual psychotherapy by a juvenile court (i.e., treatment-as-usual, TAU). We assessed adolescents' behavior problems and social functioning before and after treatment. We also assessed recidivism 24 months after treatment completion.

We expected that adolescents in both the AFAM and TAU conditions would display significant reductions on behavior problems and increases in social skills over time. Furthermore, we expected youths' psychosocial outcomes and recidivism to be similar across groups. These findings would suggest that AFAM is a viable alternative to individual counseling as it is typically administered by mental health practitioners working in a juvenile justice setting.

METHOD

Participants. Fifty adolescents (56% boys) involved in the juvenile justice system and living in the community participated in this study. Adolescents ranged in age from 12 to 17 years (M=15.69, SD=1.56). All but one youth reported European-American ethnicity. Adolescents were classified based on severity of their most recent offense: police involvement only (2%), unruly behavior (8%), misdemeanor (86%), and felony (4%). The most common offenses were physical assault (24%), disorderly conduct (14%), domestic violence (14%), and theft (12%).

Measures. The Problem Oriented Screening Instrument for Teenagers (POSIT; Rahdert, 1991) was used to assess psychosocial functioning among adolescents who participated in AFAM. The POSIT is 139-item self-report instrument designed to measure behavior problems and competence (e.g., "*Do you get into fights a lot?*"). Adolescents answer items dichotomously (i.e., yes/no). Two scales were used in this study: the Mental Health Status Scale, a measure of behavioral and socioemotional problems, and the Social Skills Scale, a measure of social competence. Higher scores on the Mental Health Status Scale indicate more severe problems; higher scores on the Social Skills Scale indicate greater social competence. The POSIT demonstrates adequate internal consistency (αs = .70 - .88) and temporal stability over one week (rs = .72-.88). Convergent validity is supported by associations with other measures of psychological functioning. The POSIT differentiates youths with and without psychosocial problems, such as substance abuse and delinquency. Normative data from a large, nonclinical sample are available (Knight, Goodman, Pulerwitz, and DuRant, 2001).

The Ohio Youth Problem and Functioning Scales (Ohio Scales; Ogles et al., 2000) were used to assess psychosocial functioning among adolescents who participated in TAU. These scales consist of 40 self-report items designed to measure behavior problems and competence (e.g., "*Do you get into fights?*"). Adolescents rate items using a six-point Likert scale ranging from 0 (Not at all) to 5 (All of the time). A composite score is created by summing the ratings. Higher scores on the Problem Scale signify more severe problems; higher scores on the Functioning Scale indicate greater social competence. The Ohio Scales show adequate internal consistency (αs = .86 - .93) and temporal stability over two weeks (rs = .63-.72). Factorial validity is supported by exploratory factor analysis. Convergent validity is supported by correlations with other measures of adolescent functioning. Evidence of discriminative validity is provided by studies showing differences in scores between youths with and without behavior problems. Normative data from a large sample of youths from the community are reported.

Portions of the Ohio Youth Assessment System (OYAS; Latessa, Lovins, and Ostrowski, 2009) were administered to therapists to assess adolescents' risk of reoffending and attitudes toward treatment. The OYAS consists of a battery of questionnaires completed by youths, caregivers, and human-service personnel for adolescents referred to the Ohio Department of Youth. The risk assessment portion of the OYAS consists of "yes/no" items that predict likelihood of reoffending among youths referred to the juvenile justice system such as substance use history, gang membership, and association with delinquent peers (e.g., "History of substance abuse?"). Items are tallied to generate a risk score with higher values indicating greater risk for recidivism. The attitudes portion of the OYAS consists of four items, each scored on a 10-point Likert scale, which assess adolescents' attitudes toward treatment, supervision, and the criminal justice system (e.g., "Attitudes/beliefs toward the criminal justice system?"). Items are summed to generate a total score indicating more positive attitudes. Data supporting the ability of the OYAS to predict recidivism come from studies involving approximately 2500 court-involved youths.

Procedure. The evaluation was conducted by reviewing data collected by a juvenile court in central Ohio. Inclusionary criteria included (a) adolescent was 12-18 years of age at time of treatment, (2) adolescent became involved in the juvenile court because of antisocial, aggressive, or delinquent behavior, (3) adolescent participated in either AFAM or traditional individual psychotherapy provided by the juvenile court, (4) treatment was successfully completed more than 24 months prior to review, and (5) complete pretreatment, posttreatment, and recidivism data were available.

Adolescents were recruited by administrators and other personnel at the juvenile court. Parents provided consent and adolescents provided assent prior to their participation. The evaluation was approved by the university IRB.

Adolescents were randomly assigned to either AFAM or traditional individual therapy. Both interventions were provided by the juvenile court. AFAM consisted of 10 sessions, each consisting of group meetings for adolescents and caregivers.

The duration of individual therapy was determined by therapists and families. Therapists described their approach as "cognitive-behavior" or "eclectic" with the primary goals of establishing rapport, improving social functioning, and reducing displays of anger and aggression.

All adolescents completed a demographics measure and OYAS before treatment. Adolescents referred to AFAM completed the POSIT before treatment (baseline) and at termination. Adolescents referred to TAU completed the Ohio Scales before treatment (baseline) and at termination. Procedural changes at the juvenile court precluded using the same measure for youths in both groups.

To compare outcomes across groups, youths' scores were converted to z-scores, using norms for each measure. Z-scores are standardized scores that reflect the number of standard deviation individuals fall above or below the mean of the standardization sample, in this case, a large sample of non-referred youths.

Recidivism was defined as any court involvement within 24 months after completion of treatment. Recidivism was determined by court records and classified according to the same scale as pretreatment offenses. Time to recidivism was calculated by determining the interval between the end of treatment and the date of the youths' next court involvement, if any.

RESULTS

We performed a series of analyses examining possible differences across treatment conditions at baseline. There were more boys in the AFAM condition (63%) compared to the TAU condition (45%). However, a two-way contingency analysis indicated that the relationship between gender and treatment condition was not significant, Pearson $\chi^2(1, N=50)=1.64$, $p>.05$, $\varphi=.18$. Independent-samples t tests indicated no differences in age, $t(48)=.380$, $p>.05$, offense severity, $t(48)=1.58$, $p>.05$, psychosocial risk factors, $t(48)=1.50$, $p>.05$, or attitudes toward treatment, $t(48)=.067$, $p>.05$. However, youths in the AFAM condition participated in significantly fewer treatment sessions than youths in the TAU condition, $t(48)= -2.56$, $p=.014$, $d= -.47$ (Table 2). At baseline, there were no differences in behavior problems shown by youths in the AFAM ($M=1.13$, $SD=1.41$) and TAU ($M=1.06$, $SD=1.48$) conditions, $t(48)=.183$, $p>.05$. There were also no differences in youths' social competence across the AFAM ($M=-.684$, $SD=.844$) and TAU ($M=-.645$, $SD=.878$) conditions, $t(48)= -.159$, $p >.05$. We performed a one-away analysis of covariance (ANCOVA) to examine youths' behavioral outcomes as a function of treatment. The independent variable was condition with two levels: AFAM and TAU.

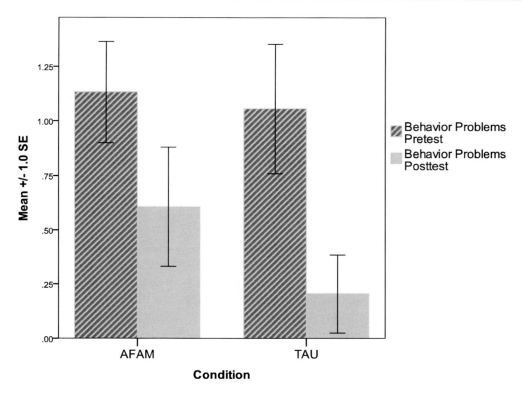

Figure 1. Behavior problems as a function of treatment condition. Both interventions resulted in significant reductions of behavior problems. There were no differences across interventions. The ordinate axis shows z-scores, which reflect standard deviations from the mean of the standardization sample.

The dependent variable was problem behaviors after treatment. Covariates included gender, severity of offense, and problem behaviors at baseline. Results indicated no differences in behavior outcomes across treatment conditions, $F(1,45)=.325$, $p>.05$, $\eta^2=.01$. Youths in both the AFAM, $t(29)=2.09$, $p=.045$, $d=.38$, and TAU, $t(19)=2.62$, $p=.017$, $d=.57$, conditions showed significant reductions in behavior problems over time (Figure 1). We performed a second ANCOVA to examine youths' social competence outcomes as a function of treatment. The independent variable was treatment condition. The dependent variable was social competence after treatment. Covariates included gender, severity of offense, and competence at baseline. As before, results showed no differences in competence outcomes across conditions, $F(1,45)=.225$, $p>.05$, $\eta^2=.01$. Youths in both the AFAM, $t(29)=-2.66$, $p=.013$, $d=.60$, and TAU, $t(19)=-2.25$, $p=.036$, $d=.58$, conditions showed significant increases in competence over time (Figure 2). We also performed a two-way contingency analysis examining differences in recidivism as a function of treatment. Twenty-four months after treatment, 36% of youths reoffended. However, results showed no differences in the number of youths who reoffended in the AFAM (40%) and TAU (30%) conditions, Pearson $\chi^2(1, N=50)=.470$, $p>.05$, $\varphi=.10$. Youths assigned to AFAM ($M=3.08$, $SD=.512$) and TAU ($M=3.00$, $SD=0.00$) showed similar severity of reoffending, $t(16)=.390$, $p>.05$. Furthermore, youths assigned to AFAM ($M=8.08$ months, $SD=6.58$ months) and TAU ($M=9.00$ months, $SD=7.29$ months) showed comparable time to recidivism, $t(16)=-.269$, $p>.05$.

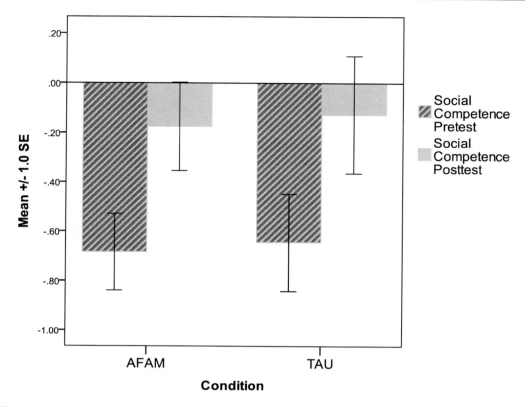

Figure 2. Social competence as a function of treatment condition. Both interventions resulted in significant improvements in social skills. There were no differences across interventions. The ordinate axis shows z-scores, which reflect standard deviations from the mean of the standardization sample.

DISCUSSION

Our findings suggest that AFAM is a viable means to reduce behavior problems, improve social functioning, and decrease recidivism among court-involved adolescents. Adolescents who participated in AFAM with their parents showed significant reductions in behavioral and socioemotional problems and significant increases in social skills. The magnitude of these effects was moderate (Lipsey and Wilson, 2001) and is comparable to the effect sizes produced by other behaviorally-based interventions for disruptive youths (Lipsey and Wilson, 1998; Wilson and Lipsey, 2007). Furthermore, adolescents who participated in AFAM moved from a state of clinically elevated behavior problems (i.e., >1SD) to within normal limits after treatment. Taken together, these findings suggest that AFAM is effective as it is typically delivered in a juvenile justice setting.

Our findings also indicate that the benefits of AFAM are comparable to those yielded by individual therapy. After controlling for baseline functioning and demographic/psychosocial risk, we observed no differences in youths' outcomes as a function of treatment type. We also observed similar recidivism among youths assigned to both treatments. These findings are important because they speak to the clinical utility of AFAM. First, they suggest that AFAM is at least as effective as other interventions used by mental health practitioners working for juvenile courts. Second, our data indicate that AFAM might yield benefits in a more time- and cost-efficient manner. Youths assigned to AFAM participated in significantly fewer sessions than youths assigned to TAU. Furthermore, AFAM was administered in group format, whereas TAU was individually-administered. Given the high costs of psychosocial interventions, and the difficulty families experience coordinating travel to and from sessions, AFAM might be an attractive alternative to traditional counseling.

Our study also suggests that the components of social skills training, anger control training, and character education can be successfully administered to groups of adolescents and their caregivers. Our data support the notion that a family-based approach to ART can be implemented to help this at-risk population. We believe group-based interventions that capitalize on the multimodal, cognitive-behavioral components of ART can be especially effective because they address systemic risk factors that often cause or maintain adolescents' defiant and aggressive behaviors. Because caregivers were introduced to the same skills as their adolescents, caregivers may be better able to recognize and reinforce their adolescents' attempts to use these skills at home. Perhaps more importantly, it is likely that many of the caregivers who participated in AFAM benefited themselves from the social skills training, emotional-regulation techniques, and prosocial strategies that were components of the program. Indeed, AFAM joins an increasing number of multimodal, evidence-based interventions which target the social problem-solving, anger management, and coping strategies of both adolescents and parents (Lochman and Wells, 2004; Stern and Azar, 1998).

Psychologists, social workers, and administrators working in juvenile justice settings have long recognized the merits of traditional ART as a means of reducing adolescent delinquency (Glick and Gibbs, 2011). The results of our study stress the importance of involving parents, as well as adolescents, in structured interventions involving skillstreaming, anger management training, and moral education (Stern and Azar, 1998). AFAM, and other family-based ART programs, join an ever-growing list of multimodal interventions designed for disruptive adolescents and their parents, such as Functional Family Therapy (FFT; Alexander and Robbins, 2010) and Multisystemic Therapy (MST; Sawyer and Borduin, 2011). Etiological models for adolescent aggression based on intrinsic variables have been abandoned in favor of more systemic models (Henggeler, 2011). It is certainly time for interventions to reflect these changes and to target not only adolescents, but families and communities as well.

Unfortunately, few mental health agencies (and still fewer independent clinicians) can offer expensive and time-intensive interventions such as FFT and MST. Furthermore, very few professionals have training and experience using these interventions. For these clinicians and their agencies, family-based ART is a viable method for helping disruptive youths. ART is time-limited in focus, straightforward in delivery, and cognitive-behavioral in orientation, making it accessible to most mental health practitioners who work with children.

Furthermore, ART can be effectively administered in group format, thereby increasing its utility in clinical settings already taxed by limited resources (Barnoski, 2004). Finally, our findings indicate that clinicians can effectively incorporate parents and other caregivers into ART from the beginning. By emphasizing the role families can play in the alleviation of adolescents' behavior problems, clinicians convey a sense of hope to parents that they can take an active role in promoting their children's social-emotional outcomes.

Table 2. Descriptive Statistics for Treatment Conditions at Baseline

	Condition	
Variable	AFAM (*n* = 30)	TAU (*n* = 20)
Age (years)	15.56 (1.45)	15.58 (1.74)
Offense Severity	3.00 (0.37)	2.80 (0.52)
Psychosocial Risk	1.27 (0.78)	1.70 (1.26)
Attitude to Treatment	22.77 (6.75)	22.90 (7.22)
Treatment Sessions	10.00 (0.00)	16.06 (13.04)

Note. AFAM = Adolescent and Family Anger Management, TAU = Treatment as Usual (individual psychotherapy); Offense severity: Most recent offense classified as 1 = police involvement only, 2 = unruly behavior, 3 = misdemeanor, 4 = felony.

The chief limitation of our study was its relatively small sample size and homogeneity of participants. A larger sample of more socio-demographically and behaviorally diverse adolescents would address the generalizability of our findings. A related threat to our study's external validity was our decision to study court-involved youths in the community. Future research should be directed at investigating the effectiveness of similar family-based interventions for youths in other juvenile justice settings.

Finally, additional research is needed to determine the mechanisms by which AFAM benefits adolescents and caregivers. For example, carefully controlled efficacy studies are needed to determine whether caregivers' (in addition to adolescents') emotion-regulation or social problem-solving skills improve as a function of treatment. Nevertheless, the available outcomes suggest that ART and family-based interventions that rely on its components, are viable approaches to helping adolescents and caregivers in need.

REFERENCES

Alexander, J.F., and Robbins, M.S. (2010). Functional family therapy: A phase-based and multi- component approach to change. In R.C. Murrihy (Ed.), *Clinical handbook of assessing and treating conduct problems in youth* (pp. 245-271). New York: Springer.Amendola, M., and Oliver, R. (2010). ART stands the test of time. *Reclaiming Children and Youth,* 19, 47-50.

Arbuthnot, J., and Gordon, D.A. (1986). Behavioral and cognitive effects of a moral reasoning development intervention for high-risk behavior-disordered adolescents. *Journal of Consulting and Clinical Psychology,* 54, 208-216.

Barnoski, R. (2004). *Outcome evaluation of Washington State's research-based programs for juvenile offenders.* Olympia, WA: Institute for Public Policy.

Barto, J.A. (1995). *The use of ART with adult offenders.* Unpublished dissertation. Louisville, KY: Spalding University.

Billings, F.C. (2003). *The effects of the violence and aggression reduction training program on African American adolescent males.* Unpublished dissertation. Athens, GA: University of Georgia.

Byrne, D.L. (2008). *The effects of participative goal setting on ART for middle school students with emotional and behavioral disorders.* Unpublished dissertation. Denver, CO: University of Denver.

Calame, R., Barile, S., Brown, D., Colantonia, M., Konopa, K., Maas, K., ...and Williams, C. (2001). Too angry to learn? *Journal of Child and Youth Care Work,* 16, 82-94.

Calame, R., and Parker, K. (2003). Reclaiming youth and families with "Family ART." *Reclaiming Youth and Families,* 12, 154-157.

Calame, R., and Parker, K. (2004). : A learning process for the whole family. In A.P. Goldstein, R. Nensen, B. Daleflod, and M. Kalt (Eds.), *New perspectives on Aggression Replacement Training* (pp. 197-229). New York: Wiley.

Cleare, M.J. (2000). *Effects of social cognitive skills training with angry, aggressive adolescent females.* Unpublished dissertation. Keene, NH: Antioch University.

Coleman, M., Pfeiffer, S., and Oakland, T. (1992). ART with behaviorally disordered adolescents. *Behavioral Disorders,* 18, 54-66.

Conger, R.D., Neppl, T., Kim, K.J., and Scaramella, L. (2003). Angry and aggressive behavior across three generations. *Journal of Abnormal Child Psychology,* 31, 143-160.

Currie, M.R. (2010). *ART: An Australian youth justice evaluation.* Unpublished dissertation. Hawthorn, Australia: Swinburne University of Technology.

Curulla, V.L. (1991). *ART in the community for adult learning-disabled offenders.* Unpublished dissertations. Seattle, WA: University of Washington.

Dishion, T.J., Poulin, F., and Burraston, B. (2001). Peer group dynamics associated with iatrogenic effects in group interventions with high-risk young adolescents. *New Directions for Child and Adolescent Development,* 91, 79-92.

Feindler, E.L., and Engel, E.C. (2011). Assessment and intervention for adolescents with anger and aggression difficulties in school settings. *Psychology in the Schools,* 48, 243-253.

Gibbs, J.C. (2010). *Moral development and reality: Beyond the theories of Kohlberg and Hoffman (2nd ed.).* Boston: Pearson.

Glick, B. (2006). ART: A comprehensive intervention for aggressive youth. In B. Glick (Ed.), *Cognitive behavioral interventions for at-risk youth* (pp. 11.1-11.27). Kingston, NJ: Civic Research Institute.

Glick, B., and Gibbs, J.C. (2011). *Aggression replacement training (3rd ed).* Champaign, IL: Research Press.

Goldstein, A.P. (1997). *Skillstreaming the adolescent.* Champaign, IL: Research Press.

Goldstein, A.P. (2002). *The psychology of group aggression.* New York: Wiley.

Goldstein, A.P., and Glick, B. (1987). *Aggression replacement training.* Champaign, IL: Research Press.

Goldstein, A.P., and Glick, B. (1994). *The prosocial gang.* New York: Sage.

Goldstein, A.P., Glick, B., Irwin, M.J., Pask-McCartney, C., and Rubama, I. (1989). *Reducing delinquency.* New York: Pergamon.

Goldstein, A.P., and Martens, B.K. (2008). *Lasting change: Methods for enhancing generalization of gain.* Champaign, IL: Research Press.

Gonzalez, B.R. (2010). *ART to improve the criminogenic need of increasing communication among Latino family members.* Unpublished thesis. Sacramento, CA: California State University.

Gundersen, K., and Svartdal, F. (2006). ART in Norway: Outcome evaluation of 11 Norwegian student projects. *Scandinavian Journal of Educational Research,* 50, 63-81.

Gundersen, K., and Svartdal, F. (2009). ART: Decreasing behavior problems by increasing social competence. In C. Cefai and P. Cooper (Eds.), *Promoting emotional education* (pp. 161-168). Philadelphia, PA: Kingsley.

Gundersen, K., and Svartdal, F. (2010). Diffusion of treatment interventions. *Psychology, Crime, and Law,* 16, 233-249.

Hatcher, R.M., Palmer, E.J., McGuire, J., Hounsome, J.C., Bilby, C.A.L., and Hollin, C.R. (2008). ART with adult male offenders within community settings. *Journal of Forensic Psychiatry and Psychology,* 19, 517-532.

Henggeler, S.W. (2011). Efficacy studies to large-scale transport: The development and validation of multisystemic therapy programs. *Annual Review of Clinical Psychology,* 7, 351-381.

Henggeler, S.W., and Schaeffer, C. (2010). Treating serious antisocial behavior using multisystemic therapy. In A.E. Kazdin (Ed.), *Evidenced-based psychotherapies for children and adolescents* (pp. 259-276). New York: Guilford.

Hollin, C.R. (2004). ART: The cognitive-behavioral context. In A.P. Goldstein, R. Nensen, B. Daleflod, and M. Kalt (Eds.), *New perspectives on Aggression Replacement Training* (pp. 3-19). New York: Wiley.

Hollin, C.R., and Bloxsom, C.A.J. (2007). Treatments for angry aggression. In T.A. Gannon, T. Ward, A.R. Beech, and D. Fisher (Eds.), *Aggressive offenders' cognition* (pp. 215-229). New York: Wiley.

Holmqvist, R., Hill, T., and Lang, A. (2009). Effects of ART in young offender institutions. *International Journal of Offender Therapy and Comparative Criminology,* 53, 74-92.

Hornsveld, R.H. (2004). Aggression control therapy for forensic psychiatric patients. In L.H. Goldstein and J.E. McNeil (Eds.), *Clinical neuropsychology* (pp. 189-196). New York: Wiley.

Hornsveld, R.H., Nijman, H.L.I., Hollin, C.R., and Kraaimaat, F.W. (2008). Aggression control therapy for violent forensic psychiatric patients. *International Journal of Offender Therapy and Comparative Criminology,* 52, 222-233.

Hosley, C. (2005). *Uniting Networks for Youth evaluation highlights 2003-2004.* Saint Paul, MN: Wilder Research.

Jackson, N.C. (1991). *Aggression control training for adolescents in acute care inpatient psychiatric treatment.* Unpublished dissertation. Starkville, MS: Mississippi State University.

Kazdin, A.E. (2010). Problem-solving skills training and parent management training for oppositional defiant disorder and conduct disorder. In A.E. Kazdin (Ed.), *Evidenced-based psychotherapies for children and adolescents* (pp. 211-226). New York: Guilford.

Kennedy, S.M. (1990). *Anger management training with adult prisoners.* Unpublished dissertation. Ottawa, Canada: University of Ottawa.

Kimonis, E.R., and Frick, P.J. (2010). Etiology of oppositional defiant disorder and conduct disorder: Biological, familial and environmental factors identified in the development of disruptive behavior disorders. In R.C. Murrihy, A.D. Kidman, and T.H. Ollendick (Eds.), *Clinical handbook of assessing and treating* (pp. 49-76). New York: Springer.

Knight, J.R., Goodman, E. Pulerwitz, T., and DuRant, R.H. (2001). Reliability of the POSIT in adolescent medical practice. *Journal of Adolescent Health,* 29, 125-130.

Latessa, E., Lovins, B., and Ostrowski, K. (2009). *The Ohio Youth Assessment System.* Cincinnati, OH: University of Cincinnati.

Leeman, L.W., Gibbs, J.C., and Fuller, D. (1993). Evaluation of a multi-component group treatment program for juvenile delinquents. *Aggressive Behavior,* 19, 281-292.

Lipsey, M.W., and Wilson, D.B. (1998). Effective intervention for serious juvenile offenders. In R. Loeber and D.P. Farrington (Eds.), *Serious and violent juvenile offenders* (pp. 313-345). Thousand Oaks, CA: Sage.

Lipsey, M.W., and Wilson, D.B. (2001). Practical meta-analysis. Thousand Oaks, CA: Sage.

Lochman, J.E., Boxmeyer, C.L., Powell, N.P., Barry, T.D., and Pardini, D.A. (2010). Anger control training for aggressive youths. In A.E. Kazdin (Ed.), *Evidenced-based psychotherapies for children and adolescents* (pp. 227-242). New York: Guilford.

Macgowan, M.J., and Wagner, E.F. (2005). Iatrogenic effects of group treatment on adolescents with conduct and substance use problems. *Journal of Evidence Based Social Work,* 2, 79-90.

McGuire, J. (2008). A review of effective interventions for reducing aggression and violence. *Philosophical Transitions of the Royal Society,* 363, 2577-2597.

McGuire, J., and Clark, D. (2004). A national dissemination program. In A.P. Goldstein, R. Nensen, B. Daleflod, and M. Kalt (Eds.), *New perspectives on Aggression Replacement Training* (pp. 139-150). New York: Wiley.

Metz, K.Y. (1996). *Increasing prosocial behavior, anger control, and moral development in juvenile delinquents.* Unpublished dissertation. Athens, OH: Ohio University.

Mitchell, C. (2010). Aggregate program performance report. Sacramento, CA: California Institute of Mental Health.

Moynahan, L., and Stromgren, B. (2005). Preliminary results of ART for Norwegian youth with aggressive behavior and with a different diagnosis. *Psychology, Crime, and Law,* 11, 411-419.

Nathan, P.E., and Gorman, J.M. (2002). *A guide to treatments that work.* New York: Oxford University Press.

Nodarse, M.V. (1997). *The effects of ART on adolescents with an emotional handicap.* Unpublished dissertation. Miami, FL: Miami Institute of Psychology.

Novaco, R. W. (1975). *Anger control: The development and evaluation of an experimental treatment.* Lexington, MA: Heath.

Nugent, W.R., Bruley, C., and Allen, P. (1999). The effects of ART on male and female antisocial behavior in a runaway shelter. *Research on Social Work Practice,* 9, 466-482.

Nugent, W.R., and Ely, G. (2010). The effects of ART on periodicities in antisocial behavior in a short-term shelter for adolescents. *Journal of the Society for Social Work Research,* 1, 140-158.

Ogles, B.M., Dowell, K., Hatfield, D., Melendez, G., and Carlston, D.L. (2004). The Ohio Scales. In M.E. Maruish (Ed.), *The use of psychological testing for treatment planning and outcomes assessment* (pp. 275-304).Mahwah, NJ: Erlbaum.

Palmer, E.J. (2007). Moral cognition and aggression. In T.A. Gannon, T. Ward, A.R. Beech, and D. Fisher (Eds.), *Aggressive offenders' cognition* (pp. 199-214). New York: Wiley.

Quinn, M.M., Kavale, K.A., Mathur, S.R., Rutherford, R.B., and Forness, S.R. (1999). A meta-analysis of social skill interventions for students with emotional or behavioral disorders. *Journal of Emotional and Behavioral Disorders, 7*, 54-64.

Rahdert, E.R. (1991). *The adolescent assessment/referral system manual.* Rockville, MD: National Institute on Drug Abuse.

Ramsey County Community Corrections. (2005). *Ramsey County community corrections 2006/2007 comprehensive plan.* Saint Paul, MN: Author.

Reddy, L.A., and Goldstein, A.P. (2001). ART: A multimodal intervention for aggressive adolescents. *Residential Treatment for Children and Youth, 18*, 47-62.

Roberts, J.M. (2009). *The effectiveness of as determined by the attitudes toward guns and violence questionnaire.* Unpublished dissertation. Fresno, CA: Alliant University.

Sawyer, A.M, and Borduin, C.M. (2011). Effects of multisystemic therapy through midlife: A 21.9-year follow-up to a randomized clinical trial with serious and violent juvenile offenders. *Journal of Consulting and Clinical Psychology, 79*, 643-652.

Stern, S.B., and Azar, S.T. (1998). Integrating cognitive strategies into behavioral treatment for abusive parents and families with aggressive adolescents. *Clinical Child Psychology and Psychiatry, 3*, 387-403.

Sukhodolsky, D.G., Kassinove, H., and Gorman, B.S. (2004). Cognitive-behavioral therapy for anger in children and adolescents: A meta-analysis. *Aggression and Violent Behavior, 9*, 247-269.

Torchin, S. (2003). *ART: Evaluation of a program for young offenders.* Unpublished thesis. Montreal, Canada: McGill University.

Webster-Stratton, C., and Reid, M.J. (2010). The Incredible Years parents, teachers, and children training series. In A.E. Kazdin (Ed.), *Evidenced-based psychotherapies for children and adolescents* (pp. 194-210). New York: Guilford.

Weiss, B., Caron, A., Ball, S., Tapp, J., Johnson, M., and Weisz, J.R. (2005). Iatrogenic effects of group treatment for antisocial youths. *Journal of Consulting and Clinical Psychology, 73*, 1036-1044.

Wilson, S.J., and Lipsey, M.W. (2007). School-based interventions for aggressive and disruptive behavior. *American Journal of Preventative Medicine, 33*, S130-143.

Zimmerman, D.L. (1987). *The effects of ART with juvenile delinquents.* Unpublished dissertation. Syracuse, NY: Syracuse University.

In: Youth: Practices, Perspectives and Challenges
Editor: Elizabeth Trejos-Castillo

ISBN: 978-1-62618-067-3
© 2013 Nova Science Publishers, Inc.

Chapter 11

WHEN WORDS FAIL – A ROLE SPECIFIC PERSPECTIVE ON THE TREATMENT OF YOUTHS

*Nikolas Anastasiadis**
Gesellschaft für Psychische Gesundheit, pro mente Tirol, Austria

ABSTRACT

The current text aims to introduce Psychodrama techniques as a well-established method in the treatment of psychologically malaffected youths. Initially, the theoretical framework will be discussed, in order to underline and justify the need for psychodramatic techniques. Within this method, I will be discussing certain key factors such as Moreno's Role Theory.

In addition, more recent theoretical perspectives will be presented, in order to emphasize the development of childhood and adolescence from a role-specific standpoint.

The discussion lays particular weight on Verhofstadt-Deneve's Phenomenological-Dialectical personality model as well as Schacht's developmental theory, which can be described by means of various developmental layers.

The principles introduced in the first part will be examined in detail, using a number of examples that equally cover both Anglo-Saxonian and German speaking countries. The examples refer to work carried out in schools, homes, youth facilities, residential homes, psychiatric establishments, youth detention centers and such places.

From these collected experiences, valuable conclusions can be drawn with regard to youth Psychodrama.

Psychodrama techniques can become especially relevant in cases where traditional conversational methods are difficult, or where the developmental age of the young person does not match their expected maturity.

---

[*] Address correspondence to: Nikolas Anastasiadis, Austria, Email: anastasiadis@karachalios.at.

1. Personality and Development

1.1. Role Theory

According to Hutter and Schwehm (2009), three parts (or structure theories, in the broader sense) are of major relevance to the method of Psychodrama: (1) Sociometry, (2) the Creative Circle and (3) Role Theory, the latter of which lays one of the corner stones for Moreno's (1946, 1953, 1960, 1961, 1962a, 1962b) developmental theory. Role Theory describes the origin and the formation of roles, how they evolve over time, and how their interplay leads to human interaction and finally identity.

Moreno classified as "roles" the present and manifest forms taken on by the Self. As such, roles represent the final crystallization of all situations in a specific observation period experienced by the subject (Moreno, 1946). Moreno believed that the formation of roles precedes the Self. He named early childhood roles, occurring before the formation of speech, "psychosomatic roles", including, for example, the Eating, the Sleeping, the Noisy and the Walking roles. He concluded furthermore, that roles are initially perceived (Role-Perception) and then learned through enactment (Role-Enactment). Repeated Role-Enactment resulted in Roleplay (or Role-Taking), which is essentially the fixed end-product, a "frozen position" or, in Moreno's own expression, "Conserve" (Moreno, 1960). In Moreno's world, Conserves represented a great deal of our everyday life and of our habits: they enable us to interact with each other, but they can also lead to psychological distress and even maladaption.

Describing a person, Moreno avoided reference to the Self or the Ego. He described these terms as less concrete, and cloaked in meta-psychological secrecy (Moreno, 1960). He was rather of the opinion that very few parts of a person are of a purely private nature. Roles are a fusion of private and collective elements, where the collective contributes the greater part (Moreno, 1943). Each of a person's roles could in fact be stripped away like the layers of an onion (Moreno, 1943).

Those roles which stem from collective thought and experience, Moreno named "sociodramatic".

Those stemming from individual sources, he named "psychodramatic". In reality, though, both role-types are interwoven into the whole. Moreno was of the opinion that the only attributes to be classified as individual were those which present the individual to a group, and those which are ultimately determined by an individual (Moreno, 1950). Moreno (1953) saw the role-pathology of regressive behavior not as an actual regression, but rather as a particularly distinct form of role-play. With paranoid behavior for example, the role-repertoire had been reduced to a contorted operation of one single role.

The patient was incapable of appropriate role-practice – either exaggerating, or inadequately fulfilling, the role. Moreno (1961) concluded that roles could be developed i) primitively, normally or excessively, ii) almost or totally absently or iii) pervertedly or corruptly, leading to psychological malfunction. In the following section, I will introduce some additional and more recent concepts, which recommend a specific approach to personality theory and development. Particular emphasis shall be placed on work with children and youths.

1.2. Verhofstadt-Deneve's Existential-Dialectical Personality Model

In her book, Verhofstadt-Deneve (2000) presents a concept of personality, as seen from an existential-dialectical point of view. By "dialectical" the author describes both a method and a process. She argues that progress from childhood to adulthood consists of a continuous process, in which the experience of conflict, and the dialectical synthesis of elements which are experienced as contradictory, arise in a constant flow. Successful resolution or integration of conflict, leading to synthesis, represents a further step in the constant process of formation of the Self. In this context, there is much discussion of the ever-fluctuating balance between (Ideal-)Self, (Ideal-)Other and (Ideal) Meta-Self. Successful or incomplete development (defined as the realization of potential present in one's own being, leading to developed self-awareness, greater interactive powers, personal freedom, independence and responsibility – and ultimately to active relationships with others and with the physical world) depends on a child's resilience, his ability to bear internal tension, and to accommodate its opposing poles. Verhofstadt-Deneve considers this resilience as, for one thing, demonstrating a sufficient degree of self-esteem. However a person's level of maturity, as well as current situation in life, plays the greatest role.

In her personality-model, Verhofstadt-Deneve (2000) distinguishes between the "Ego" and the "Self". Here, the Ego plays the part of describing and reflecting about the "Self". The Ego is also, essentially, our intuitive element; the Self, on the other hand, is the actual subject of description. The Ego is process, while the Self is content. The author adds that the Self can never be fully comprehended by the Ego. This relationship of Self and Ego, on the one hand, and dimensions of time, reference and level of abstraction, on the other, can be brought together to form Self Constructs. The "time"-dimension comprises past, present and future; the "reference"-dimension refers to intrapersonal and interpersonal connections; and the "abstraction"-dimension comprises real-, ideal-, or meta-image. From combining these dimensions, the following six Self Concepts can be drawn: (1) Who am I (self-image)? (2) Who do I wish to be (Ideal-Self)? (3) What are others like (Alter-image)? (4) How should others be (Ideal-Alter)? (5) How do others see me (Meta-Self)? (6) How should others see me (Ideal-Meta-Self)? Each of these so-called Self-Constructs are strongly affected by the way in which a child grows up. For example, a child who grows up in an abusive family learns already at the pre-speech stage, that his environment can only be threatening or unsafe (Alter-image). The abuse experienced by the child would also damage his Self-image, leading to feelings of worthlessness. Ultimately, the experience of abuse would through the years have an effect on the child's Meta-Self. In his later development, such a child would probably possess poor powers of self-reflection (poor interaction between Ego and Self); and have a detrimental view of the external world, viewing other persons as either purely good or purely bad.

Although Verhofstadt-Deneve's (2000) personality-model attributes less significance to role-principle as Moreno's original Role-Theory, it still manages very well to draw out every intangible element which Moreno (1943, 1950) described as "individual" (which, in other words, presents the individual to a group). By virtue of the six Self-Constructs, such elements can be altered down to a manageable field of reference and, through description, made accessible. The model also allows one to deduce concrete possibilities of intervention. One downside of the personality-model, however, is that it has not yet been sufficiently validated.

Moreover, the six Self-Constructs leave a lot of room for interpretation, which is a hindrance when comparing descriptions of various subjects.

1.3. Schacht's Developmental Layer-Theory

Schacht (2009), in his description of role-development, focuses on Moreno's psychosomatic, psychodramatic and social role-levels (Moreno, 1960). Here, he describes each level through the agency of the following four questions: 1. How are role-related expectations handled? 2. How is the Self experienced? 3. Through what form of knowledge do experiences make their mark? 4. How does the person make sense of his experiences?

1) *Psychosomatic role-level*. Operational competence on the psychosomatic level develops in the first fifteen to eighteen months, while the infant exists in the "First Universe" (world of psychosomatic role-level; experience and operation are directly related to immediately recognizable internal and external stimuli). Role-related expectations are handled through gesture, mime, and other signals. The infant is not yet able to view himself as object, because the Self exists initially purely as subject. Experiences are registered purely through implicit (procedural) awareness. The infant interprets through her experience of emotional sensation. At this stage the infant still turns to the Helping-Ego-skills of the attachment-figure.

2) *Psychodramatic role-level*. Operational competence on the psychodramatic level develops between fifteen to eighteen months and four to six years, the pre-eminence of First Universe increasingly giving way to the child's inner perceptions. She is becoming able, through her own fantasy, to perceive things which are not actually there. The Self becomes in its simplest form an object, which the child can recognize in a mirror. Role-related expectations are processed through speech (expression of wishes, intentions, etc.). Self-awareness and an initial self-image emerge, the latter based on concrete features. Those terms which the child uses to describe his own experience, must first be provided by the attachment-figure. The child's consciousness makes use of tangible, concrete thought, he understands the nature of wishes, needs, preferences and targets. Each occurrence that befalls the child gains meaning partially through speech, but principally through pictorial representation. At this stage the child does not yet understand that his reflections on occurrences in his environment are mere mental images. There is no alternative way to view things.

3) *Sociodramatic role-level*. On the sociodramatic role-level, the child develops an altered understanding of others. She has now passed the age between four and six. She has perceived that people are able to look differently at one and the same thing. Language becomes the tool of self-instruction. Role-related expectations are increasingly negotiated through the medium of perspective-assumption. Own feelings and thoughts are now recognized to be subjective, the child can reflect on herself. By this point, at the latest, she is able to consider herself from the viewpoint of others. Complex thought processes are now possible (in Piaget's terms "concrete, or Formally Operational Stage"). Meaning is expressed through language (discursive symbolic). Apart from the three role-levels, Schacht (2009) also attributes to (1) experienced immediate environment (the field of tensions between approach and

avoidance), (2) attachment (secure bonding to the attachment-figure), (3) successful autonomy (independent universal discovery) and (4) identity (positioning of own person among the family system) great significance in the development of personality.

Regarding role-reversal (internal adoption of a position from one's own role-repertoire or of an opponent's position), Schacht (2009) concludes that a child on the psychosomatic role-level cannot undertake this. It will only become possible with time, as through internal perspective-assumption, another's experiences (and not only by emotional engagement with, or imitation of the other) come to hold a central position. One must also learn how to handle those emotions which are triggered by others, or they can later become a threatening experience. On the psychodramatic role-level, however, the child already possesses the imaginative ability to put himself in another's place. But the author emphasizes that this type of role-reversal is mainly associated with cognitive perspective-adoption.

Role-reversal is only possible on the sociodramatic role-level, and proceeds by the following stages: At the first stage (five to ten years of age) the child appreciates that her own views are subjective, and that others have their own opinions. Nevertheless, her understanding of relationships remains one-sided, and in conflict-resolution there can only be victory or submission. At the second stage (ten to fifteen years of age) the youth is aware that other people appraise her through her individual features and qualities (internal role-reversal). She also, in turn, recognizes the importance to others of her appraisal of them (reciprocal role-reversal). Through internal role-reversal, intimacy becomes possible. At the third stage (15 to 20 years of age), role-reversal with a "generalized other" becomes possible, and opposing personal positions can be acknowledged and integrated. At this stage, youths accept the nature of collective norms, and of political, religious and philosophical world-views. There is, however, no potential for inner perspective while reflecting on these – which is why personal opinions are held as absolute. This restriction at the third stage is finally overcome at the fourth stage (pan-systemic perspective). A society's perspectives can then be developed through a wealth of global views, and in the face of personal interpretation of norms, values and global conviction, take on altered form. This fourth stage of development is not achieved by all. Schacht's (2009) approach is very successful in making connections between role-theoretical concepts and more modern elements of research into infant-to-adult personality development. He is thereby able to preserve Moreno's opinion (1940, 1947b), that a person should be seen as a distinct participant in his environment, at first inspired, then until death constantly influenced and altered by it. A possible disadvantage of this model lies in its complexity – making it difficult to form concrete practical solutions in the treatment of children and youths. In the following section, I will give a number of practical examples of how psychodramatic and sociometric techniques were applied to children and youths in the past. The theoretical perspectives presented in the first section lead to the conclusion that youth therapy requires an adaptation of therapeutic techniques. This holds especially true when, due to psychological malfunction, a child's developmental age does not match her physical age. The studies I will present all utilize psychodramatic methods to address youths' specific needs on a technical level. Practitioners will thereby have access to alternative and powerful approaches to working with youths. Moreover, the readers will come to understand the reasons that lie behind the adaptation of certain techniques. The examples will refer both to Anglo-Saxonian and German speaking countries.

2. Practical Examples of Psychodrama with Children and Youths

2.1. Psychodrama in Youth Facilities and in Residential Settings

In his principal work "Who Shall Survive?", Moreno (1953) focuses on his attempts to reform a Training School for girls in Hudson, New York. Action was needed on account of the high number of young women constantly escaping from the institution. In compelling detail, he describes the community in question; a village of 500 to 600, exclusively female, inhabitants – each of whom was legally assigned to this institution by the State of New York. They remained there during their formative years, with matrons adopting a maternal role. According to Moreno (1953), the village consisted of 16 small houses to accommodate the young women, a chapel, a school, a hospital, a manufacturing plant, a grocery, a laundry and a small farm. All inhabitants were expected to contribute to the working of these facilities. Beyond this formal structure was a further sociometric hierarchy, in which every individual inhabitant had her position. In his article, Hare (1992) presents an overview of all the sociometric techniques applied by Moreno (1953) at the home between 1932 and 1938: Sociometric Tests, Tests for a woman's "emotional capacity" (measuring the frequency of social exchange), for her "emotional expansiveness" (measuring the "emotional energy", a woman's ability to create and maintain relationships), Tests of Spontaneity and Role Play Tests, as well as techniques investigating interactive skills within a small group. Moreno (1953) partly developed these techniques to reveal hidden differences in the young women's social functions. The method would also be of assistance in resolving conflicts between colored and white inhabitants, between employees and trainees and ultimately among fellow employees. Moreno (1953) encountered considerable resistance from social services, and from the staff of the home, but by the time he concluded his restructuring, the number of escapees had reduced to an acceptable number.

Bosselmann, Kindschuh-van Roje and Martin (1996) describe the use of various psychodramatic techniques at the remedial-pedagogic home "Leppermühle" in Busek in the seventies. Children and youths assigned to the program had suffered from serious neglect, from brain-organic malfunctioning, from neurotic behavior and from other emotional- and conduct-related disturbances. The authors describe three operational areas: children's groups, one-to-one sessions with youths and in Psychodrama group work with parents. During their work, therapists paid particular attention to diagnostic elements such as the levels of confrontation, activity, and inhibition as well as conflict-resolution skills. (1) Play consisted of hand-puppet representation, with one child acting and the others watching. The therapists guided the children in both structuring and handling their scenes, from amongst the audience and from behind the curtain, performing the function of Auxiliary Ego, and never giving an evaluation of the play (e. g. "antisocial play"). (2) Regarding one-to-one work with youths, the authors consider this age group to be more guarded when voicing internal processes. They argue that psychodramatic techniques are a means to get in touch with youths, who, in turn, become able to face and actively resolve their difficulties in a non-literal manner. To build the scenes, the authors used coins, chairs or building bricks, whether the thematic matter were reality, dream or invention. Psychodrama techniques were often better applied outside the boundaries of the treatment room, for example while taking a walk. (3) The authors see their advisory and explanatory work with parents as particularly important. A sample case shows how strikingly a mother's attitude to her son can change through exploring the child's role.

Stamenkovic (2006) describes her experiences using Psychodrama with traumatized refugee youths in the Laura Gatner House in Vienna. The house accommodates up to 44 persons from 13 to 19 who left their homes under threat or due to war. Many of the underaged were prosecuted, witnessed torture and violence or were victims of torture themselves. In order to help the refugees overcome their trauma, the House offers – besides assistance in covering some of the most basic needs like housing, clothing, school and education – a weekly Psychodrama group, with attendance on a voluntary basis. The youths were introduced in small steps to the psychodramatic process, with special emphasis placed on making the rules and the structure of the groups clear (specifically, the three stages of Warm-Up, the scene and the Sharing). Sociodrama was the preferred method of choice. Very often, the scenes depicted everyday life and conflicts among the residents. Role Reversal was used to further understanding of each other and to resolve conflict. Stamenkovic (2006) emphasizes the strong need for stabilizing techniques in the work with traumatized patients. In Psychodrama, this can be accomplished by building "a secure place" on the stage, which helps the client re-establish a sense of being safe.

2.2. Psychodrama in Psychiatric Youth Facilities

Gröschner (1996) reports on her attempts to apply Psychodrama techniques in a psychiatric residential home. Groups were held once a week. Due to the duration of therapy (approximately two years), group consistency changed over time. The clients, not strictly youths (aged between 18 and 35), had formerly been admitted to psychiatric units following a psychotic episode. Some of these residents had also been diagnosed with a Personality Disorder, many of which were considered Borderline. The author emphasizes Doubling as an effective method in treating these psychotic patients. In this method, the client is provided with one or more Auxiliary-Ego(s), whose role is to enhance communication with others as well as the self. It was also possible to apply Doubling in the clients' everyday life, for example outside the facility, at the supermarket or during physical health care. According to the author, the Role Reversal method is not advisable when treating psychotic patients, as the latter have weak Egos and fear loss of identity. On the other hand, she supports Role Reversal as a method, where the patient has not experienced an acute psychotic episode and when actual personal difficulties can be overcome "in the here and now". Gröschner (1996) also considers work with Sociometric exercises, hand-puppets, the Empty-Chair Technique and the Magic Shop to be highly effective. The author describes that after applying Psychodrama, the group's members became livelier and that this had a direct influence on the facility's atmosphere. Relationships between residents became more trustful, and the patients' fear of presenting themselves in front of the group was reduced. In summary, Gröschner (1996) believes that this modified form of Psychodrama can enhance Ego-stability and improve spontaneity and creativity.

Adriaenssens and Schrans (2000) describe their experiences with youth Psychodrama at a psychiatric hospital, where – in addition to Psychodrama techniques – other approaches like Psychodynamic and Family Therapy were used. The authors cite the following techniques: (1) Social Atom: in one-to-one sessions, persons important to the client can be represented by an empty chair or by a puppet. (2) Family Tree: its branches are drawn, and the patient's relationship with each family member can be explored on a deeper level (again, this method can be of value in one-to-one sessions). (3) Sociogram: depicts a diagram of all persons who play an important role in the patient's life (e. g. the school class, other youths at the hospital, youth organizations etc.). (4) Work with chairs: this method can be applied whenever a youth has two or more opposed views of the same situation and can be of assistance in decision taking (e. g. the choice between returning home and a host family, repetition of the same class in school, etc.). (5) Intra-Psychic Psychodrama: differentiates and explores the inner aspects of a person; conflictual inner standpoints or perspectives can be represented by chairs or objects. (6) Symbol-Drama: can be used in Group Therapy, in Couples Counseling and in one-to-one sessions; the youth is asked to imagine a willow, a brook, a mountain or a house; later, images that arose can be discussed, but without interpretation. (7) Magic Shop: at an imaginary store, the youth gets the opportunity to buy personal qualities like humor, understanding or even common sense; in return, he can leave behind unwanted qualities. (8) The Empty Chair: by this technique, the client can address an empty chair as if a significant person in her life were sitting in it. The Empty Chair can be used during one-to-one sessions or as a Warm-Up in Group Therapy.

Anastasiadis and Meller (2011) describe how techniques of Psychodrama were applied in a psychiatric youth facility in Tyrol, Austria (the Residential Home SPACE). The facility provided 24-hour care for up to 12 youth residents who had been diagnosed with a psychiatric disorder, including suicidality, Social Maladjustment, Psychosis and Personality Disorder. Before their acceptance for treatment, most clients had experienced serious neglect and physical or sometimes sexual abuse. As most residents had quit school before 15, the facility offered a highly structured daily program, consisting of one-to-one sessions, therapeutic groups and a variety of other group activities such as sports or cooking. Psychodrama techniques were applied in one-to-one sessions as well as in groups. (1) Regarding one-to-one work, sessions were held on a weekly basis. In these sessions, clients could bring up any topic of their choice, including personal issues and thoughts, feelings and even dreams. Sometimes, those topics were used for the creation and in-depth-exploration of a small psychodramatic stage. Role Reversal was used whenever necessary. At the end of each session, there was always a Sharing or at least some feedback from the therapist. (2) In regard to group sessions, the leaders used Sociometry as a method. Another exercise was to let the youths choose among pre-defined locations in order to show and express their personal emotional state. Psychodrama group work was combined with other therapeutic elements such as creative self-expression through sculptural arts. Here, aerated and light-weighted concrete elements were used, usually used for house construction (YTONG blocks). With these blocks, the residents created simple sculptures and beautiful reliefs. Group sessions were always closed by a Sharing. The authors conclude that the methods of Doubling and of Role Reversal seem appropriate in youth therapy, as long as the leaders' instructions are highly directive and if youths' resistance to play is respected at all times.

2.3. Children and Youth Psychodrama in Schools

Goldman and Goldman (1968) report on "Upward Bound", a program developed by the United States government in the late 1960s with the aim of motivating urban disadvantaged youths to attend college or at least some further education beyond high school level. The program consisted of a full-time summer residential period, during which high school students from deprived backgrounds spent a period of six to eight weeks on their college campus, attending courses in English, history, chemistry, math, and reading. Afterwards, the students were offered Tutoring, Counseling, and various activities, all of which were later continued until the students graduated from school. Socio- and Psychodrama were used to address difficulties that came up among group members, including covert racism, discipline problems or stealing. Through the method of Sociodrama, three main relationship areas were worked on: Student – teacher, parent – child, and peer. As participants gained more trust and confidence, the sociodramatic sessions could progress into personal Psychodramas. By applying techniques such as Role Reversal and Doubling, both students and teachers could see each other in a new light. The students could discover some of the reasons behind their own feelings and behaviors, bonds between students and staff members could be established, old patterns and expectations could be overcome. Taken together, "all participants [...] became acutely aware that the innate human problems that prevent the realization of potentials are the same for everyone, regardless of whether they are black or white, rich or poor, or come from the suburbs or the slums." (1968, p. 207).

Verhofstadt-Deneve (1988) gives an example of Psychodrama in a classroom and of work on youths' relationships with the elderly. The author suggests that, at the beginning, one of the youths can be chosen and asked to tell the others about his relationship with his own grandparents. Or a fictitious situation (such as a dialogue between a youth and a senior) can serve as the starting point in building a scene. Verhofstadt-Deneve (1988) emphasizes that the scene must always depict the subjective view of the youth(s). Sometimes, opposing ideals (such as the "helpful and understanding", as opposed to the "hostile and contemptuous" youth) will come into conflict. In such cases, the Psychodrama therapist can create an "intermediate role", paving the way for the mediation. Such an intermediate role is close to a youth's actual behavior in reality, and each participant can easily identify with it. At the same time, the youth can openly communicate his perceptions and emotions, for – in his peers' eyes – he speaks in the role and not as himself. This setting differs from classical Psychodrama in that there is no co-conductor, that the group is larger than usual, that personal involvement is reduced and that there is no emphasis on Catharsis.

Kruczek and Zagelbaum (2004) investigate whether Psychoeducational Drama can increase adolescent awareness of at-risk behaviors. This method combines elements of both Psychodrama and theatrical performance. At a public school in the Midwest, narratives of parents whose child had been killed in a drunk driving accident as well as of a 20-year-old college freshman who was in recovery from alcohol and marijuana dependence were presented to middle and high school children. The narratives, presented by role players who had been instructed prior to the program, did not reflect their real-life problems, but were typical of someone who had actually experienced the situation. By such means, the investigators hoped to engage the children at an affective, cognitive and behavioral level, as these three elements are considered to be crucial in developing improved insight, increased awareness of feelings, and greater awareness of feelings associated with certain behaviors (Fink, 1990). The results of the study indicated that Psychoeducational Drama can be an effective tool for increasing adolescent awareness of at-risk behaviors. The analysis of a feedback questionnaire, given to the audience afterwards, indicated that middle school-aged and female participants were most susceptible to Psychoeducational Drama, suggesting that this kind of intervention might lead to future change of at-risk behaviors, especially with regard to substance abuse.

Amatruda (2006) describes how Psychodrama techniques were used in a classroom. The author believes that, when applied to schoolchildren, Psychodrama can lead to better conflict resolution skills; furthermore, that children can train their social skills and increase self-esteem. The study was conducted in a public school, at special classes attended only by children whose behavior indicated the existence of some disorder, covering the range from Depression to Conduct Disorder, Oppositional-Defiant Disorder (ODD), Attention Deficit Disorder (ADD), Attention Deficit Hyperactive Disorder (ADHD) and behavior disorders with impulse and/or control deficit. Groups took place twice a week and lasted approximately 30 to 40 minutes. For the Warm-Up, Amatruda used sociometric exercises like the Spectrogram (imaginary scale, on which each child must take a position in respect to some pre-defined criterion), name games (participants call out their peers' names, varying speech speed or the emotional tone of their voice), games where characteristic adjectives are attached to the participants' names or "Weather as Mood Barometer" (participants are asked "which weather they are today"). After this Warm-Up, the children were asked to recall a recent instance when they experienced a sudden emotional shift. Through methods of Role Reversal and Doubling, participants could experience the impact that their emotions made on people around them. To increase social skills, the author used the Mirror Technique. For this exercise, two players sit on chairs opposing each other. While the first player chooses a certain facial expression, the other tries to imitate it. Interpersonal conflicts could be resolved by means of sociodramatic exercises. In addition, the author used "Locograms" (pre-defined positions, defining certain feelings or reactions, from which the students had to make a choice). Finally, Amatruda used psychodramatic sculptures, as well as the imagination of one's future self ("What are you going to be like in the future?").

2.4. Children and Youth Psychodrama with Special Target Groups

Baum (1973) reports on her work over a one-year period with emotionally disturbed, broken-home children aged between six and eight. Most of them had lived in welfare institutions; only a minority had lived at home. The author describes two main characteristics of the children: first, their developmental age did not match their biological age; and, second, these children could not restrain their needs or defer satisfaction. Baum refers to a wide variety of techniques she applied to the children: making noise or keeping quiet upon a pre-defined signal, introducing oneself in the manner the child desired (e. g. as a "good boy" or a "good girl"), drawing, expressing "large and small" in a non-verbal way, the Magic Shop – but always changing medium (i. e., drawing, drama, dance, sculpture, etc.), consequently reducing the "act-hunger". By acting out little dramas, the children could slip into different roles, thereby gaining new perspectives. Baum used Role Reversal and the Auxiliary Ego as a method. Her conclusion is that "words fail these children [...] in expressing their fantasy-filled internal world" (1973, p. 61). They can, however, express this internal world through other means. Psychodrama, for example, can help children express and cultivate their feelings and anxieties. The author writes that, at the end of the year, the children were more capable of verbal expression in a conversation.

Trussell (1973) catalogues a variety of group experiences offered in a particular setting devoted to providing mental health services to middle-class, drug-using young people, the Carriage House Project. This was a nontraditional mental health facility in the 1970s, treating young drug-users. Drug-related problems were not the primary focus of therapy, as one might expect. Instead, the adolescents brought typical struggles to work on: difficulties in negotiating the school system, family tensions and disruptions, boy-girl hassles, identity problems, uncertainty about career choice and concern about military obligation. Besides such methods as Group Therapy, Guided Affective Imagery, Meditation, creative writing and art, Psychodrama groups were an important element in the Carriage House Program. These were conducted by an experienced psychodramatist. The author emphasizes that professionals in the field need a conviction that they can do their particular work any place, anytime, and under practically any conditions.

Elliot (1987) describes how Psychodrama could be applied in a secure treatment program, at the Judge J. Connelly Youth Center in Massachusetts. The center, specializing in work with criminal offenders, accommodated up to 15 seriously delinquent young men aged between 13 and 18, who had committed crimes like murder, child and adult rape, kidnapping or armed robbery. The youths were assigned to the program after a full assessment procedure. The methods utilized at the center were mainly psychodynamic. Psychodrama was only applied for those who did not have the intellectual capacity to gain insight into their own personal dynamics. The main topics being worked on were normative values, dealing with conflict, family issues, separation and individuation.

Carbonell and Parteleno-Barehmi (1999) report on treating girls in a middle school setting who had been sexually abused. The sample consisted of 26 girls, whose age ranged from 11 to 13 years. The Warm-Up phase was a time for the girls to become familiar with each other and with Psychodrama techniques. During the Action Phase, each participant was given the opportunity to create a stage to show the others what had happened to her. During this re-enactment, the girls could create a positive ending to the scene if they wished, different from what had happened in reality. By such means, the clients were given a sense of personal control over themselves, as well as over their traumatic experiences. Whenever the intensity of a scene became too overwhelming, alternative methods were applied in order to avoid re-traumatization. Finally, there was a Sharing where each participant could tell the others what she had experienced in the previous scene. During this last phase, any kind of judgment or interpretation by the therapists was avoided. Post-Tests showed that after treatment, the girls were more open, less anxious, their depression had decreased and self-efficacy had increased.

Braet (2000) presents an example of how to work psychodramatically with overweight youths and, more specifically, how to increase their self-esteem. The author refers to past findings that suggest some correlation between negative self-attribution and obesity. Moreover, overweight children and youths turned out to have a negative self-image, as compared to controls. Braet believes that one of the main goals in treating obesity is to help the youth realize eventual discrepancies between his self-image and ideal Self. In order to achieve this goal, the author had youths draw self-images, watch their reflection in a mirror or record themselves on video. Other methods involved puppets (when working with small children) and role play. (1) With the help of puppets, a challenging situation was re-enacted (e. g. a visit to an auntie). Afterwards, the child got the opportunity to try out her ideal Self (e. g. by dancing). In a third step, the child was asked to present some free play. (2) Regarding the use of role play, the children were asked to play a key situation related to their maladaptive eating behavior (e. g. Christmas, a party or feelings of sadness). Another participant was then chosen to play the role of someone offering the child food or sweets. While trying to resist the offer, the protagonist was asked to think aloud: "I know that I can accept the offer and eat now, but I decide not to!". Or: "Even if I can't resist, there might be a third option!". The author refers to typical situations as the playground, trying on new clothes, leaving the water at a public swimming pool, the tramway or a mobbing situation. Common to all applied methods was the creation of some alternative self-image.

Melbeck-Thiemann (2002) describes the effects of Group-Centered Psychodrama, a method already studied in a variety of settings, on children from broken homes. The study was conducted with a total of five children who attended elementary school and whose parents had been divorced less than one year. Therapeutic sessions lasted 90 minutes and were conducted over a period of 20 weeks. Children with delayed Ego-development, aggressive behaviors, poor frustration tolerance and severe pathology were excluded from the study. Pre- and post-measures were applied, combining quantitative methods, such as frequency-counting of recurrent roles or topics during scenes on one hand and personality testing on the other, with qualitative methods, such as the observation of certain interaction- and contact-behaviors as well as of the childrens' social position among their peers. The author comes to the conclusion that Group-Centered Psychodrama can help children to (1) allow negative feelings related to their parents' divorce to arise and find expression; (2) work through disturbed family relations and patterns, where they feel used as a partner surrogate or drawn into a loyalty conflict between parents; (3) enhance self-confidence; (4) find a way to deal with their own aggression and (5) create positive and supportive peer relations.

Conclusion

The previous sections afforded an overview of Moreno's (1946, 1953, 1960, 1961, 1962a, 1962b) Role-Theory, as well as two more recent concepts which build on Role-Theory, allowing for more exploration in certain areas. Practical examples were given of how psychodramatic techniques were applied in various settings, including residential homes, psychiatric youth facilities and schools.

Moreno (1953, 1961) assumed that a person operates through roles, and that these develop through time, with the individual's interaction with his environment. In time, each role becomes established in the role-self via so called role-clusters. Moreno believed that role-development was a life-long process, never to be considered as complete – which made him a pioneer of the age. By association with the specific elements of a person's life, Moreno (1947a, 1953) put his role-concept into an inter-subjective context ("Social Atom"). Similarly, he saw the "Cultural Atom" as part of a more generalized socio-cultural framework, reflecting socially accepted role-patterns or behaviors (Moreno, 1939; 1953).

Moreno's (1960) understanding of roles was later taken up and widely varied by various researchers. Verhofstadt-Deneve's (2000) Phenomenological-Dialectical Personality Model thus turns to the nature or quality of the relationship between the Ego and the Self. From this relationship, the author draws six dimensions, each of which provide the answer to a key-question addressing the (ideal) Self-image, the (ideal) Alter-image and ultimately the (ideal) Meta-Self. Verhofstadt-Deneve and Verhofstadt (2007) write that the six core questions could form the basis of a therapeutically practical and "living" personality-model, which consists of six personality-dimensions. Especially noteworthy is how Verhofstadt-Deneve (2000), in her practical work with children, assigned a high importance to the potential for reflection.

Schacht (2009) regards an infant's progress to adulthood as gradual, proceeding through several stages. Where the infant essentially perceives through his emotions, the adult ideally has the ability to unite others' perceptions of him with his own self-image, and form his self-conduct accordingly. Regarding role-reversal in a child, Schacht finds this only gradually possible with the passing of years. While the author makes no specific suggestion of a minimum age for participation in psychodramatic sessions, a late-developing skill for Role-Reversal processes is clearly implied with regard to the practical treatment of young people.

The examples presented in the second part aim to demonstrate the richness and usefulness of Psychodrama techniques in the treatment of youths. In residential settings, sociometric exercises can be applied in order to reveal hidden differences in the the residents' social functions, to explore closeness and distance between persons and to identify outsiders or specific group configurations. A variety of therapeutic techniques like Role Reversal and Doubling can be used, and this applies not to only to residential homes, but also to psychiatric establishments, to jails and even to classrooms. The techniques used in treatment can easily be adjusted to a person's age or mental maturity. In other words, whereas it seems appropriate to use hand puppets or Playmobil in one case, Role Reversal seems to be the method of choice in another instance. Throughout the examples presented, diagnosis seems to play a rather secondary role, for Psychodrama techniques were effectively used in the treatment of most disorders. In general, the examples reported in the current text suggest that, in the treatment of psychotic patients, Doubling should be the method of choice. This does not exclude Role Reversal for such clients. Instead, the guiding question in choosing the right approach should always be the main goal that lies behind a given intervention. Regarding therapy and trauma, it applies to both youths and adults that the techniques used in treatment should never cause re-traumatization. It should be added that, at the time of writing, I know of no study advising against role play in traumatized children.

The significance of Psychodrama methods in intervention programs cannot be overestimated. Therapeutic work with youths can be a highly demanding task, where conversational methods fail all too often. This failure is not due to resistance or the child's attempt to challenge the therapist (as observed in classical approaches), but due to substantially altered developmental needs, and limited function of a personality still under development. Through Psychodrama, the therapist can avoid the conversational-semantic level of speech, and activate fundamental mechanisms whose operational mode does not depend on conscious reflection or mental abstraction. Where in traditional approaches words are the means for change, in Psychodrama the situation itself becomes the vehicle, and the youth a part of it. Psychodrama sets up the framework in which youth and therapist together can experience and explore new situations. I have sometimes been amazed to realize how much the Therapeutic Bond between a youth and myself improves after successful work on a psychodramatic scene. I have also observed that, after only a few psychodramatic sessions, many youths can significantly enhance their social competence and behaviors. This, in turn, enhances their relationships with other youths, and as a consequence the peer group becomes much more stable and cooperative as a whole.

In contrast with other psychotherapists, psychodramatists can in certain circumstances work on a non-verbal level. The method is especially successful in work with youths with migration backgrounds. An example was given by Stamenkovic (2006), who describes her experience of Psychodrama with traumatized refugee youths in the Laura Gatner House in Vienna. It is self-evident that a refugee youth from Nepal, China, Georgia or Afghanistan does not understand the language spoken in her host country. Psychodrama can be easily adapted across cultural divides when communication becomes difficult. I personally have limited experience in treating refugee youths, but recall a surprising occurrence with an Armenian woman who's German was too weak for dialogue. In a scene depicting a face-to-face encounter with the son that war had forced her to abandon, Psychodrama enabled her to reconcile herself with this experience. The woman, incidentally, chose to play the scene in Armenian.

It is however important to keep in mind how strong the emotional impact of Psychodrama can be. I have witnessed a number of situations where group members reacted in a highly emotional way to certain psychodramatic interventions. Therapists must always remember, never to take a youth beyond her personal limits. This can result in incidents where, for example, a person suddenly leaves the room, leaving behind a group in turmoil. I have also experienced a youth jumping out of the window, and another leaving the room, slamming the door and smashing all the plates and glasses in the kitchen. It is always advisable to have a second leader present who can assist when a situation becomes dangerous. A second obstacle lies in the fear felt by some youths to disclose or embarrass themselves in the presence of their peers. (How "uncool" must it be for a 15 year old boy to play the role of a teacher, a newspaper or a wardrobe!) There are some youths who never overcome their fear of being humiliated, which must ultimately exclude them from the target group for such interventions.

The use of alternative therapeutic approaches in intervention programs such as Psychodrama cannot be discussed in isolation from questions regarding finance and policy making: well trained psychodramatists (and other psychotherapists) cost more than social workers and other professionals without psychotherapeutic training. Over the past years, there has been a steady reduction in public welfare spending. In Austria, Germany and other European countries, the professional identity of mental-care-givers has been constantly altered (or downgraded), partly due to contractual agreements. As a consequence, many psychodramatists (and other psychotherapists) prefer to work independently, where they are better rewarded for their work. For public intervention programs, this results in a loss of expertise and quality. Given the efficiency, effectiveness and flexibility of Psychodrama methods, social policy makers would be well advised to shift focus from short-term cost to long-term benefit. This could ultimately help reduce expenses and enhance quality.

I would like in conclusion to underline the strong need for more research into the use of Psychodrama in youth intervention programs. I selected the practical examples introduced in the second part of the current text with the help of the PsyCLIT database. In an extensive search through existing literature, a combination of various key-words such as "Psychodrama" and "youth" returned not more than a few dozen entries. This is surprising, given the benefits of the method and its long tradition. Future research should focus on whether Psychodrama techniques benefit youths more than other therapeutic approaches. In a study conducted by Tschuschke (2011), data of 244 adult clients from Psychodynamic groups and of 91 clients from Psychodrama groups were analyzed and compared. The results suggest a strong relationship between psychotherapeutic treatment and the reduction of psychological distress, independent of approach. I know of no such study focusing specifically on youths. Mann and Mann (2011) showed that extended role-play experience leads to an increase in a person's overall ability to play a role, independent of context or situation. Under the assumption that the ability for playing roles is a strong indicator for mental health, no age group would benefit more than youth from Psychodramatic interventions. Unfortunately, Mann and Mann's study does not permit conclusions regarding the influence of role-playing abilities on mental health. Further studies will be needed to associate these variables. Another interesting perspective regards possible influences of Psychodrama on personality development. Extensive studies will be needed to clarify this intriguing question.

REFERENCES

Adriaenssen, K., and Schrans, J. (2000). Self-Reflective Techniques in Individual Therapy with Adolescents in a Residential Setting. In L. Verhofstadt-Deneve (Ed.), Theory and Practice of Action and Drama Techniques. Developmental Psychotherapy from an Existential-Dialectical Viewpoint (pp. 255-277). London: Jessica Kingsley Publishers Ltd.

Amatruda, M.-J. (2006). Conflict Resolution and Social Skill Development With Children. *Journal of Group Psychotherapy, Psychodrama and Sociometry*, 58 (4), 168-181.

Anastasiadis, N., and Meller, H. (2011). Psychodrama in einer Österreichischen Jugendwohngemeinschaft. *Zeitschrift für Psychodrama und Soziometrie*, 10, 297-308.

Baum, N. (1973). Psychodrama and multi-media therapy with emotionally disturbed children. *Group Psychotherapy and Psychodrama*, 26 (1-2), 48-66.

Bosselmann, R., van Roje, E. K., and Martin, M. (1996). Einige Einsatzmöglichkeiten des Psychodramas im therapeutischen Heim. In R. Bosselmann, E. Lüffe-Leonhardt, and M. Gellert (Eds.), *Variationen des Psychodramas* (pp. 292-300). Kiel: Christa Limmer.

Braet, C. (2000). Action Techniques for Boosting Self-Esteem in Obese Children. In L. Verhofstadt-Deneve (Ed.), Theory and Practice of Action and Drama Techniques. Developmental Psychotherapy from an Existential-Dialectical Viewpoint (pp. 233-253). London: Jessica Kingsley Publishers Ltd.

Carbonell, D. M., and Parteleno-Barehmi, C. (1999). Psychodrama groups for girls coping with trauma. *International Journal of Group Psychotherapy*, 49 (3), 285-306.

Elliot, J. G. (1987). The treatment of serious juvenile delinquents in Massachusetts. *Educational Psychology in Practice*, 3 (2), 49-52.

Fink, S. O. (1990). Approaches to emotion in psychotherapy and theatre: Implications for drama therapy. *The Arts in Psychotherapy*, 17, 5-18.

Goldman, E., and Goldman, S. (1968). Sociodrama and psychodrama with urban disadvantaged youth. *Group Psychotherapy: A Quarterly*, 21 (4), 206-210.

Gröschner, U. (1996). Das Drama der Psychose – Gruppentherapeutische Erfahrung mit dem Psychodrama in einer psychiatrischen Übergangseinrichtung. In R. Bosselmann, E. Lüffe-Leonhardt, and M. Gellert (Eds.), Variationen des Psychodramas (pp. 76-94). Kiel: Christa Limmer.

Hare, A. P. (1992). Moreno's Sociometric Study at the Hudson School for Girls. *Journal of Group Psychotherapy, Psychodrama and Sociometry*, 45 (1), 24-39.

Hutter, C., and Schwehm, H. (Eds.). (2009). *J. L. Morenos Werk in Schlüsselbegriffen*. Wiesbaden: VS Verlag für Sozialwissenschaften.

Kruczek, T., and Zagelbaum, A. (2004). Increasing adolescent awareness of at risk behaviors via psychoeducational drama. *The Arts in Psychotherapy*, 31, 1-10.

Mann, J. H., and Mann, C. H. (2011). The effect of role-playing experience on role-playing ability. *Zeitschrift für Psychodrama und Soziometrie*, 10, 9-20.

Melbeck-Thiemann, K. (2002). Die Wirkung von gruppenzentrierter Psychodrama-Therapie in der Behandlung von Kindern aus Trennungs- und Scheidungsfamilien. Unpublished doctoral dissertation, Universität Bremen.

Moreno, J. L. (1939). Creativity and cultural conserves. *Sociometry*, 2, 1-36.

Moreno, J. L. (1940). Psychodramatic treatment of psychoses. *Sociometry*, 3 (2), 115-132.

Moreno, J. L. (1943). The Concept of Sociodrama. A New Approach to the Problem of Inter-Cultural Relations. *Sociometry*, 6 (4), 434-449.

Moreno, J. L. (1946). *Psychodrama, Vol. I.* New York: Beacon House Inc.

Moreno, J. L. (1947a). Organization of the social atom. *Sociometry*, 10, 287-293.

Moreno, J. L. (1947b). The social atom and death. *Sociometry*, 10 (1), 80-84.

Moreno, J. L. (1950). Group psychotherapy: Theory and practice. *Group Psychotherapy*, 3, 142-188.

Moreno, J. L. (1953). Who shall survive? A new approach to the problem of human interrelations. New York: Beacon House Inc.

Moreno, J. L. (1960). The Sociometry Reader. Illinois: The Free Press of Glencoe.

Moreno, J. L. (1961). The Role Concept. A Bridge Between Psychiatry and Sociology. *American Journal of Psychiatry*, 118, 518-523.

Moreno, J. L. (1962a). Role theory and the emergence of the self. *Group Psychotherapy*, 15, 114-117.

Moreno, J. L. (1962b). The united role theory and the drama. *Group Psychotherapy*, 15, 253-254.

Schacht, M. (2009). *Das Ziel ist im Weg*. Wiesbaden: VS Verlag für Sozialwissenschaften.

Stamenkovic, M. (2006). Psychodramatische Stabilisierungstechniken. *Zeitschrift für Psychodrama und Soziometrie*, 5, 239-244.

Trussell, W. D. (1973). Groups for young people from the drug using community. *Group Process*, 5, 63-68.

Tschuschke, V. (2011). Effectiveness of psychodrama group therapy – Results from the PAGE-study. *Zeitschrift für Psychodrama und Soziometrie*, 10, 45-56.

Verhofstadt-Deneve, L. (1988). Persoon en psychodrama. Toepassingsmogelijkheden in het onderwijs' [Person and Psychodrama. Practicability in Educational Settings]. *Handboek leerlingbegeleiding* 6, *6540*, 1-41.

Verhofstadt-Deneve, L. (2000). An Existential-Dialectical Developmental Psychology: Basic Principles and Underlying Personality Model. In L. Verhofstadt-Deneve (Ed.), Theory and Practice of Action and Drama Techniques. Developmental Psychotherapy from an Existential-Dialectical Viewpoint (pp. 67-114). London: Jessica Kingsley Publishers Ltd.

Verhofstadt-Deneve, L., and Verhofstadt, M. (2007). Psychodrama with the `Children's Psychodrama-Puppets Kit'. *Forum. Journal of the International Association of Group Psychotherapy*, 2, 95-112.

Chapter 12

EARNING GRADES WITH EXCELLENT INTELLIGENCE ASSESSED BY RAVEN'S MATRICES

Chau-kiu Cheung and Elisabeth Rudowicz*
City University of Hong Kong, China

ABSTRACT

Although the student's intelligence commonly predicts grades in school, theoretical and empirical bases for the prediction are uncertain. A theoretical mechanism is that intelligence promotes learning effort to get grades and another theoretical elaboration is that excellence in intelligence particularly contributes to better grades. Investigation of the contributions due to excellence in intelligence and learning effort is the aim of this study. The study measured intelligence with Raven's Standard Progressive Matrices, school grades, and learning effort from 2,545 Hong Kong Chinese students. It identified intelligence that embodied the hierarchical structure as proposed for the assessment. With this identification, results show that excellent intelligence based on the most difficult items contributed to grades, partly through mediation by learning effort. In contrast, intelligence indexed on less difficult items had no contribution to grades and effort. Students who cannot solve the most difficult items are therefore most in need of improvement in grades and the improvement partly relies on raising the students' effort.

Despite some research showing the contribution of young people's intelligence on school grades (Pind et al. 2003; Raven and Raven 2003), research and theory have not been overwhelmingly uniform and cogent in justifying the contribution (Mills and Ablard 1993; Kohn 1996). On the one hand, null and weak findings about the contribution are present (Chamorro-Premazic and Furnham 2006; Cote and Levine 2000; Hickman et al. 2000). On the other hand, theory and research have not ascertained the basis and mechanism for the contribution. In theory, a possible mechanism is mediation by study effort, which serves as a mediator between intelligence and grades (Cassidy and Lynn 1991; Opdenakker and Van

---

* Address Correspondence to: Chau-kiu Cheung, Ph.D., Associate Professor, City University of Hong Kong, China. Email: ssjacky@cityu.edu.hk.

Damme 2007). However, research and theory have not elucidated the relative contributions of intelligence, effort, and the mediation process. More fundamentally, research has not illustrated the contribution of intelligence in its theoretically coherent way, that is, as a latent trait. With respect to Raven's Standard Progressive Matrices, a latent trait is one that differentiates people who correctly answer different compositions of items with differential discrimination and difficulty, according to the theoretical design for measuring intelligence. Substantiating the empirical and theoretical grounds of such a latent trait is the impetus for the present study. This study involved eighth and ninth graders in Hong Kong, China, by identifying the latent trait of Raven's Standard Progressive Matrices.

School grades are an important criterion for calibrating intelligence because of its theoretical relevance to intelligence and success if life. Empirically, grades are commonly a consequence or manifestation of intelligence (Chamorro-Premazic and Furnham 2008; Johnson et al. 2007). The relationship simply illustrates consistency between grades and intelligence due to their common function as a demonstration of ability and cognitive development (Bradley et al. 1988; Sims and Sims 1995). Similar to intelligence, grades are therefore an indicator of competence (Furstenberg et al. 1999; Luthar et al. 2006). Moreover, grades are crucial for social stratification (de Bruyn et al. 2003), attaining success in society (Wilson et al. 1997), maintaining personal and social health or well-being (Sacker et al. 2002), and myriad social activities (Hynd et al. 2000), including those in work (Cooksey and Rindfuss 2001; Rich 1999) and leisure (Adams and Stone 1977). Hence, societal pressure on students' achievement in school grades is evident (Broh 2002; Dehejia et al. 2009). The pressure is particularly high and vital on students' getting high grades, which are difficult to get and therefore provides a publicly recognized indication of performance and competence.

CONTRIBUTIONS OF INTELLIGENCE AND EFFORT

Although the thesis of consistency tends to explain the contribution of intelligence to grades, this thesis is not entirely convincing because of the presence of inconsistency in practice between intelligence and grades. Notably, while intelligence such as Raven's Standard Progressive Matrices typically taps reasoning ability by multiple-choice items, grades obtained in school cover abilities in various subjects. The assessment of subject ability typically involves a plurality of methods, including teachers' assessment of students' essay writing and other performances. That is, both the coverage and assessment methods of grades are different from the test of intelligence and conceptual inconsistency between grades and intelligence is evident. Hence, the ability assessed in the intelligence test does not directly translate into school grades. The translation would rather require the student's learning effort, which applies intelligence to studying to get grades. This mediating process of effort involves the effect of intelligence on effort and the effect of effort on grades. The former effect reflects the social-cognitive or self-efficacy mechanism in which the student's belief about competence or intelligence leads the student to put effort into studying (Gadzella et al. 1997; Verkuyten et al. 2001). A basis for the effect is the student's expectation about getting grades based on the competence of the effort or outcome expectancy (Levpuscek et al. 2009; Murdock and Miller 2003). When a student finds oneself to have competence in making rewarding study effort, the student is likely to make the effort (Hau and Salili 1996). This effect furthermore hinges on the student's realization of his or her actual intelligence, possibly by learning and self-reflection through experience in study and testing (Tompson and Dass 2000). The intelligence is thus a basis for forming study effort to earn grades. Obviously, study effort is part of the assessment for grades, as the teacher tends to emphasize the student's perseverance in completing classroom and homework assignments (George et al. 1998; Ho 2003). Accordingly, rather than relying on tests, the teacher requires the student to demonstrate effort and competence in the learning process, including individual and collective engagement in exercises and projects. Without doubt, studying effort is an essential means to acquire learning and thereby grades, simply because the student cannot learn a substantive subject just with a quick glance (Brookhart 1998; Singh et al. 2007). Learning the grammar, formulae, and ways of reasoning is clearly required for studying in secondary school.

Suspicion about the contribution of intelligence to school grades largely evolves from research and theory about academic achievement in higher education, where the contribution fails to materialize (Cote and Levine 2000; Hickman et al. 2000). Explanations for the failure are fourfold, pertaining to the (1) range or selectivity effect, (2) educational expansion, (3) importance of study effort instead, and (4) declining validity or relevance (Cote and Levine 2000; Hickman et al. 2000; Laidra et al. 2007; Strenze 2007; Zhang 2000). The range or selectivity effect means that students group themselves into an educational institution according to their intelligence. This grouping reduces variation in intelligence and therefore its predictive power. The second force, educational expansion, purports that intelligence becomes less important as a concern for education. Consequently, demand for and difficulty in schoolwork diminish and students with low intelligence can achieve high grades. Moreover, the importance of intelligence tends to shrink because of the rising importance of study effort, which teachers treasure in grading (George et al. 1998). A further explanation is the declining relevance of intelligence, in terms of analogical reasoning and spatial ability, to studying in substantive subjects in school. Cumulative knowledge in the subjects would instead be essential for the further acquisition of knowledge to earn grades.

Clarifying the independent and related contributions of intelligence and effort to grades is of concern for this study. The concern arises because effort is not solely a product of intelligence, and effort and intelligence can contribute to grades independently (Brackney and Karabenick 1995; Schaefer and McDermott 1999). Furthermore, the concern involves the relative contributions of intelligence and effort, as effort is sometimes more predictive of grades than is intelligence (Schaefer and McDermott 1999). When grades hinge on the teacher's assessment and judgment, they are likely to depend on the student's effort. Nevertheless, some of the contribution of effort is attributable to intelligence, which is partly an antecedent to effort. To be fair, the total effect of intelligence on grades, including the mediated effect through effort and the direct effect, deserves examination.

Intelligence may not be equally predictive of grades in various subjects. Theory and research have suggested that intelligence is more predictive of mathematical achievement than language achievement (Pind et al. 2003; Raven and Raven 2003). The differential predictability may stem from the stronger relationship between mathematical achievement and nonverbal analogical reasoning tapped by Raven's Standard Progressive Matrices. Apparently, verbal intelligence is distinct from nonverbal ability assessed by the Matrices (Kuttala and Lehto 2008; Mackintosh and Bennett 2005).

EXCELLENCE THEORY

Going beyond assessing the contributions of intelligence and effort to grades, this study aims to test an *excellence theory* of the acquisition of grades. The excellence theory posits that the upper end of intelligence, identified by ability to solve the most difficult reasoning problems, is particularly a contributor of grades. This theory stems from the need to put the contribution of intelligence into the context of getting school grades. Under such a context, intelligence is unlikely to translate directly into school grades. The context in practice is one in which the teacher awards grades preferably to a few outstanding students, who benefit from their excellent intelligence and their classmates' support.

In the first place, the teacher would offer privileged treatment to a few outstanding students by giving them extraordinarily higher grades to allow them to get scholarships and other awards. This practice is partly to promote outstanding students as paragons for the school and partly to stem from comparative assessment, which grades one's performance with reference to others' performance (Natriello and McPartland 1999; Soodak and Podell 1994). The grading approach simply reflects the logic that when something is scarce or exceptionally in a positive way, it is most valuable. This preference for excellent intelligence rests on the interpersonal theory of academic achievement, which emphasizes the student's relationship with the teacher as a decisive determinant of grades (Mpofu 1997). Accordingly, the teacher's liking for the student is the prime cause of the student's getting good grades (Dijkstra et al. 2004; Magnuson et al. 2006). The teacher's preference for the excellent student, moreover, reflects the case that the winner takes all. This case suggests that students compete for their grades in school and the winner is the top excellent student whom the teacher likes.

Secondly, excellent intelligence reflected by ability to solve the very difficult reasoning problems would indicate comprehensive and versatile competence, which is most conducive to school achievement, as well as success in other aspects. This is because solving the very difficult reasoning problems requires mastery of an integrated set of analytic skills (Mackintosh and Bennett 2005; van der Ven and Ellis 2000). Such mastery is categorically superior to ability to solve problems of lower difficulty and is likely to determine success in school and other places. A condition for the success is that the synergy of abilities required to solve difficult problems can engender multiplicative and much more valuable benefits than can singular abilities (Ford 1996; Sternberg and Grigorenko 1993).

Thirdly, the student with superior intelligence would enjoy admiration and support from classmates, as well as the teacher, because of the desire for affiliation with the excellent and successful person (Prinstein and La Greca 2002). The admiration and affiliation also reflect students' tendency of clustering themselves around excellent, attractive, and similar students (Snijders and Baerveldt 2003). Evidently, whereas low-achievers like to form a clique of their own, high-achievers like to admire and support the most outstanding achiever. The high-achievers' support would further contribute to the top achiever's grades by collaboration and offering other favors in school. According to the logic of division of labor, collaboration is beneficial by allowing partners to exercise their best to earn the greatest (Lou et al. 2000). The merit of collaboration clearly happens in school, which requires the division of labor to tackle different problems collaboratively (Chauvet and Blatchford 1993; WIlczenski and Coomey 2007). Notably, collaborative learning and exercises are a component of schoolwork that is conducive to grades (Jarvis et al. 1997; Muscott and O'Brien 1999). When the top intelligent student gets other achievers' support and collaboration, his or her grades are likely to elevate further.

LATENT TRAIT OF INTELLIGENCE

A necessary basis for the test of the intelligence effect is the identification of the latent trait of intelligence that is consonant with the underlying theory about the assessment of intelligence. Essential in the latent trait is the hierarchical property differentiating intelligence items of varying levels of difficulty. The response to an item is then a function of the respondent's intelligence and the difficulty and discrimination of the item (Baker 1992; Muthen and Muthen 2006). Clearly, Raven's Standard Progressive Matrices comprise items of differential levels of difficulty, grouped into five sets to assess intelligence or its eductive reasoning component (Raven 2000; Raven and Raven 2003). Eductive reasoning means the ability to draw meaning from an array of objects by both perceptive and analytic skills, which employ reasoning rules such as figural addition and subtraction to solve problems (Mackintosh and Bennett 2005; van der Ven and Ellis 2000). The different compositions of skills required thereby define five sets of intelligence with clear-cut difficulty or ability levels.

Apart from its internal hierarchical structure, the latent trait of intelligence would demonstrate relationships with external factors according to pertinent theory and research. Age, grade in school (i.e., education level), and gender can be three such external factors. Based on the developmental perspective of maturation, age would raise intelligence (Brouwers et al. 2006; Gormley et al. 2005). This expectation would also apply to grade in school (Ceci 1996; Halpern 1996).

However, because this study only covers students of two consecutive grades, variation in grade may not be sufficient to illustrate the grade effect on intelligence. As such, the effect of grade on intelligence would not be prominent. Further, gender would not make a difference, as the boy and girl are too young to manifest differential development in intelligence (Lynn and Irwing 2004).

The above review thus unfolds several loopholes for the current study to address. These loopholes include the verification the excellence facet of intelligence measured by Raven's Standard Progressive Matrices and the exploration of its relationships with age, grade in school, gender, study effort, and school achievement. Filling these loopholes would essentially champion the excellence theory of intelligence to register the excellence facet as particularly crucial for school achievement.

RELEVANCE OF THE HONG KONG STUDY

As a place somewhat different from the West and others, Hong Kong is apt for updating knowledge about intelligence that is of international interest. Principally, intelligence, as based on Raven's Progressive Matrices, has involved research and practice that are comparable internationally (Mills and Ablard 1993; Pind et al. 2003). Adaptation of knowledge about intelligence across places, such as Hong Kong (Chan 1984; Raven 2000), is feasible. This happens because of many similarities between Hong Kong and other places, including the Westernized political and educational structure (Kennedy 2004; Sweeting 1990), educational expansion (Shive 1992), and emphasis on internalization (Adamson and Lai 1997). Nevertheless, distinct features in Hong Kong particularly make it a valuable place for testing and generalizing knowledge. Such features include ability stratification in schooling (Marsh et al. 2000; Marsh and Hau 2003), collectivistic emphasis in schooling (Chan 2005; Marsh et al. 2000), and de-emphasis on standardized tests in routine schooling (Fok 2004). These features make the study important for examining how the function of intelligence traverses differences across places.

The Current Study

The aim of the study is to examine the contribution of intelligence and effort to school grades, with particular reference to the excellence theory, based on the latent trait of intelligence. For this aim, the following research tasks will be completed:

1. Identifying the latent trait that follows the theory about the constitution of intelligence, that is, reasoning ability based on Raven's Standard Progressive Matrices
2. Identifying a latent trait to represent the excellence facet of intelligence based on the most difficult items (i.e., those of Set E) and another latent trait to represent intelligence based on less difficult items (i.e., those of Sets A to D)
3. Examining the effects of age, grade in school, and gender on the latent traits
4. Examining the effects of various latent traits of intelligence on study effort and grades
5. Examining the effects of study effort on grades

Methods

In 1998, we conducted a survey of 2,545 eighth and ninth graders attending 23 secondary schools in Hong Kong to complete Raven's Standard Progressive Matrices and questions about studying in school. They completed the assessment of intelligence and the survey in a classroom setting, with research personnel's invigilation.

The schools represented a randomly selected random sample solicited from the government, which provided funding for all schools, except a few private schools. As such, the secondary schools covered those located in different parts of Hong Kong and those of different bands of ability standing (i.e., based on grades in primary school).

The presence of the different bands happened when the government classified secondary school entrants into different ability bands and assigned different bands of entrants to different schools.

Among the student participants, 60.0% were eighth graders and 40.0% were ninth graders. Their average age was 14.3 years (see Table 1). Slightly more (52.1%) of them were boys than were girls (47.9%). They attended one of the 72 different classes (i.e., fixed groupings) of the schools.

Table 1. Means and standard deviations

	Scoring	M	SD
Chinese grades	0-100	61.7	15.5
English grades	0-100	58.7	17.4
Math grades	0-100	58.7	21.3
Core grades	0-100	59.7	14.3
Intelligence	0-60	48.2	8.3
Intelligence (normalized)	-	95.3	16.8
Effort	0-100	55.8	16.0
Grade	8-9	8.4	0.5
Age	years	14.3	1.0
Female	0, 100	47.9	50.0

MEASUREMENT

Each of the students completed Raven's Standard Progressive Matrices and answered questions about study effort and latest grades. Raven's Standard Progressive Matrices, the instrument for measuring intelligence, consisted of 60 multiple-choice questions ordered in five sets (Sets A to E).

The Matrices, consisting of nonverbal, pictorial patterns, had evolved since 1936 (Raven and Raven 2003).

Table 2. Standardized factor loadings of effort and grades

Item	Loading
Effort	
I work hard to do well in this class even if I don't like what we are doing.	.427
When course work is difficult, I give up. (-)	.531
Even when course materials are dull, I manage to keep working until I finish.	.549
I often feel so bored when I study that I quit before finish what I planned to do. (-)	.464
Grades	
Chinese	.544
English	.635
Math	.712
Intelligence based of the most difficult items (Set E)	
E05	.922
E06	.837
E07	.649
E08	.779
E09	.671
E10	.712
E11	.588
E12	.613

Note: (-): reversed scoring.

This study eventually retained 30 items to identify a latent trait of intelligence that conformed to the theoretical structure of increasing difficulty across the five sets. Among these 30 items, the eight most difficult items in Set E identified the latent trait of excellent intelligence, whereas the other 22 items reflected non-excellent intelligence based on items of lower difficulty.

Study effort comprised four five-step rating items (Pintrich et al. 1991), giving an internal consistency reliability (α) coefficient of .548 (see Table 2).

For the ease of interpretation and without distortion, the five steps generated scores of 0 for "strongly disagree," 25 for "disagree," 50 for "neutral," 75 for "agree," and 100 for "strongly agree." The latest grades were in a range from 0 to 100, with 100 representing the maximum. They included those for Chinese, English, and mathematics. The average of these three grades represented the grades of the three core subjects, which were common in all secondary schools in Hong Kong.

ANALYTIC APPROACHES

Whereas the conventional approach technique applied linear regression analysis to composites (i.e., simple averages) of items representing intelligence, study effort, and grades, the unprecedented latent-clustering analytic approach pioneered in this study identified latent factors based on the items of intelligence, effort, and grades. The latter was the preferred and standard approach, which aptly identified the latent traits or factors, taking consideration of differential discrimination and difficulty of different items. In identifying the latent factors, the approach recognized the clustering nature of the sample, which grouped students into 72 classes. Students within each class are interdependent, due to their exposure to the common contextual effect of the class. Adjustment for the clustering effect was viable by M*plus*, which also identified the latent trait of intelligence based on dichotomous items in a confirmatory factor analysis plus a structural relation analysis framework (Muthen and Muthen 2006).

Identification of the latent trait of intelligence aimed to reveal the difficulty of items in five levels, ranging from Set A to Set E. Furthermore, the aim was to avoid overlap or reversal in difficulty among items of different sets, such that the difficulties of all items in Set A were lower than were those of any item in Set B and so on. To meet such an identification requirement, the analysis eventually needed to reduce the number of items to obtain a refined set of items. The identification would only be credible when the latent trait model fitted the data. In this connection, Mplus displayed the likelihood-ratio chi-square (L^2), root-mean-square error of approximation (RMSEA), Comparative Goodness-of-Fit Index (CFI), and Tucker-Lewis Fit Index (TLI) to indicate the fit. The rule of thumb for a model with 15 input variables suggested a good fit with the RMSEA below .07 and CFI or TLI above .95 (Hu and Bentler 1999). Relaxation of the rule was appropriate for more input variables (Marsh et al. 2004), as in the models examined in this study. To attain a good fit, the models needed to identify sources of relationships other than the proposed latent trait of intelligence. An alternative source pertained to the five sets (Set A to E), which were likely to impose contextual effects on items within each of the sets (Tourangeau et al. 2000). The contextual effect of each of the sets would result in residual correlations among items of the same set.

Specification of such contextual effects was necessary to identify the latent trait with a good fit.

In addition to identifying the latent traits of intelligence, the integrated model of structural equation modeling identified the latent factors of effort and grades as well. Whereas the latent factor of effort comprised four items, the latent factor of grades encompassed grades in Chinese, English, and mathematics. Moreover, the integrated model included age, grade in school, and gender as background predictors.

Essentially, the latent-clustering approach fitted six models: Model 1 was a confirmatory factor model of one intelligence trait based on all sixty items. Model 2 was another confirmatory factor model of one intelligence trait based on a reduced set of items. Model 3 identified an intelligence trait and effort factor for a structural relation analysis. Model 4 identified a grades factor for the structural relation analysis, in addition to those specified in Model 3. Model 5 differentiated a latent trait of intelligence based on the most difficult items and another latent trait based on less difficult items, together with the factor of effort in the structural relation analysis. Model 6 identified the factor of grades, in addition to those specified in Model 5.

RESULTS

On average, the students' grades ranged from 58.7 to 61.7 and the average grades of the three core subjects were 59.7 (see Table 1). The average study effort was 55.8. Based on the count of correct items in Raven's Standard Progressive Matrices, the average was 48.2. The average intelligence, as normalized according to age, was 95.3 (Chan 1984). All of these findings indicated that the average had a modest level of grade, effort, and intelligence.

Application of the latent-clustering analytic approach showed that all the six models attained a good fit (see Table 3). Model 1, which represented the confirmatory factor model using all the 60 intelligence items, attained a lower Comparative Goodness-of-Fit Index (CFI) of .848, than did those of the other models. Nevertheless, Model 1 still received a good fit, according to other goodness-of-fit indicators. Because of the good fit of the models, estimates from the models were credible. These findings therefore endorsed all the confirmatory factor models and integrated structural relation models, including varying numbers of latent traits or factors.

Table 3. Goodness of fit

Model	Input variables	Latent variables	L^2	df	RMSEA	CFI	TLI
1.	60	1 (IQ)	1673	231	.048	.848	.939
2.	30	1 (IQ)	114	38	.028	.952	.975
3.	36	2 (IQ, effort)	177	48	.033	.915	.947
4.	36	3 (IQ, effort, grades)	181	48	.034	.912	.945
5.	36	3 (IQ1, IQ2, effort)	179	30	.033	.914	.947
6.	36	4 (IQ1, IQ2, effort, grades)	172	49	.032	.918	.950

Note: IQ1 = intelligence based on the most difficult (Set E) items; IQ2 = intelligence based on less difficult items.

IDENTIFICATION OF LATENT FACTORS

All the 60 items of intelligence specified in Model 1 manifested substantial discrimination or factor loadings, thus indicating the convergent validity of the items in identifying the latent trait of intelligence (see Table 4). However, the difficulties of the 60 items did not demonstrate the hierarchical structure as maintained by the theory that separated the items into five levels of difficulty. For instance, the difficulty of Item A12 was higher than were those of some items in Set B and the difficulty of Item B12 was higher than were those of some items in Set C. Hence, even though Model 1 found a good fit and convergent validity, it did not bolster the hierarchical structure in item difficulty.

To attain a hierarchical structure consonant of the theory, a series of analysis culminated in Model 2 to retain 30 of the 60 items. Model 2 manifested convergent validity in terms of discrimination or factor loadings and hierarchical structure in item difficulty. The latter condition maintained that item difficulty in a set of lower difficulty was all lower than that in a set of higher difficulty.

A drawback in Model 2 was the somewhat lower discrimination of the two most difficult items. The finding might be an indication that the most difficult items tended to identify a latent trait other than that identified by the less difficult items.

In addition, identification of the two more factors for study effort and grades was successful. As the involved items demonstrated substantial loadings on their respective factors (see Table 2), their convergent and discriminant validity held in view of the good fit of the overall model (see Table 3).

A further confirmatory factor model were able to differentiate a latent trait based on the most difficult items of Raven's Matrices from another latent trait based on less difficult items.

Table 4. Standardized discrimination and difficulty of intelligence items

Item	Original composition		Refined composition	
	Discrimination	Difficulty	Discrimination	Difficulty
A01	.546	-2.029	.576	-2.029
A02	.584	-2.045	.580	-2.045
A03	.548	-1.992	.550	-1.992
A04	.591	-2.104	.565	-2.104
A05	.780	-2.132	.736	-2.132
A06	.749	-2.095	.723	-2.095
A07	.724	-1.907	.737	-1.907
A08	.524	-1.665	.482	-1.665
A09	.749	-1.957	.745	-1.957
A10	.680	-1.741	.661	-1.741
A11	.556	-1.212	-	-
A12	.448	-.784	-	-
B01	.778	-2.078	-	-
B02	.761	-1.971	-	-
B03	.809	-2.086	-	-
B04	.781	-1.964	-	-

Item	Original composition		Refined composition	
	Discrimination	Difficulty	Discrimination	Difficulty
B05	.753	-1.871	-	-
B06	.434	-1.404	.507	-1.404
B07	.492	-1.303	.566	-1.303
B08	.518	-1.111	.584	-1.111
B09	.511	-1.245	.570	-1.245
B10	.629	-1.638	.686	-1.638
B11	.541	-1.152	.595	-1.152
B12	.586	-.728	-	-
C01	.895	-1.866	-	-
C02	.725	-1.612	-	-
C03	.579	-1.531	-	-
C04	.595	-1.254	-	-
C05	.745	-1.627	-	-
C06	.672	-.990	.700	-.990
C07	.850	-1.479	-	-
C08	.605	-.491	-	-
C09	.601	-1.041	.587	-1.041
C10	.615	-.433	-	-
C11	.602	-.198	-	-
C12	.584	.666	-	-
D01	.813	-1.838	-	-
D02	.725	-1.528	-	-
D03	.724	-1.378	-	-
D04	.750	-1.348	-	-
D05	.819	-1.595	-	-
D06	.665	-1.111	-	-
D07	.625	-.961	.624	-.961
D08	.561	-.877	.542	-.877
D09	.634	-.817	.619	-.817
D10	.708	-.946	.654	-.946
D11	.381	.413	-	-
D12	.437	.851	-	-
E01	.706	-.946	-	-
E02	.680	-.767	-	-
E03	.680	-.802	-	-
E04	.656	-.563	-	-
E05	.708	-.710	.627	-.710
E06	.626	-.422	.569	-.422
E07	.515	-.177	.409	-.177
E08	.591	-.110	.528	-.110
E09	.485	.174	.404	.174
E10	.524	.369	.436	.369
E11	.379	.737	.269	.737
E12	.420	.756	.328	.756

Notably, the discriminations or factor loadings of the most difficult items of intelligence (Set E) were stronger than were those estimated for the latent trait based on all items (compare Table 2 and Table 4). This factor of excellent intelligence involved only eight items embedded in Set E of Raven's matrices. The correlation between the latent trait based on the most difficult intelligence items and the latent trait based on the less difficult intelligence items was .634. Nevertheless, the correlation was not strong enough to imply that the two latent traits were redundant or collinear.

PREDICTING GRADES

Intelligence based on the latent trait was significantly but weakly predictive of grades in Chinese ($\beta = .105$) and English ($\beta = .183$) (see Table 5). In contrast, the direct contribution of intelligence to grades in mathematics was stronger ($\beta = .273$).

Table 5. Standardized effects on grades

Predictor	Latent-clustering				Conventional			
	Chinese	English	Math	Core	Chinese	English	Math	Core
Intelligence	.105*	.183***	.273***	.311***	.143***	.205***	.281***	.280***
Effort	.259***	.261***	.277***	.414***	.178***	.182***	.188***	.232***
Grade	-.060	.043	-.142**	-.092	-.043	.058*	-.126***	-.058**
Age	.115**	-.065	.104*	.071	.103***	-.071**	.093***	.056*
Female	.163***	.190***	.030	.208***	.168***	.193***	.039	.155***
R^2	.123	.157	.183	.348	.095	.124	.139	.170

*: $p < .05$; **: $p < .01$; ***: $p < .001$.

Table 6. Standardized effects on grades

Predictor	Chinese	English	Math	Core
Intelligence (Set A – D)	-.015	.020	.051	.016
Intelligence (Set E)	.151*	.214***	.270***	.369***
Effort	.249***	.248***	.264***	.391***
Grade	-.063	.029	-.146***	-.098
Age	.103*	-.082*	.085	.040
Female	.169***	.199***	.040	.223***
R^2	.131	.173	.199	.388

*: $p < .05$; **: $p < .01$; ***: $p < .001$.

Table 7. Total effects on grades

Predictor	Chinese	English	Math	Core
Intelligence (Set A – E)	.138**	.173***	.216***	.364***
Intelligence (Set A – D)	-.025	.009	.040	-.004
Intelligence (Set E)	.199**	.262***	.321***	.449***
Female	.173***	.196***	.032	.216***

*: $p < .05$; **: $p < .01$; ***: $p < .001$.

This contrast is in line with the expectation about the differential predictability of grades by intelligence. Whereas the direct contribution to the grades of each of the individual subjects was weak, the contribution to the factor of grades of the three core subjects was stronger ($\beta = .311$). Importantly, similar findings evolved from analysis based on the conventional approach, which employed composites without identifying the latent factors and adjusting for the clustering effect (see Table 5). Nevertheless, the direct effect of intelligence on the overall grades of the three core subjects was weaker as estimated by the conventional approach. By identifying the latent factor of grades or academic achievement, the latent-clustering approach thus detected a stronger contribution by intelligence. Intelligence appeared to emit a weaker direct effect on grades than did study effort, as estimated by the latent-clustering approach (see Table 5). Notably, the direct effect of effort on the grades factor was .414, whereas that of intelligence was only .311. These findings evolved from the analysis that allowed for effects of background predictors. Significant findings about background predictors showed that grades in mathematics were higher with advancing age but lower with advancing grade in school. Grades in Chinese were higher in an older student or a female student and grades in English were higher in a girl. Notably, tests based on the latent-clustering approach were more conservative than were those based on the conventional approach, because of adjustment for the clustering effect in the former. Identification of excellent intelligence based on the most difficult items obtained stronger direct effects on grades than before (compare Table 6 with Table 5). Notably, the direct effect of excellent intelligence on the grades factor was .391, which was noticeably stronger than .311 due to the intelligence factor based on all 30 items. In contrast, intelligence based on less difficult items did not yield a significant direct effect on any of the grades. Hence, intelligence based on the eight most difficult items outperformed intelligence based on the 22 less difficult items in predicting grades. Nevertheless, the direct effect of intelligence was generally inferior to that of study effort, except on grades in mathematics ($\beta = .270$ vs. 264). The total effects of intelligence on grades were stronger, as they incorporated the part mediated by study effort. As such, the total effect of intelligence based on 30 items on the grades factor was .364 and the total effect of intelligence based on the eight most difficult items was .449 (see Table 7). The latter was stronger than the direct or total effect of study effort ($\beta = .391$) and the total effect of gender ($\beta = .216$).

PREDICTING EFFORT AND INTELLIGENCE

The mediation role of study effort was clear in view of the significant effect ($\beta = .127$) of intelligence (based on 30 items in Sets A to E) on effort (see Table 8). Particularly, intelligence based on the eight most difficult items (Set E) led a stronger effect ($\beta = .206$) on study effort, whereas intelligence based on the 22 less difficult items did not pose a significant effect ($\beta = -.053$). Study effort was also significantly predictably by age and gender such that the younger and female student made more effort. Intelligence, based on either all 30 items or the 8 most difficult items, was significantly a function of age. The age effects ($\beta = .090$ and .150), nevertheless, were weak. In contrast, intelligence based on the 22 less difficult items did not significantly depend on age. Grade in school and gender also did not exhibit a significant effect on any latent trait of intelligence.

Table 8. Standardized effects on effort and intelligence

Predictor	Effort	Effort	Intelligence	Intelligence (Set A – D)	Intelligence (Set E)
Intelligence (Set A – E)	.127*	-	-	-	-
Intelligence (Set A – D)	-	-.053	-	-	-
Intelligence (Set E)	-	.206**	-	-	-
Grade	.059	.055	.076	.067	.082
Age	-.067*	-.084**	.090*	.057	.150**
Female	.064*	.071*	-.051	-.038	-.078
R^2	.024	.037	.022	.012	.045

*: $p < .05$; **: $p < .01$; ***: $p < .001$.

DISCUSSION

The study identifies latent traits of intelligence based on 30 items of Raven's Standard Progressive Matrices and illustrates the contributions of the traits and study effort on school grades. Importantly, the illustration highlights the value of the excellence theory of grades attainment by demonstrating the contribution of intelligence based on the most difficult items to grades. The findings thereby elucidate some remarkable features of intelligence, grades, and their relationship as follows.

Sets A to E of Raven's Matrices, which order items with ascending difficulty, converged to identify a latent trait embodying such a hierarchical structure. The trait, nevertheless, was identifiable by 30 of the original 60 items, meaning that half of the items did not conform to the hierarchical structure. This finding happened as the solution to the Matrices involves abilities other than those for eductive, analogical reasoning, and the multiplicity of abilities can overshadow eductive reasoning. Consequently, only 30 items best reflected the ability proposed for the development of the instrument.

Furthermore, intelligence reflected in Raven's Matrices can consist of an excellent facet based on the most difficult items in Set E and other less outstanding facets. This possibility echoes effects due to the contexts of the five sets, which produce correlations among items within the same set.

The various facets of intelligence identified from different sets were clearly related, but not redundant. Notably, excellent intelligence based on the most difficult items differed a lot from intelligence based on easier items in relation to school grades, study effort, and background characteristics. Whereas excellent intelligence contributed to grades and effort and was predictable by age, intelligence based on easier items had none of the relationships. Hence, excellent intelligence was the effective facet of intelligence as a whole that displayed relationships with grades, efforts, and age.

Findings thus clearly support the excellence theory about the attainment of school grades due to excellent performance, as indexed by intelligence based on the most difficult items. As such, the underlying processes of the theory in the teacher's privileged grading, the gifted student versatile ability, and the student's earning support from admirers are plausible. Such plausibility largely relies on the secondary school context supportive of teachers' grading approach, coursework complexity, and students' social dynamics. The complexity of this context would make intelligence of a lower caliber ineffective for earning school grades (Brown 2001). Meanwhile, a way out of the complexity is attention to excellent intelligence demonstrated by the ability to solve the few most difficult problems. Apparently, the ability to solve the eight most difficult items of Raven's Matrices is conspicuous enough to attract support from both teachers and classmates.

Nevertheless, the contribution of intelligence or its excellent facet to school grades was at best moderate or modest, comparable to findings from some studies (Laidra et al. 2007; Meijer and van den Wittenboer 2004).

However, the contribution was weaker than that noted by some other studies (Chamorro-Premazic and Furnham 2006, 2008; Deary et al. 2007; Johnson et al. 2006, 2007; Rindermann and Neubauer 2004).

The contribution was particularly low to grades of singular language subjects, reflecting the lack of consistency between nonverbal reasoning in the intelligence assessment and language achievement (Deary et al. 2007; Pind et al. 2003). However, the contribution of intelligence as measured to grades in mathematics was not decidedly strong (total effect < .321). All these findings reveal the lack of strong consistency or similarity between the assessments of intelligence and school subject performance. Hence, intelligence assessed by Raven's Matrices could not directly translate into school grades. Furthermore, the findings purport that intelligence based on eductive reasoning does not appeal to the concern in school, which is instead dedicated to the promotion of subject knowledge and skills (Adamson and Lai 1997; Natriello and McPartland 1999).

Another explanation for the weak contribution of intelligence is the importance of learning effort and strategy (Schaefer and McDermott 1999; Zhang 2000). Accordingly, effort generally appeared to have a stronger contribution to grades than did intelligence and the contribution was mostly independent of that of intelligence. To attain good grades in language, learning effort was especially beneficial. Essentially, effort functions to bridge the gap between intelligence and grades. Effort also partly explained the girl's higher grades, because the girl made more effort than did the boy. This explanation concurs with the view about gender socialization (Duckworth et al. 2006; van Houtte 2004).

IMPLICATIONS

Although intelligence in terms of nonverbal analogical reasoning had a certain contribution to grades, the contribution is not strong. As intelligence is not a decisive predictor of grades, its role in the identification of underachievement is in need of caution. When the identification regards underachievement as achieving a level lower than that predicted by intelligence (McCall et al. 1992), the identification presumes a decisive prediction by intelligence. If the prediction were not decisive, the identification of underachievement would not be conclusive.

Rather than underachievement, achievement in terms of grades would be important for promotion. A crucial promotional message is that intelligence is not so deterministic of grades and learning effort is often more helpful than intelligence for earning grades. Crucially, discouragement of an entitative or fatalistic view about the contribution of intelligence to grades would be vital to motivate effort (Stipek and Gralinski 1996). Accordingly, the entitative view holds that as intelligence is stable, school performance would have little room for improvement. In contrast, an incremental view of school performance, which expects an increase in performance due to effort, is worth promotion.

Promotion of grades is especially necessary for students who are not excellent or able to solve the most difficult analogical problems. Such students would not achieve outstanding grades possibly because they are unable to appeal to teachers' favor and classmates' support. Assisting these students to excel in some way may be conducive to their improvement in grades. Such assistance, basing on the interpersonal theory of grading and the collaborative approach to school achievement, needs to set an aim at strengthening relationships between the students and their teachers and classmates. The assistance would benefit from the promotion of multiple opportunities for excellence (Catalano et al. 2003; Mettetal et al. 1997).

Essentially, different levels of reasoning measured by Raven's Progressive Matrices offer different implications for policy and practice. While the lower levels of reasoning measured by Matrices A to D appear to have minimal effects on learning effort and grades, advanced reasoning tapped by Matrix E is predictive the effort and grades. Hence, advanced reasoning particularly deserves attention, promotion, and scrutiny, just as intelligence and its resultant performance are of popular concern for meritocratic reasons (Guo and Steerns 2002; van der ven and Ellis 2000).

The above implications are relevant to the use Raven's Progressive Matrices in the international context, since the Matrices represent a nonverbal test that is free of cultural constraint. Essentially, the study highlights an excellence facet of just eight items of the Matrices that is particular relevant to students' grades, especially those in mathematics, which is not culturally dependent. Moreover, the prediction of grades in both English and Chinese by the excellence facet of the Matrices purports that the findings are clearly relevant to a spectrum of cultures affiliated with the two languages.

FURTHER RESEARCH

The present findings show that the excellence theory is a promising theory for further research, in both corroborating and substantiating the findings. As the excellence theory relies on the mechanisms of teacher grading, complicated coursework, and classmates' support, the three mechanisms deserve further research for illuminating the causal path from excellent intelligence to grades. Regarding teachers' grading, factors for research include the teacher's detection of, preference for, and desire to award the student's excellent intelligence. Research is to verify the interpersonal theory of grade attainment (Mpofu 1997), such that the relationship between the teacher and student is decisive on grades awarded to the student and the relationship builds on the student's excellent intelligence. Meanwhile, further research needs to verify students' competitiveness in getting grades, such that grades register relative accomplishment. Research would examine if prominent intelligence gives the edge in the competition. Regarding coursework complexity, further research needs to investigate if excellence intelligence particularly contributes to the solving of difficult academic problems. As such, research would examine the link between high levels of eductive, analogical, abilities and their synthesis to abilities required to tackle academic problems. Regarding classmates' support, further research needs to scrutinize the formation and contribution of classmates' network to the excellent student's grades. The essential condition for the contribution is the requirement for collaborative learning and accomplishment to earn grades. A crucial basis for the contribution in need of study is students' gravitation around and lending support to the top intelligent student. Conceivably, the support is only sustainable in a mutually beneficial students' network, such that all network members can find the network rewarding. However, further research needs to verify that the reward in terms of grades is more to the top intelligent student than to other students. An explanation in need of research is that the excellently intelligent student is better than are others in capitalizing on others' support to raise grades.

For generalizing the present and further research findings, further research needs to employ diverse samples and measurements. As such, research needs to include something more than Hong Kong Chinese students' responses to Raven's Matrices. Moreover, further research can cover a diverse set of contexts, including schooling, cultural and temporal or historical ones, to determine influences due to contexts. Notably, students' educational level would make a difference in the contribution of intelligence according to range and differential validity effects. In this case, a more selective setting that results in the concentration of students of high intelligence would reduce the contribution of intelligence. Meanwhile, the relevance of intelligence to school assessment is another parameter for contextual examination. With regard to cultural influence, the student's intelligence would be influential more in an individualist culture than in a collectivist culture, because the individualist culture prizes the individual's ability more than the collectivist culture. Furthermore, intelligence may have differential effects between the short term and the long term, depending on the tendency of adaptation and effort to make compensation (Strenze 2007). Further research can examine the impact of the self-fulfilling prophecy on the increasing effect of intelligence over time and the impact of remediation on the decreasing effect of intelligence over time. Essentially, the goal of the contextual analysis is to explore the limit of generalizing findings about the intelligence effect.

REFERENCES

Adams, Arthur J., and Thomas H. Stone. 1977. "Satisfaction of Need for Achievement in Work and Leisure Time Activities." *Journal of Vocational Behavior,* 11:174-181.

Adamson, Bob, and Winnie Auyeung Lai. 1997. "Language and the Curriculum in Hong Kong: Dilemmas of Triglossia." *Comparative Education,* 33(2):233-246.

Baker, Frank B. 1992. Item Response Theory: Parameter Estimation Techniques. New York: Marcel Dekker.

Brackney, Barbara E., and Stuart A. Karabenick. 1995. "Psychopathology and Academic Performance: The Role of Motivation and Learning Strategies." *Journal of Counseling Psychology,* 42(4):456-465.

Bradley, Robert H., Bettye M. Caldwell, and Stephen L. Rock. 1988. "Home Environment and School Performance: A Ten-Year Follow-up and Examination of Three Models of Environmental Action." *Child Development,* 59:852-867.

Broh, Beckett A. 2002. "Linking Extracurricular Programming to Academic Achievement: Who Benefits and Why?" *Sociology of Education,* 75(1):69-91.

Brookhart, Susan M. 1998. "Determinants of Student Effort on Schoolwork and School-based Achievement." *Journal of Educational Research,* 91(4):201-208.

Brouwers, Symen A., Ramesh C. Mishra, and Fons J.R. Van de Vijver. 2006. "Schooling and Everyday Cognitive Development among Kharwar Children in India: A Natural Experiment." *International Journal of Behavioral Development,* 30(6):559-567.

Brown, David K. 2001. "The Social Sources of Educational Credentialism: Status Cultures, Labor Markets, and Organizations." Sociology of Education Extra Issues:19-34.

Cassidy, Tony, and Richard Lynn. 1991. "Achievement Motivation, Educational Attainment, Cycles of Disadvantage, and Social Competence: Some Longitudinal Data." *British Journal of Educational Psychology,* 61:1-12.

Catalano, Richard F., James J. Mazza, Tracy W. Harachi, Robert D. Abbott, Kevin P. Haggerty, and Charles B. Fleming. 2003. "Raising Healthy Children through Enhancing Social Development in Elementary School: Results after 1.5 Years." *Journal of School Psychology,* 41:143-164.

Ceci, Stephen J. 1996. On Intelligence: A Bioecological Treatise on Intellectual Development. Cambridge, MA: Harvard University Press.

Chamorro-Premazic, Tomas, and Adrian Furnham. 2008. "Peronality, Intelligence and Approaches to Learning as Predictors of Academic Performance." *Personality and Individual Differences,* 44:1596-1603.

Chamorro-Premuzic, Thomas, and Adrian Furnham. 2006. "Self-assessed Intelligence and Academic Performance." *Educational Psychology,* 26(6):769-779.

Chan, David W. 2005. "Self-perceived Creativity, Family Hardiness, and Emotional Intelligence of Chinese Gifted Students in Hong Kong." *Journal of Secondary Gifted Education,* 16(2/3):47-56.

Chan, J. (1984). Raven's Progressive Matrices Test in Hong Kong. New Horizons, 25, 43-49.

Chauvet, Marie Josephe, and Peter Blatchford. 1993. "Group Composition and National Curriculum Assessment at Seven Years." *Educational Research,* 35(2):189-196.

Cooksey, Elizabeth C., and Ronald R. Rindfuss. 2001. "Patterns of Work and Schooling in Young Adulthood." *Sociological Forum,* 16(4):731-755.

Cote, James E., and Charles G. Levine. 2000. "Attitude versus Aptitude: Is Intelligence or Motivation more Important for Positive Higher-educational Outcomes?" *Journal of Adolescent Research,* 15(1):58-80.

de Bruyn, Eddy H., Maja Dekovic, and G. Wim Meijnen. 2003. "Parenting Goal Orientations, Classroom Behavior, and School Success in Early Adolescence." *Applied Developmental Psychology*, 24:393-412.

Deary, Ian J., Steve Strand, Pauline Smith, and Cres Fernandes. 2007. "Intelligence and Educational Achievement." *Intelligence,* 35:13-21.

Dehejia, Rajeev Thomas DeLeire, Erzo F.P. Luttmer, and Josh Mitchell. 2009. "The Role of Religious and Social Organizations in the Lives of Disadvantaged Youth." Pp.213-235 in The Problems of Disadvantaged Youth: An Economic Perspective, edited by Jonathan Gruber. Chicago, IL: University of Chicago Press.

Dijkstra, Anne Bert, Rene Veenstra, and Jules Peschar. 2004. "Social Capital in Education: Functional Communities around High Schools in the Netherlands." Pp.119-144 in Creation and Returns of Social Capital: A New Research Program, edited by Henk Flap and Beate Volker. London: Routledge.

Duckworth, Angela Lee, and Martin E.P. Seligman. 2006. "Self-discipline Gives Girls the Edge: Gender, Self-discipline, Grades, and Achievement Test Scores." *Journal of Educational Psychology*, 98(1):198-208.

Fok, Shui Che. 2004. "Values Orientations of Hong Kong's Reform Proposals." *Social Effectiveness and School Improvement,* 15(2):201-214.

Ford, Martin E. 1996. "Motivated Opportunities and Obstacles Associated with Social Responsibility and Caring Behavior in School Contexts." Pp.126-153 in Social Motivation: Understanding Children's School Adjustment, edited by Jeana Juvonen, and Kathryn R. Wentzel. Cambridge: Cambridge.

Furstenberg, Frank F., Jr., Thomas D. Cook, Jacquelynne Eccles, Glen H. Elder, Jr., and Arnold Sameroff. 1999. Managing to Make It: Urban Families and Adolescent Success. Chicago, IL: University of Chicago Press.

Gadzella, Bernadette M., Dean W. Ginther, G. Bryant, and Wendell, G. 1997. "Prediction of Performance in an Academic Course by Scores on Measures of Learning Style and Critical Thinking." *Psychological Reports,* 81(2):595-602.

George, Paul, Gordon Lawrence, and Donna Bushnell. 1998. Handbook for Middle School Teaching. New York: Longman.

Gormley, William T., Jr., Ted Gayer, Deborah Phillips, and Brittany Dawson. 2005. "The Effects of Universal Pre-K on Cognitive Development." *Developmental Psychology,* 41(6):872-884.

Guo, Guang, and Elizabeth Stearns. 2002. "The Social Influences on the Realization of Genetic Potential for Intellectual Development." *Social Forces* 80(3):881-1010.

Halpern, Diane F. 1996. "Changing Data, Changing Minds: What the Data on Cognitive Sex Differences Tell Us and What We Hear." *Learning and Individual Differences,* 8(1):73-82.

Hau, Kit-tai, and Farideh Salili. 1996. "Motivational Effects of Teachers' Ability versus Effort Feedback on Chinese Students' Learning." *Social Psychology of Education,* 1:69-85.

Hickman, Gregory P., Suanne Bartholomae, and Patrick C. McKenry. 2000. "Influence of Parenting Styles on the Adjustment and Academic Achievement of Traditional College Freshmen." *Journal of College Student Development,* 41(1):41-54.

Ho, Wai-chung. 2003. "Democracy, Citizenship, and Extra-musical Learning in Two Chinese Communities: Hong Kong and Taiwan." *Compare,* 33(2):155-171.

Hu, Li-tze, and Peter M. Bentler. 1999. "Cutoff Criteria for Fit Indexes in Covariance Structure Analysis: Conventional Criteria versus New Alternatives." *Structural Equation Modeling,* 6(1):1-55.

Hynd, Cynthia, Jodi Holschuh, and Scherrie Nist. 2000. "Learning Complex Scientific Information in Motivation Theory and Its Relation to Student Perceptions." *Reading and Writing Quarterly,* 16(1):23-57.

Jarvis, Sara V., Liz Sheer, and Della M. Hughes. 1997. "Community Youth Development: Learning the New Story." *Child Welfare*, 76(5):719-741.

Johnson, Wendy, Matt McGue, and William G. Iacono. 2006. "Genetic and Environmental Influences on Academic Achievement Trajectories During Adolescence." *Developmental Psychology,* 42(3):514-532.

Johnson, Wendy, Matt McGue, William G. Iacono. 2007. "Socioeconomic Status and School Grades: Placing Their Association in Broader Context in a Samof Biological and Adoptive Families." *Intelligence,* 35:526-541.

Kennedy, Peter. 2004. "The Politics of Lifelong Learning in Post-1997 Hong Kong." *International Journal of Lifelong Education,* 23(6):589-624.

Kohn, Melvin L. 1996. "The Bell Curve from the Perspective of Research on Social Structure and Personality." *Sociological Forum,* 11(2):395-411.

Kuttala, Minna, and Juhuni E. Lehto. 2008. "Some Factors Underlying Mathematical Performance: The Role of Visuospatial Working Memory and Non-verbal Intelligence." *European Journal of Psychology of Education,* 23(1):77-94.

Laidra, Kaia, Helle Pullmann, Juri Allik. 2007. "Personality and Intelligence as Predictors of Academic Achievement: A Cross-sectional Study from Elementary to Secondary School." *Personality and Individual Differences,* 42:441-451.

Levpuscek, Melita Puklek, and Maja Zupancic. 2009. "Math Achievement in Early Adolescence: The Role of Parental Involvement, Teachers' Behavior, and Students' Motivational Beliefs about Math." *Journal of Early Adolescence,* 29(4):541-570.

Lou, Yiping, Philip C. Abrami, and John C. Spence. 2000. "Effects of Within-class Grouping on Student Achievement: An Exploratory Model." *Journal of Educational Research,* 94(2):101-112.

Luthar, Suniya S., and Karen A. Shoum, and Pamela J. Brown. 2006. "Extracurricular Involvement among Affluent Youth: A Scapegoat for Ubiquitous Achievement Pressures?" *Developmental Psychology,* 42(3):583-597.

Lynn, Richard, and Paul Irwing. 2004. "Sex Differences in the Progressive Matrices: A Meta-analysis." *Intelligence,* 32:481-498.

Mackintosh, N.J., and E.S. Bennett. 2005. "What Do Raven's Matrices Measure? An Analysis in terms of Sex Differences." *Intelligence,* 33:663-674.

Magnuson, Katherine, Greg J. Suncan, and Ariel Kalil. 2006. "The Contribution of Middle Childhood Contexts to Adolescent Achievement and Behavior." Pp.150-172 in Developmental Contexts in Middle Childhood: Bridges to Adolescence and Adulthood, edited by Aletha C. Huston, and Marika N. Ripke. Cambridge, UK: Cambridge Univesity Press.

Marsh, Herbert W., Kit-tai Hau, and Zhonglin Wen. 2004. "In Search of Golden Rules: Comment on Hypothesis-testing Approaches to Setting Cutoff Values for Fit Indexes and Dangers in Overgeneralizing Hu and Bentler's (1999) Findings." *Structural Equation Modeling,* 11(3):320-341.

McCall, Robert B., Cynthia Evahn, and Lynn Kratzer. 1992. High School Underachievers. Newbury Park, CA: Sage.

Meijer, Anne Marie, and Godfried L.H. van den Wittenboer. 2004. "The Joint Contribution of Sleep, Intelligence and Motivation to School Performance." *Personality and Individual Differences,* 35:95-106.

Mettetal, Gwendolyn, Cheryl Jordan, and Sheryll Harper. 1997. "Attitudes toward a Multiple Intelligences Curriculum." *Journal of Educational Research,* 91(2):115-122.

Mills, Carol J., and Karen E. Ablard. 1993. "The Raven's Progressive Matrices: Its Usefulness for Identifying Gifted/talented Students." *Roeper Review,* 15(3):183-186.

Mpofu, Elias. 1997. "Children's Social Acceptance and Academic Achievement in Zimbabwean Multicultural School Settings." *Journal of Genetic Psychology,* 158(1):5-25.

Muscott, Howard S., and Sara Talis O'Brien. 1999. "Teaching Character Education to Students with Behavioral and Learning Disabilities through Mentoring Relationships." *Education and Treatment of Children,* 22(3):373-390.

Muthen, Linda K., and Bengt O. Muthen. 2006. *Mplus User's Guide.* Los Angeles, CA: Muthen and Muthen.

Natriello, Gary, and James M. McPartland. 1999. "Beyond the Battle of the Requirements: Accommodation and Motivation in Adjustments in High School Teachers' Grading Criteria." *Research in Sociology of Education and Socialization,* 12:165-184.

Opdenakker, Marie-Christine, and Jan Van Damme. 2007. "Do School Context, Student Composition and School Leadership Affect School Practice and Outcomes in Secondary Education?" *British Educaitonal Research Journal,* 33(2):179-206.

Pind, Jorgen, Eyrun K. Gunnarsdottir, Hinrik S. Johannesson. 2003. "Raven's Standard Progressive Matrices: New School Age Norms and a Study of the Test's Validity." *Personality and Individual Differences,* 34:375-386.

Pintrich, P. R., Smith, D. A. F., Garcia, T., and McKeachie, W. J. (1991). *A manual for the use of the Motivated Strategies for Learning Questionnaire (MSLQ).* Ann Arbor, MI: University of Michigan.

Prinstein, Mitchell J., and Annette M. La Greca. 2002. "Peer Crowd Affiliation and Internalizing Distress in Childhood and Adolescence: A Longitudinal Follow-back Study." *Journal of Research on Adolescence,* 12(3):325-351.

Raven, John, and Jean Raven. 2003. "Raven Progressive Matrices." Pp.223-237 in Handbook of Nonverbal Assessment, edited by R. Steve McCallum. New York: Kluwer.

Raven, John. 2000. "The Raven's Progressive Matrices: Change and Stability over Culture and Time." *Cognitive Psychology,* 41:1-48.

Rich, Lauren M. 1999. "Family Welfare Receipt, Welfare-benefit Levels, and the Schooling and Employment Status of Male Youth." *Social Science Research,* 28:88-109.

Rindermann, H., and A.C. Neubauer. 2004. "Processing Speed, Intelligence, Creativity, and School Performance: Testing and Causal Hypotheses Using Structural Equation Models." *Intelligence,* 32:573-589.

Sacker, Amanda, Ingrid Schoon, and Mel Barttey. 2002. "Social Inequality in Educational Achievement and Psychosocial Adjustment throughout Childhood: Magnitude and Mechanisms." *Social Science and Medicine,* 55:863-880.

Schaefer, Barbara A., and Paul A. McDermott. 1999. "Learning Behavior and Intelligence as Explanations for Children's Scholastic Achievement." *Journal of School Psychology,* 37(3):299-313.

Shive, Glenn. 1992. "Educational Expansion and the Labor Force." Pp.215-231 in Education and Society in Hong Kong: Toward One Country and Two Systems, edited by Gerard A. Postiglione. Hong Kong: Hong Kong University Press.

Sims, Serbrenia J., and Ronald R. Sims. 1995. "Learning and Learning Styles: A Review and Look to the Future." Pp.193-210 in The Importance of Learning Styles: Understanding the Implications for Learning, Course Design, and Education, edited by Ronald R. Sims and Serbrenia J. Sims. Westport, CT: Greenwood.

Singh, Knsum, Mido Chang, and Sandra Dika. 2007. "Effects of Part-time Work on School Achievement during High School." *Journal of Educational research,* 101(1):12-22.

Snijders, T.A.B., and Chris Baerveldt. 2003. "A Multilevel Network Study of the Effects of Delinquent Behavior on Friendship Evolution." *Journal of Mathematical Sociology,* 27:123-151.

Soodak, Leslie C., and David M. Podell. 1994. "Teachers' Thinking about Difficult-to-teach Students." *Journal of Educational Research,* 88(1):44-51.

Sternberg, Robert J., and Elena L. Grigorenko. 1993. "Thinking Styles and the Gifted." *Roeper Review,* 16(2):122-130.

Stipek, Deborah, and J. Heidi Gralinski. 1996. "Children's Beliefs about Intelligence and School Performance." *Journal of Educational Psychology,* 88(3):397-407.

Strenze, Tarmo. 2007. "Intelligence and Socioeconomic Success: A Meta-analytic Review of Longitudinal Research." *Intelligence,* 35:401-426.

Sweeting, Anthony. 1990. Education in Hong Kong Pre-1841 to 1941: Fact and Opinion: Materials from a History of Education in Hong Kong. Hong Kong: Hong Kong University Press.

Tompson, George H., and Parshotam Dass. 2000. "Improving Students' Self-efficacy in Strategic Management: The Relative Impact of Cases and Simulations." *Simulation and Gaming,* 31(1):22-41.

Tourangeau, Roger, Lance J. Rips, and Kenneth Rasinski. 2000. The Psychology of Survey Response. Cambridge: Cambridge University Press.

van der Ven, A.H.G.S., and J.L. Ellis. 2000. "A Rasch Analysis of Raven's Standard Progressive Matrices." *Personality and Individual Differences,* 29(1):45-64.

van Houtte, Mieke. 2004. "Why Boys Achieve Less at School than Girls: The Difference between Boys' and Girls' Academic Culture." *Educational Studies,* 30(2):159-173.

Verkuyten, Maykel, Jochem Thijs, and Kadir Canatan. 2001. "Achievement Motivation and Academic Performance among Turkish Early and Young Adolescents in the Netherlands." *Genetic, Social, and General Psychology Monographs,* 127(4):378-408.

WIlczenski, Felicia L., and Susan M. Coomey. 2007. A Practical Guide to Service Learning: Strategies for Positive Development in Schools. New York*: Springer.*

Wilson, Melvin N., Deanna Y. Cooke, and Edith G. Arrington. 1997. "African-American Adolescents and Academic Achievement: Family and Peer Influences." Pp.145-155 in Social and Emotional Adjustment and Family Relations in Ethnic Minority Families, edited by Ronald D. Taylor and Margaret C. Wang. Mahwah, NJ: Lawrence Erlbaum.

Zhang, Li-fang. 2000. "University Students' Learning Approaches in Three Cultures: An Investigation of Biggs's 3P Model." *Journal of Psychology,* 134(1):34-55.

In: Youth: Practices, Perspectives and Challenges
Editor: Elizabeth Trejos-Castillo

ISBN: 978-1-62618-067-3
© 2013 Nova Science Publishers, Inc.

Chapter 13

FAMILY DYSFUNCTION IN PEDIATRIC BIPOLAR DISORDER AND ASSOCIATED FAMILY-BASED INTERVENTIONS

Brendan A. Rich and Heather R. Rosen*

Department of Psychology, The Catholic University of America, Washington, DC, US

ABSTRACT

Pediatric bipolar disorder (PBD) is one of the most controversial areas of child psychopathology research and practice. The rate at which BD is being diagnosed in youth has substantially increased over the past decade: one study found a forty-fold increase in the diagnosis of BD in youth in outpatient settings (Moreno et al., 2007). Onset of bipolar illness in childhood can have a devastating impact on the emotional, cognitive, and social functioning of youth (Miklowitz, Biuckians, and Richards, 2006). Given the family environment's permeating influence on child development, family processes are important psychosocial factors to consider when evaluating the development and maintenance of severe psychopathology among youth (Repetti, Taylor, and Seeman, 2002).

This chapter reviews emerging empirical efforts to understand the causes, longitudinal outcomes, and optimal treatments for PBD by focusing on family functioning. Research has shown that having a child with BD adversely impacts the family (Schenkel, West, Harral, Patel, and Pavuluri, 2008). Conversely, family dysfunction has been shown to negatively impact the course of bipolar symptomatology in BD youth (Townsend, Demeter, Youngstrom, Drotar, and Findling, 2007).

In addition to reviewing this bi-directional causal relationship between PBD and family dysfunction, this chapter will focus on empirically supported family-based treatments for youth with BD. Identification of optimal psychosocial treatments of PBD increasingly focuses on the family system. This chapter will detail family-based approaches to treating PBD and identify shared psychotherapeutic approaches for

---

* Corresponding Author: Brendan A. Rich, Ph.D. Department of Psychology, The Catholic University of America, 620 Michigan Ave., NE, Washington, DC 20064, Phone / Fax: 202-319-5823 / 202-319-6263, Email: richb@cua.edu

ameliorating core PBD symptomatology and family dysfunction. Future directions for research, policy implications and recommendations for the field are also discussed.

INTRODUCTION

Bipolar disorder (BD) is one of the most severe and impairing psychiatric illnesses. Individuals with BD vary between extreme states of mania (a highly euphoric, energized or irritable mood state) and depression (a severe withdrawn, sad and often suicidal state) (Miklowitz, 2007). Among all medical illnesses, BD is the sixth leading cause of disability worldwide (Murray and Lopez, 1996). Approximately 2% of the U.S. population suffers from bipolar I or bipolar II disorder, and an additional 2.4% is affected by subsyndromal forms of the disorder (Merikangas et al., 2007). The diagnosis of BD in youth was traditionally considered rare (Biederman et al., 2003; Faedda, Baldessarini, Glovinsky, and Austin, 2004), and epidemiologic studies suggest that approximately 1-2% of children are diagnosed with BD (Lewinsohn, Klein, and Seeley, 1995; Merikangas and Pato, 2009; Merikangas et al., 2010). However, the past decade has witnessed substantially increased diagnosis of BD in youth (Harris, 2005; Moreno et al., 2007). For example, two studies find a four-fold increase in the diagnosis of BD in youth discharged from U.S. community hospitals (Blader and Carlson, 2007; Case, Olfson, Marcus, and Siegel, 2007). Even more alarming, a recent study finds a 40-fold increase in the diagnosis of BD in youth in outpatient settings (Moreno et al., 2007).

Bipolar disorder is associated with high rates of morbidity and mortality: between 25% and 50% of BD patients attempt suicide at least once and up to 15% die by suicide (Miklowitz and Johnson, 2006). Early-onset BD (i.e., onset of illness before late adolescence) may be a particularly insidious form of the illness. Youth who develop BD in childhood or early adolescence experience a more severe and longer course of illness than individuals who develop BD in adulthood (Geller and Luby, 1997). They have poorer response to treatment, decreased rates of recovery, greater rates of relapse in comparison to individuals with adult-onset BD (Geller et al., 2001), and have a 10-fold increased risk of suicide relative to the general population (Joshi and Wilens, 2009). Importantly, early-onset of bipolar illness greatly interferes with critical developmental tasks, especially in adolescence, including identity development, psychological independence, the formation of romantic relationships, and academic achievement (Miklowitz et al., 2006). Thus, due to the severity, complexity and chronicity of symptoms, pediatric BD (PBD) is an important public health concern.

In attempting to understand the factors that both cause and may improve the treatment of BD in youth, one domain of great interest to researchers and clinicians is family functioning. Broadly speaking, given the family environment's permeating influence on child development, family processes are important psychosocial factors to consider when evaluating the development and maintenance of severe psychopathology among youth (Repetti, Taylor, and Seeman, 2002). This chapter reviews emerging empirical efforts to understand the causes, longitudinal outcomes, and optimal treatments for PBD by focusing on family functioning. We discuss evidence demonstrating a bi-directional causal relationship between PBD and family dysfunction; that is, while having a child with BD impacts family and parental functioning, family factors also impact the course of BD in youth. Further, we will detail empirically supported family-based psychotherapeutic treatments for youth with

BD and identify shared components of psychotherapeutic approaches that ameliorate core PBD symptomatology and family dysfunction. Finally, future directions for using the family to identify predictors of psychopathology in at-risk youth and preventative interventions will be discussed.

EVIDENCE FOR DYSFUNCTION IN FAMILIES WITH BIPOLAR YOUTH

As noted the above, empirical data strongly support a bi-directional relationship between PBD and family dysfunction: while having a child with BD causes substantial adversity within the family environment, a family environment characterized by conflict can adversely impact the development and course of BD in youth. Given the severity of impairments associated with PBD, considerable demands are often placed on family members, impacting the overall functioning of the family unit (Schenkel, West, Harral, Patel, and Pavuluri, 2008). The family environments of BD youth are typically under tremendous strain, including high levels of emotional, economic, and pragmatic burdens and distress (Morris, Miklowitz, and Waxmonsky, 2007; Perlick, Hohenstein, Clarkin, Kaczynski, and Rosenheck, 2005). Caregivers often feel overwhelmed and isolated in their struggles to cope with their child's disorder and are in dire need of support (Miklowitz et al., 2004). Frequently, parents of BD adults and children develop depression themselves and seek psychiatric treatment (Perlick et al., 2005).

Additionally, Sullivan and Miklowitz (2010) found that increased severity of depressive symptoms in BD youth was related to decreased cohesion of parent-child relationships as reported by parents. Findings also indicated that the greater severity of manic symptoms, the higher familial conflict parents reported and the lower levels of cohesion reported by adolescents. Furthermore, family conflict may be greatest among BD adolescents with comorbid diagnoses [e.g., attention deficit hyperactivity disorder (ADHD) or oppositional defiant disorder (ODD)] (Sullivan and Miklowitz, 2010).

Expressed emotion (EE) is an important construct to consider when characterizing the family context in that it measures the emotional attitudes of caregiving relatives toward a mentally ill family member (Morris et al., 2007). Relatives with high-EE express high levels of critical comments, hostility, and/or emotional overinvolvement (i.e., overprotective behaviors, exaggerated emotional responses) when describing their interactions with the ill family member (Fristad, Gavazzi, and Mackinaw-Koons, 2003; Morris et al., 2007).

There is a greater tendency for high-EE relatives to attribute negative behaviors of their ill family member to internal and controllable aspects, such as personality or a lack of effort. High-EE relatives are particularly likely to display negative verbal and nonverbal interactions toward the patient following an acute episode of illness (Miklowitz, 2004), i.e., when most in need of support from family members. In contrast, low-EE relatives are more likely to attribute the patient's behaviors to uncontrollable factors, such as external stressors or illness (Barrowclough and Hooley, 2003), thus minimizing the extent to which they blame the patient for his/her difficulties.

Although there is limited research on the relationship between PBD, high-EE parents, and family functioning, one study found that BD adolescents with at least one high-EE parent, compared to BD teens with low-EE parents, have decreased family cohesion and adaptability, along with increased conflict during or shortly following a mood episode (Sullivan and Miklowitz, 2010).

While PBD can result in family dysfunction, conversely, family dysfunction has been shown to negatively impact the course of bipolar symptomatology in BD youth. Research overwhelmingly indicates an association between family environmental factors and the course of recurrent mood disorders (Miklowitz et al., 2004). In particular, discord, criticism, and conflict within the family environment are strongly related to recurring episodes of BD (Miklowitz, 2007). Townsend, Demeter, Youngstrom, Drotar, and Findling (2007) found that weaker problem solving ability within the family predicted greater depressive symptoms among BD adolescents. Additionally, impaired family functioning is also related to poor medication adherence among BD youth, which causes more rapid recurrences of illness episodes (Miklowitz et al., 2004).

Finally, there is evidence for long-term impact of family dysfunction on BD youth: lower maternal warmth has been associated with higher rates of relapse in BD adolescents at 8-year follow-up (Geller, Tillman, Craney, and Bolhofner, 2004).

Previous research also indicates that EE strongly influences the course of illness among patients with BD and other psychiatric disorders (Butzlaff and Hooley, 1998). In the adult BD literature, family environments with high-EE are strongly associated with poorer outcomes and increased relapse rates (Butzlaff and Hooley, 1998). For example, studies have shown that adults with BD are two to three times more likely to experience relapse in the nine months following an acute episode when they return home to high-EE family environment than patients who return to low-EE family environments (Barrowclough and Hooley, 2003; Miklowitz, 2004). Interestingly, a meta-analysis conducted by Butzlaff and Hooley (1998) found that this relationship between high-EE and relapse is greater in mood disorders including BD than in schizophrenia and adults with psychosis. As noted above, the literature on EE and PBD is limited. However, one study found that BD adolescents with at least one high-EE parent, compared to BD teens with low-EE parents, have significantly higher depressive and manic symptom ratings over the course of two years (Miklowitz et al., 2006). In summary, the research presented here strongly highlights the bi-directional relationship between family dysfunction, including factors related to EE, and PBD symptomatology and long-term outcome.

GENERAL TREATMENT APPROACHES

Pharmacological Interventions

With the tremendous amount of scholarly attention the field of PBD has received over the past decade and with the significant increase in the rate at which it is being diagnosed, there has correspondingly been a growth in the number of drug trials for children and adolescents with BD (Miklowitz et al., 2008). Pharmacotherapy is the first step of treatment for BD to assist with more immediate reduction of symptoms and to stabilize the patient for engagement in psychotherapy (Miklowitz et al., 2004). In particular, pharmacological treatment is used to address acute mood episodes, continuous relapse prevention, and bipolar symptom control (Morris et al., 2007). According to the treatment guidelines of the American Academy of

Child and Adolescent Psychiatry, mood stabilizers (e.g., lithium carbonate, divalproex sodium, topiramate, valproate) and atypical antipsychotics (e.g., quetiapine, risperidone, aripiprazole, olanzapine) are typically the first line of treatment for PBD (McClellan, Kowatch, and Findling, 2007). Monotherapy (i.e., use of a single drug) versus combination therapy (i.e., simultaneous use of multiple drugs) is also based on the presence of psychosis: monotherapy with mood stabilizers or atypical antipsychotics is the first step for youth presenting without psychosis, whereas combination therapy is the recommended first step for youth presenting with psychosis (Kowatch et al., 2005).

Although pharmacotherapy is the first line of treatment for PBD, it is of limited efficacy: 55% to 70% of individuals with child-onset BD experience relapse within a two- to four-year period even when taking medication (Geller et al., 2004). Furthermore, there is a serious problem of medication adherence among both adults and youth with BD, which causes more rapid recurrences of illness episodes (Miklowitz et al., 2004; Morris et al., 2007). Poorer adherence to drug treatment has been associated with younger age in BD populations (Miklowitz et al., 2004). Miklowitz, Goldstein, Nuechterlein, Snyder, and Mintz (1988) found that only about 30% of BD youth with recent-onset mania adhered to their medication regimens on a regular basis at a nine-month follow-up. Individuals with BD often discontinue their use of medications due to pharmacological side effects, belief that they will not experience another mood episode, perceived loss of control, and societal stigma. As noted earlier, a negative family environment is associated with poor adherence to medication treatment (Miklowitz et al., 2004). The sudden termination of medication, however, typically results in relapse (Morris et al., 2007). While medications are implicated as the first course of treatment, their limited efficacy, concerns about side effects, and poor compliance requires that researchers identify non-pharmacological interventions that can aid in the treatment of PBD.

Psychosocial Interventions

While progress has been made in the treatment of young patients with BD via pharmacological interventions, little empirical attention has focused on adjunctive psychosocial interventions for early-onset BD (Fristad et al., 2003; Miklowitz et al., 2004). Medication alone does not sufficiently address the important psychosocial issues that accompany bipolar illness (Morris et al., 2007). For example, it is unlikely that medications will be effective in reducing the intensity of environmental stressors or in buffering against stress after the BD individual discontinues their medication (Miklowitz, Mullen, and Chang, 2008).

Psychosocial interventions aimed at increasing youth's adherence to pharmacological treatments may also contribute considerably to improving the course of the illness (Morris et al., 2007). Additionally, psychosocial treatments may help to alleviate the adverse effects of environmental pressures (e.g., family, social, academic, etc.) on mood cycling by increasing the child's understanding of BD and teaching the child skills to effectively communicate and solve problems (Miklowitz et al., 2004). Thus, psychosocial interventions have the potential to effectively decrease the severity of contextual risk factors and increase resiliency and coping skills of the BD patient (Miklowitz et al., 2008). Although there are a limited number of randomized controlled trials examining psychosocial treatments for the early-onset BD phenotype, there is growing evidence suggesting that psychosocial interventions play a critical role in improving patient outcomes.

FAMILY TREATMENT APPROACHES

It is crucial to focus psychosocial treatment of BD youth on the family unit since children typically live with their parents and greatly depend on their families (Miklowitz et al., 2004; Miklowitz et al., 2008). Evidence suggests that in conjunction with pharmacotherapy, psychosocial interventions incorporating the family lead to more positive outcomes, including an improved course of illness, greater adherence to medication, and fewer relapses among BD youth (Morris et al., 2007). In fact, a family therapy approach is typically implicated for most forms of psychopathology in youth and has shown to be an effective method of treatment (Repetti et al., 2002).

Drawing from a biopsychosocial approach, family treatments of BD are based on the notion that family environments have the ability to protect individuals who are at-risk for mood disorders (Morris et al., 2007). Thus, children with psychopathological vulnerabilities may never develop BD if compensatory influences are present within the child and the environment (Miklowitz et al., 2006). In particular, the family environment can serve as a buffer against mental illness if members of the family are adept in their ability to alter and adapt their reactive behaviors in ways that are developmentally appropriate for the at-risk or mentally ill child. Alternatively, the family environment can also aggravate the child's vulnerabilities and fuel psychopathology. For example, a family that does not modify and adapt their interactional patterns and fails to provide external structure and consistency may restrict the at-risk child from learning emotional self-regulation and successfully forming relationships outside of the family (Miklowitz et al., 2006).

Therefore, family treatment for early-onset BD brings balance to both protective and threatening factors within the family and social contexts. This type of treatment is most implicated when family conflict and criticism have the greatest impact on the child's development of emotional competence (Miklowitz, 2007). Family-based treatments assist the child in enhancing internal controls and emotional self-regulation skills through stable routines and consistent caretaking within the family structure. By incorporating family psychoeducation, family treatment of early-onset BD provides families with strategies for managing bipolar illness. With stability and consistency, families are capable of increasing patients' adherence to medication, which will ultimately decrease the number of relapses (Miklowitz et al., 2006). Furthermore, children with BD have an increased likelihood of having a parent or sibling with BD or another mood disorder due to the high heritability rates of BD. Therefore, approaching treatment from a family-based perspective may be beneficial for all members of the family (Young and Fristad, 2007).

Reducing EE among families with mood disordered youth and altering the emotional response of parents may moderate the impact of these environmental stressors on the child and decrease considerably the severity of the child's symptoms (Fristad et al., 2003; Miklowitz et al., 2004). The EE literature has spawned the development of psychoeducational interventions (Fristad et al., 2003). All empirically supported psychosocial interventions for BD youth are family-based and contain a psychoeducation component (Young and Fristad,

2007). At the core of the psychoeducational approach is teaching children and their families to recognize bipolar symptoms, understand the course of illness, develop strategies for early intervention in response to recurrent mood episodes, and encourage consistency with the management of the disorder and adherence to medication regimens (Fristad et al., 2003; Miklowitz, 2007). Treatments utilizing psychoeducation allow parents to respond to their child in a more consistent and positive way, which could improve parenting skills, enhance overall family functioning, and lead to a healthier environment for the child (Fristad et al., 2003). Moreover, clinicians attend to affective reactions to the illness of both patients and family members and assist the family in developing coping skills specifically for their family's situation (Miklowitz, 2007). Most importantly, psychoeducation promotes understanding among family members that BD is not the affected youth's fault and encourages the family to differentiate the child from his or her symptoms (Young and Fristad, 2007).

In this chapter, we review the four evidence-based treatments for PBD: I. Family-Focused Treatment for Adolescents (FFT-A), II. Child- and Family-Focused Cognitive-Behavioral Therapy for Pediatric Bipolar Disorder (CFF-CBT), III. Multifamily Psychoeducation Groups (MFPG), and IV. Individual Family Psychoeducation (IFP).

I. FAMILY-FOCUSED TREATMENT FOR ADOLESCENTS (FFT-A)

Various types of family interventions have been highly effective as adjuncts to pharmacotherapy among adult BD patients (Young and Fristad, 2007). Originally developed for treating BD adults, Family-Focused Treatment (FFT) has been adapted and developed into a manual-based version for use in BD adolescents (ages 13-17) who have experienced a recent episode of mania, mixed mood, or depression (FFT-A; Miklowitz et al., 2004). The primary goals of FFT-A are to reduce the degree of psychosocial impairment, enhance the family's knowledge of PBD, strengthen communication and coping skills among the family, and increase adherence to medication. In addition, FFT-A seeks to decrease levels of EE among family members, improve caregivers' understanding and coping strategies, and encourage a family environment that offers stability and consistency (Miklowitz et al., 2004).

FFT-A includes three primary components: psychoeducation, communication enhancement training, and problem solving skills training. These three phases also comprise FFT for BD adults; however, they have been modified to meet the developmental needs of BD youth and their families. For example, parents of BD adolescents often feel that they lack control over their child's behavior and believe the BD adolescent holds a great deal of power within the family system. Therefore, FFT-A assists parents in developing plans to control the rapid-onset of brief mood episodes that typically characterize the early-onset form of BD. In addition, adolescents struggle deeply with issues of identity and autonomy in relation to BD, such as acceptance of their disorder and adherence to their medication regimens (Miklowitz et al., 2006). Thus, FFT-A helps the adolescent patient make sense of his or her disorder, come to an acceptance of the illness, and achieve autonomy from parents through medication adherence (Miklowitz et al., 2006; Pavuluri, Birmaher, and Naylor, 2005).

Treatment Format

Similar to FFT for BD adults, FFT-A consists of 12 weekly family sessions, six biweekly family sessions, and then three once-a-month family sessions (21 fifty-minute sessions over the course of nine months). Following the nine months, families may receive maintenance sessions every three months for the following 15 months (Miklowitz et al., 2004). Psychoeducation, which typically occurs in the first nine sessions, focuses on increasing the family's knowledge about the etiology, course, treatment, risk factors (e.g., changes in sleep/wake patterns, nonadherence to medication, family disagreements) and protective factors (consistent and regulated sleep/wake rhythms, medication compliance, minimal family conflict), and management of BD. In addition, the adolescent is encouraged to keep track of his or her mood and, together with the therapist, the family develops a plan to prevent relapse of mood episodes. The communication enhancement stage of treatment (typically sessions 10-15) uses role-playing techniques to focus on strengthening positive and effective communication and decreasing negative affect among the family by practicing such skills as active listening, positive feedback, constructive negative feedback, and positive requests for changes in behavior. The final phase of treatment (typically sessions 16-21) incorporates cognitive-behavioral therapy to improve problem-solving skills and resolve family disagreements. Parents are taught behavioral management strategies and, together with their children, collaboratively identify areas of conflict, generate solutions, evaluate potential outcomes of each solution, and finally choose and execute a solution (Miklowitz et al., 2004; Miklowitz et al., 2006; Morris et al., 2007).

Outcome Research

Miklowitz and colleagues (2004) conducted an open treatment trial with 20 BD adolescents and found that FFT-A, in conjunction with mood stabilizers, reduced adolescents' manic symptoms by approximately 38% and improved symptoms of depression and mania at 12-month follow-up.

In a later study examining the effectiveness of FFT-A and pharmacotherapy, Miklowitz et al. (2008) conducted a randomized controlled trial with two-year follow-up. BD adolescents were randomly assigned to FFT-A and pharmacotherapy or enhanced care (EC) and pharmacotherapy. Enhanced care consisted of three weekly family sessions of psychoeducation that focused on relapse prevention, increasing adherence to medication, and reducing conflict among the family environment. While there were no differences in rates of recovery from baseline mood episodes, patients who received FFT-A had a faster recovery from their baseline depressive symptoms than patients who received EC. Additionally, although there were no differences in time to subsequent episodes of depression or mania between groups, patients in the FFT-A group spent less time in depressive episodes and had more positive outcomes in terms of decreased depressive symptoms over the course of two years than patients in the EC group. Therefore, in conjunction with pharmacotherapy, FFT-A appears to be effective in stabilizing depressive symptomatology among BD adolescents.

II. CHILD- AND FAMILY-FOCUSED COGNITIVE-BEHAVIORAL THERAPY FOR PEDIATRIC BIPOLAR DISORDER (CFF-CBT), OR THE RAINBOW PROGRAM

Pavuluri and colleagues (2004) developed the manual-based Child- and Family-Focused Cognitive- Behavioral Therapy for Pediatric Bipolar Disorder (CFF-CBT). This program is an adaptation of the FFT model and is structured around the acronym RAINBOW: *Routine; Affect Regulation; I Can Do It!; No Negative Thoughts and Live in the Now; Be a Good Friend and Balanced Lifestyle for Parents; Oh, How Can We Solve the Problem?;* and *Ways to get Support.* Similar to FFT-A, the RAINBOW Program integrates cognitive-behavioral principles, interpersonal therapies, empathic validation, and psychoeducation to address psychosocial factors (e.g., EE, stressful life events, problem solving, coping strategies, communication skills, crisis management, relapse prevention) that impact the course of bipolar illness (Pavuluri et al., 2004).

Treatment Format

CFF-CBT consists of 12 one-hour weekly sessions with parents and their BD child (aged 8 to 12 years) as well as one session for siblings. This approach increases parents' awareness of their own unhelpful cognitions and allows parents to acquire new strategies to manage their child's illness. The session for siblings gives them the opportunity to learn about their brother or sister's disorder and the nature of BD. Empathic interactions and the development of coping skills are also encouraged (Pavuluri et al., 2004). A description of each step of the RAINBOW process is as follows:

Routine. This step of the process calls for the establishment of a strict and predictable routine that involves regulating sleeping patterns, eating habits, and work/play balance. A structured environment creates a sense of safety and decreases negative reactivity to changes in the child's schedule. Research on the mutual relationship of sleep-wake cycles, circadian rhythms, and mood has shown that stabilizing both sleep-wake cycles and circadian rhythms improves bipolar symptomatology (Frank, Swartz, and Kupfer, 2000).

Affect regulation. This involves self-monitoring of moods by having the child chart his/her affect throughout the day. Both parents and children use narratives to externalize the unwanted mood episode and to help children gain a sense of mastery over their affective state. In addition, parents are also taught how to appropriately respond to their child's negative reactivity.

I can do it! The goal of this step is to assist children in developing more positive self-statements by creating a positive script or self-story to be referred to during depressive episodes. Such positive self-statements also aid in increasing motivation among youth to utilize more effective problem-solving strategies. Parents are also encouraged to continuously mention positive qualities of the child.

No negative thoughts and live in the "now." This step uses cognitive restructuring techniques to identify unhelpful or harmful thoughts and then reframe them into more helpful ones, which subsequently assists the child in developing more positive problem-solving skills.

The "here and now" portion of this step provides a way for both children and parents to cope with overwhelming situations and not dwell on past challenges.

Be a good friend and balanced lifestyle for parents. This component focuses on youth building healthy and supportive peer relationships by learning what it means to be a good friend and practicing social skills in therapy. Parents assist their child in fostering these friendships by organizing play dates and other opportunities for their child to practice these skills. In addition, therapists help parents obtain a more balanced lifestyle that focuses on finding time to care for themselves, cope with the intense demands of caring for a child with BD, and recharge.

Oh, how can we solve the problem? This step of the process specifically addresses problem-solving within the family system. Parents are taught to view their children as partners and together, they practice the process of successful problem-solving, including evaluating the pros and cons of each possible solution.

Ways to get support. During this stage, children draw a support tree that names the people in their lives that can help in difficult situations and who can be trusted. The therapist and child then discuss the process through which the child can seek out the help he/she needs and what are reasonable expectations of others (Pavuluri et al., 2004).

Outcome Research

Pavuluri et al. (2004) conducted an open trial using the RAINBOW Program with 34 children and adolescents, extending the age range to include youth aged 5-17. Preliminary results indicated significant decreases in symptoms of mania, depression, psychosis, ADHD, aggression, and sleep disturbance. In addition, patients showed improved treatment adherence (i.e., attendance at scheduled sessions) and global functioning. These findings suggest that CFF-CBT is a useful tool for the treatment of BD children of various ages and reducing symptoms of BD (Pavuluri et al., 2004).

CFF-CBT has also been adapted for use in a group format (West, Henry, and Pavuluri, 2007). In a preliminary study that did not include a control comparison group, results demonstrated that 26 families of BD youth (aged 6-12 years) receiving the group treatment had greater improvement in manic symptoms and in parent-report of psychosocial functioning, and a nonsignificant improvement in parents' coping capabilities. However, no improvements were observed in the presentation of depressive symptoms (West et al., 2007).

III. MULTI-FAMILY PSYCHOEDUCATION GROUPS (MFPG)

Multi-Family Psychoeducation Groups (MFPG) is a manual-based treatment approach for families of youth with BD and depressive disorder aged 8-12 years (Fristad et al., 2003). Like FFT-A and CFF-CBT models, MFPG utilizes psychoeducation as a means of increasing the family's knowledge about pediatric BD, reducing levels of EE, and enhancing family problem solving, communication, and management of symptoms. MFPG is distinct from FFT-A and CFF-CBT in that it was developed for youth with BD and depressive spectrum disorders (Fristad et al., 2003; Young and Fristad, 2007).

The group structure of MFPG provides parents with support from other families who are also coping with a mood-disordered youth. Parents are encouraged to play more active roles in the treatment of their BD child. In addition, the child groups help to normalize the BD youth's experience with a mental disorder. They gain support from other children who share their same struggles. The group format also provides children with an opportunity to practice and improve social and problem solving skills (Young and Fristad, 2007).

Treatment Format

MFPG consists of eight 90-minute weekly sessions, where each session begins with a "check-in" meeting with both parents and children to discuss the previous week's work. Parents and youth are then separated into two groups and focus on that week's specific topic. For the last 15-20 minutes of each session children partake in recreational and group games to promote positive social interactions and relationships with peers. The sessions conclude with parents and children coming together once again to review what was done in session and introduce family projects for the upcoming week (Fristad et al., 2003; Lofthouse and Fristad, 2004).

The first half of MFPG predominately centers on family psychoeducation about mania, depression, and other disorders that commonly co-occur with PBD, including ADHD, anxiety, and ODD. Families create their own treatment goals in the first few sessions, referred to as "Fix-it Lists." Importantly, the "Naming the Enemy" exercise is used to help families separate the child from his or her diagnosis by identifying the child's symptoms as well as his or her strengths (Fristad, Gavazzi, and Soldano, 1999).

The second portion of MFPG focuses on coping skill development among both children and parents. One important component of the child groups is the "Tool Kit," where the child creates a list of pleasant and relaxing activities in four categories (i.e., creative, physical, social, and rest and relaxation) that can be used during a negative mood or interpersonal conflict (Young and Fristad, 2007). MFPG also consists of a therapeutic technique called "Thinking-Feeling-Doing" (TFD) as a way of applying CBT strategies to the treatment of BD youth. The primary objective of TFD is to enhance the parent and child's awareness of their own negative thoughts and behaviors that coincide with negative mood states. Increasing a family's insight into the interrelationship between their feelings, thoughts, and behaviors allows for the later development of other thoughts and behaviors that produce more positive mood states among the family (Fristad, Davidson, and Leffler, 2008). The sequence, "Stop-Think-Plan-Do-Check" is used to teach parents and children problem-solving skills for family problems typically associated with mood disorders. At the end of the program, families are provided with feedback, recommendations for future growth, and resources in their community, and then "graduate" (Lofthouse and Fristad, 2004; Young and Fristad, 2007).

Outcome Research

In a pilot study with 35 families of children (ages 8-11 years) with BD or a depressive disorder [MDD or dysthymic disorder (DD)], children and parents were randomly assigned to either immediate MFPG with protocol pharmacotherapy or a six-month wait-list control

(WLC) group with protocol pharmacotherapy. At four months following treatment, both BD and MDD/DD families receiving immediate MFPG displayed significantly greater knowledge about mood disorders and more positive family interactions than families in the WLC sample. Four-month post treatment results also showed that children in the BD and MDD/DD groups reported greater perceived parental support. These findings suggest that families of children with both BD and MDD/DD can be combined in a group format for treatment. This approach is particularly beneficial for MDD/DD families in terms of early recognition of symptoms and intervention strategies. Given that approximately one-third of depressed prepubertal children progress to a diagnosis of BD by early adolescence and about 50% progress to a BD diagnosis by the age of 21 (Geller et al., 2001), it is important for MDD/DD families to learn about the symptoms and management of mania and gain exposure to the experiences of families with a BD child (Fristad, Goldberg-Arnold, and Gavazzi, 2002). Similarly, in a subsequent randomized controlled trial, results demonstrated increased parent knowledge about childhood mood disorders, improved parent report of parent-child relationships, and greater child report of perceived social support from parents in the BD and MDD/DD samples compared to WLC (Fristad et al., 2003).

In a larger randomized controlled trial of 165 children aged 8-12 years old with mood disorders (70% with a bipolar spectrum disorder and 30% with a depressive disorder), families receiving MFPG showed greater improvements than WLC sample at one-year follow-up. In particular, participation in MFPG resulted in greater utilization of higher quality of services, mediated by parents' beliefs about treatment, and reduced severity of child's mood symptoms, mediated by quality of services used. Therefore, these results suggest that MFPG assists parents in becoming more informed about treatment options and better consumers in seeking higher quality of services which, in turn, reduces the severity of children's mood symptoms (Mendenhall, Fristad, and Early, 2009).

IV. INDIVIDUAL FAMILY PSYCHOEDUCATION (IFP)

Treatment Format

More recently, MFPG has been modified for use in individual families when MFPG is not feasible (e.g., families do not want to receive therapy in a group format, families do not want to wait for the formation of a group, families live in geographically remote settings, etc.).

This adapted intervention is referred to as Individual Family Psychoeducation (IFP; Fristad, 2006). IFP is a manualized treatment program that originally consisted of sixteen 50-minute sessions that alternate between parent- and child-only sessions following "check-ins" at the beginning of each child-only session. Instead of the recreational and group games component of MFPG, "Healthy Habits" is used in IFP that centers on enhancing sleep hygiene practices, nutritional eating, and exercise regimens that are developmentally appropriate. In particular, "Healthy Habits" target specific side effects of mood disorders, including circadian rhythm disruption (with sleep hygiene), weight gain due to mood stabilizers and antipsychotics (with healthy eating and exercise), and overall mood (with the mental health benefits associated with exercise). IFP also includes one "in the bank" session that could be used at any time for crisis purposes.

Based on feedback from a pilot study, IFP extended to a 24 session format (IFP-24) that includes 20 sessions focusing on specific and relevant topics and four "in the bank" sessions to help cope with crisis situations or further reinforcement of a particular topic that is troublesome for the family. Further, IFP-24 includes an additional psychoeducational session that teaches parents about diagnoses and associated symptoms, an additional session focusing specifically on treatment and school-based intervention programs, an additional "Healthy Habits" session, and a session devoted to working with siblings (Fristad, 2006).

Outcome Research

In a pilot study, 20 BD children aged 8-11 years and their parents participated in a randomized controlled trial of the original 16-session IFP format. Compared to WLC, children receiving IFP experienced improved mood symptoms and such improvements were maintained at 12-month follow-up.

Results from a later study found that families receiving IFP had significantly reduced rates of high-EE compared to WLC (Fristad, 2006). Research also indicates that IFP-24 results in similar improvements for BD children and families relative to WLC families (Davidson and Fristad, 2008).

CONCLUSION

As one of the most intense and controversial areas of child psychopathology research, PBD has received considerable scholarly and clinical attention over the past decade. Given the high rates of treatment resistance and poor outcomes among children and adolescents with BD, there is a critical need for a comprehensive and immediate approach to the treatment of early-onset BD. Intervening early in the course of bipolar illness may alter the subsequent course of the disorder, lead to more positive outcomes, and reduce the likelihood of relapse (Miklowitz et al., 2008). More importantly, interventions designed for use early in the course of BD may prevent the progression from prodromal phases of the disorder (i.e., bipolar disorder not otherwise specified or cyclothymia) to bipolar I or bipolar II disorders (Post and Kowatch, 2006). Without early intervention, the developmental trajectory of individuals with early-onset BD can become severely disrupted, sometimes irreparably, and result in significant social, intellectual, and emotional impairment, particularly during the critical stages of adolescent development (Miklowitz et al., 2008).

All psychosocial interventions with empirical support that have been designed for treating children and adolescents with BD are family-based. Derived from a biopsychosocial theoretical approach, the basis of family interventions is that negativity (i.e., conflict, criticism, hostility) within the family environment is a risk factor for subsequent mood dysregulation episodes. In comparison to healthy individuals, families of BD youth are less cohesive, less organized, and have greater conflict (Sullivan and Miklowitz, 2010). Family-based interventions have shown to be effective among BD adults in relapse prevention, speeding up episode recovery, and improving medication adherence (Miklowitz, 2007).

Four psychosocial interventions that have been developed to treat youth with BD in conjunction with pharmacotherapy include FFT-A, CFF-CBT, MFPG, and IFP. While each intervention varies in its approach, all four treatments include a focus on psychoeducation and improving coping skills. Treatments for PBD utilizing psychoeducation provide families with information about the causes, course, and outcome of bipolar illness. Findings suggest that these family-based therapies in combination with pharmacotherapy help to stabilize the child, reduce bipolar symptomatology, and increase adherence to medication regimens.

Recommendations

The research covered in this chapter has significant implications for policy makers, educators, practitioners, and health care professionals working in the child and adolescent mental health field. Although medications are the first line of treatment, in light of their limitations, clinicians should strongly consider complementing pharmacotherapy with family-based psychotherapy at the outset of treatment. Importantly, clinicians should target negative affect and problem-solving and communication difficulties within the family, with particular emphasis on bolstering coping skills for all members since these families are often dealing with multiple disorders (in both the parent and child). Given that educating parents about their child's disorder results in a greater likelihood of that child receiving high-quality services which, in turn, results in reductions of symptom severity, clinicians should support parental involvement in the child's treatment and encourage parents to be active participants throughout the therapy process. Furthermore, involvement of parents in the treatment of PBD and the use of family-based interventions should also be supported and stressed by policies at the community and government levels to ensure that youth and their families are receiving the most optimal treatment available.

Further, PBD is often characterized by high rates of comorbidity with other common childhood disorders such as ADHD, conduct disorder (CD), ODD, substance abuse, and anxiety disorders (Biederman et al., 2003; Leibenluft and Rich, 2008). Due to this complex presentation of illness, children and adolescents with BD are more unresponsive to treatment than adults with BD (Biederman et al., 2003). In addition, comorbidity appears to be associated with high family conflict and low family cohesion (Esposito-Smythers et al., 2006). Therefore, it is also important for clinicians to understand the role of comorbidity in the treatment of PBD, to determine how comorbid diagnoses will be addressed and incorporated into the treatment plan, and to assess for potential barriers to treatment due to co-occurring disorders.

Future Directions for Research

While the family-based interventions discussed here show promise for reducing BD symptoms in youth, the number of overall evidence-based interventions for PBD is very small, and the research examining the efficacy of such treatments is often limited by small sample sizes and in some cases, an absence of a comparison group. Therefore, additional randomized clinical trials are needed to validate the efficacy of these approaches as manual-based interventions for PBD. Furthermore, future effort is needed to determine the degree to which these family-based treatments for PBD are effective in real-world, clinical settings. Additional research on the treatment of PBD should also focus on when psychosocial interventions are the most effective during the course of illness.

As discussed in this chapter, due to the fact that children are generally more dependent on their families than adults, EE and negative affect within the family have a significant potential to impact the child's course of illness. Therefore, family treatment of PBD and other psychiatric disorders should continue to evaluate the mechanisms through which high-EE attitudes develop, the ways in which BD youth process and respond to the negative affect of caregiving relatives, the behaviors of BD youth that instigate negative responses from family members, and the ability of BD youth to cope with adverse interactions among relatives. Ultimately, additional research will help to further clarify the directionality and the causal pathways of family dysfunction and PBD.

Finally, longitudinal studies may help to further understand the developmental course between PBD and adult BD, and determine which psychosocial interventions will be effective into adulthood. This will ultimately allow for more precise monitoring of BD in youth, improved understanding of PBD, the development of more effective treatments tailored to BD children and their families, and further investigation of the role of preventative interventions in delaying the onset of bipolar illness among at-risk youth.

REFERENCES

Barrowclough, C., and Hooley, J.M. (2003). Attributions and expressed emotion: A review. *Clinical Psychology Review,* 23, 849-880.

Biederman, J., Mick, E., Faraone, S.V., Spencer, T., Wilens, T.E., and Wozniak, J. (2003). Current concepts in the validity, diagnosis and treatment of paediatric bipolar disorder. *International Journal of Neuropsychopharmacology,* 6, 293-300.

Blader, J.C., and Carlson, G.A. (2007). Increased rates of bipolar disorder diagnoses among U.S. child, adolescent, and adult inpatients, 1996-2004. *Bipolar Disorder: Neurocircuitry and Neurodevelopment,* 62, 107-114.

Butzlaff, R.L., and Hooley, J.M. (1998). Expressed emotion and psychiatric relapse: A meta-analysis. *Archives of General Psychiatry,* 55, 547-552.

Case, B.G., Olfson, M., Marcus, S.C., and Siegel, C. (2007). Trends in the inpatient mental health treatment of children and adolescents in U.S. Community hospitals between 1990 and 2000. *Archives of General Psychiatry,* 64, 89-96.

Davidson, K.H., and Fristad, M.A. (2008). Family psychoeducation for children with bipolar disorder. In B. Geller and M. DelBello (Eds.), *Treating child and adolescent bipolar disorder* (pp. 184-204). New York, NY: Guildford Press.

Esposito-Smythers, C., Birmaher, B., Valeri, S., Chiappetta, L., Hunt, J., Ryan, N.,...Keller, M. (2006). Child comorbidity, maternal mood disorder, and perceptions of family functioning among bipolar youth. *Journal of the American Academy of Child and Adolescents Psychiatry,* 45, 955-964.

Faedda, G.L., Baldessarini, R.J., Glovinsky, I.P., and Austin, N.B. (2004). Pediatric bipolar disorder: Phenomenology and course of illness. *Bipolar Disorders,* 6, 305-313.

Frank, E., Swartz, H.A, and Kupfer, D.J. (2000). Interpersonal and social rhythm therapy: Managing the chaos of bipolar disorder. *Biological Psychiatry,* 48, 593-604.

Fristad, M.A. (2006). Psychoeducational treatment for school-aged children with bipolar disorder. *Developmental Psychopathology,* 18, 1289-1306.

Fristad, M.A., Davidson, K.H., and Leffler, J.M. (2008). Thinking-feeling-doing: A therapeutic technique for children with bipolar disorder and their parents. *Journal of Family Psychotherapy,* 18, 81-103.

Fristad, M.A., Gavazzi, S.M., and Mackinaw-Koons, B. (2003). Family psychoeducation: Adjunctive intervention for children with bipolar disorder. *Biological Psychiatry,* 53, 1000-1008.

Fristad, M.A., Gavazzi, S.M., and Soldano, K.W. (1999). Naming the enemy: Learning to differentiate mood disorder "symptoms" from the "self" that experiences them. *Journal of Family Psychotherapy,* 10, 81-88.

Fristad, M.A., Goldberg-Arnold, J.S., and Gavazzi, S.M. (2002). Multifamily psychoeducation groups (MFPG) for families of children with bipolar disorder. *Bipolar Disorders,* 4, 254-262.

Geller, B., Craney, J.L., Bolhofner, K., DelBello, M.P., Williams, M., and Zimerman, B. (2001). One-year recovery and relapse rates of children with a prepubertal and early adolescent bipolar disorder phenotype. *American Journal of Psychiatry,* 158, 303-305.

Geller, B., and Luby, J. (1997). Child and adolescent bipolar disorder: a review of the past 10 years. *Journal of the American Academy of Child and Adolescent Psychiatry,* 36, 1168-1176.

Geller, B., Tillman, R., Craney, J.L., and Bolhofner, K. (2004). Four-year prospective outcome and natural history of mania in children with a prepubertal and early adolescent bipolar disorder phenotype. *Archives of General Psychiatry,* 61, 459-467.

Harris, J. (2005). The increased diagnosis of 'juvenile bipolar disorder': What are we treating? *Child and Adolescent Psychiatry: Psychiatric Services,* 56, 529-531.

Joshi, G., and Wilens, T. (2009). Comorbidity in pediatric bipolar disorder. *Child and Adolescent Psychiatric Clinics of North America,* 18, 291-319.

Kowatch, R.A., Fristad, M., Birmaher, B., Wagner, K.D., Findling, R.L., Hellander, M., and the Workgroup Members. (2005). Treatment guidelines for children and adolescents with bipolar disorder: Child psychiatric workgroup on bipolar disorder. *Journal of the American Academy of Child Adolescent Psychiatry,* 44, 213-235.

Leibenluft, E., and Rich, B.A. (2008). Pediatric bipolar disorder. *Annual Review of Clinical Psychology,* 4, 163-187.

Lewinsohn, P.M., Klein, D.N., and Seeley, J.R. (1995). Bipolar disorders in a community sample of older adolescents: Prevalence, phenomenology, comorbidity, and course. *Journal of the American Academy of Child and Adolescent Psychiatry,* 34, 454-463.

Lofthouse, N., and Fristad, M.A. (2004). Psychosocial interventions for children with early-onset bipolar spectrum disorder. *Clinical Child and Family Psychology Review,* 7, 71-88.

McClellan, J., Kowatch, R., and Findling, R.L. (2007). Practice parameter for the assessment and treatment of children and adolescents with bipolar disorder. *Journal of the American Academy of Child and Adolescent Psychiatry,* 46, 107-125.

Mendenhall, A.M., Fristad, M.A., and Early, T.J. (2009). Factors influencing service utilization and mood symptom severity in children with mood disorders: Effects of multifamily psychoeducation groups (MFPGs). *Journal of Consulting and Clinical Psychology,* 77, 463-473.

Merikangas, K.R., Akiskal, H.S., Angst, J., Greenberg, P.E., Hirschfeld, R.M.A., Petukhova, M., and Kessler, R.C. (2007). Lifetime and 12-month prevalence of bipolar spectrum disorder in the National Comorbidity Survey replication. *Archives of General Psychiatry,* 64, 543-552.

Merikangas, K.R., He, J.P., Burstein, M., Swanson, S.A., Avenevoli, S., Cui, L., Benjet, C., Georgiades, K., and Swendsen, J. (2010). Lifetime prevalence of mental disorders in U.S. adolescents: Results from the National Comorbidity Survey Replication-Adolescent supplement (NCS-A). *Journal of the American Academy of Child and Adolescent Psychiatry,* 49, 980-989.

Merikangas, K.R., and Pato, M. (2009). Recent developments in the epidemiology of bipolar disorder in adults and children: Magnitude, correlates, and future directions. *Clinical Psychology: Science and Practice,* 16, 121-133.

Miklowitz, D.J. (2004). The role of family systems in severe and recurrent psychiatric disorders: A developmental psychopathology view. *Development and Psychopathology,* 16, 667-688.

Miklowitz, D.J. (2007). The role of the family in the course and treatment of bipolar disorder. *Current Directions in Psychological Science,* 16, 192-196.

Miklowitz, D.J., Axelson, D.A., Birmaher, B, George, E.L., Taylor, D.O., Schneck, C.D., and Brent, D.A. (2008). Family-focused treatment for adolescents with bipolar disorder: Results of a 2-year randomized trial. *Archives of General Psychiatry,* 65, 1053-1061.

Miklowitz, D.J., Biuckians, A., and Richards, J.A. (2006). Early-onset bipolar disorder: A family treatment perspective. *Development and Psychopathology,* 18, 1247-1265.

Miklowitz, D.J., George, E.L., Axelson, D.A., Kim, E.Y., Birmaher, B., Schneck, C.,…Brent, D.A. (2004). Family-focused treatment for adolescents with bipolar disorder. *Journal of Affective Disorder,* 82S, S113-S128.

Miklowitz, D.J., Goldstein, M.J., Nuechterlein, K.H., Snyder, K.S., and Mintz, J. (1988). Family factors and the course of bipolar affective disorder. *Archives of General Psychiatry,* 45, 225-231.

Miklowitz, D.J., and Johnson, S.L. (2006). The psychopathology and treatment of bipolar disorder. *Annual Review of Clinical Psychopathology,* 2, 199-235.

Miklowitz, D.J., Mullen, K.L., and Chang, K.D. (2008). Family-focused treatment for bipolar disorder adolescence. In B. Geller, and M.P. DelBello (Eds.), *Treatment of Bipolar Disorder in Children and Adolescents* (pg. 166-183). New York, NY: Guilford Press.

Moreno, C., Laje, G., Blanco, C., Jiang, H., Schmidt, A.B., and Olfson, M. (2007). National trends in the outpatient diagnosis and treatment of bipolar disorder in youth. *Archives of General Psychiatry,* 64, 1032-1039.

Morris, C.D., Miklowitz, D.J., and Waxmonsky, J.A. (2007). Family-focused treatment for bipolar disorder in adults and youth. *Journal of Clinical Psychology: In Session,* 63, 433-445.

Murray, C.L., and Lopez, A.D. (Eds.). (1996). The global burden of disease: A comprehensive assessment of mortality and disability from disease, injuries, and risk factors in 1990 projected to 2020. (GBD Series Vol. I. Harvard School of Public Health on behalf of the World Health Organization and the World Bank, Cambridge, Massachusetts).

Pavuluri, M.N., Birmaher, B., and Naylor, M.W. (2005). Pediatric bipolar disorder: A review of the past 10 years. *Journal of the American Academy of Child and Adolescent Psychiatry,* 44, 846-871.

Pavuluri, M.N., Graczyk, P.A., Henry, D.B., Carbray, J.A., Heidenreich, J., and Miklowitz, D.J. (2004). Child- and family-focused cognitive-behavioral therapy for pediatric bipolar disorder: Development and preliminary results. *Journal of the American Academy of Child and Adolescent Psychiatry,* 43, 528-537.

Perlick, D.A., Hohenstein, J.M., Clarkin, J.F., Kaczynski, R., and Rosenheck, R.A. (2005). Use of mental health and primary care services by caregivers of patients with bipolar disorder: A preliminary study. *Bipolar Disorders,* 7, 126-135.

Post, R., and Kowatch, R.A. (2006). The health care crisis of childhood-onset bipolar illness: Some recommendations for its amelioration. *Journal of Clinical Psychiatry,* 67, 115-125.

Repetti, R.L., Taylor, S.E., and Seeman, T.E. (2002). Risky families: Family social environments and the mental and physical health of offspring. *Psychological Bulletin,* 128, 330-366.

Schenkel, L.S., West, A.E., Harral, E.M., Patel, N.B., and Pavuluri, M.N. (2008). Parent-child interactions in pediatric bipolar disorder. *Journal of Clinical Psychology,* 64, 422-437.

Sullivan, A.E., and Miklowitz, D.J. (2010). Family functioning among adolescents with bipolar disorder. *Journal of Family Psychology,* 24, 60-67.

Townsend, L.D., Demeter, C.A., Youngstrom, E., Drotar, D., and Findling, R.L. (2007). Family conflict moderates response to pharmacological intervention in pediatric bipolar disorder. *Journal of Child and Adolescent Psychopharmacology,* 17, 843-851.

West, A.E., Henry, D.B., and Pavuluri, M.N. (2007). Maintenance model of integrated psychosocial treatment in pediatric bipolar disorder: A pilot feasibility study. *Journal of the American Academy of Child and Adolescent Psychiatry,* 46, 205-212.

Young, M.E., and Fristad, M.A. (2007). Evidence based treatments for bipolar disorder in children and adolescents. *Journal of Contemporary Psychotherapy,* 37, 157-164.

In: Youth: Practices, Perspectives and Challenges
Editor: Elizabeth Trejos-Castillo

ISBN: 978-1-62618-067-3
© 2013 Nova Science Publishers, Inc.

Chapter 14

ACHIEVING ACADEMIC RESILIENCE FOR MEXICAN AMERICAN STUDENTS: ISSUES AND CHALLENGES

Alfredo H. Benavides[*] *and Eva Midobuche*
Texas Tech University, Lubbock, TX, US

ABSTRACT

This paper will review the existing literature on the issue of resiliency among Mexican American students. The identification and classification of resilient and non-resilient students will be examined, including criteria such as achievement test results, grades, percentile rank, teacher identification, nominating procedures and criteria, (including teacher expectations and attitudes towards the students). In addition to the factors mentioned in this review, this chapter will also examine the issues of resiliency among this particular subset of students within American schools. Mexican American students represent a diverse set among the general Hispanic/Latino student population of the United States. These students may be native born or undocumented, English learners, bilingual or English dominant. They may also be at different stages of language acquisition or different stages of acculturation. Some of these students may also come from families that are highly mobile, and thus have attended multiple school systems in short time spans. Low socioeconomic status among other poverty factors, such as health and generational factors within the group, will also be discussed.

Teachers and school environments are extremely important in creating and fostering resilient students. Of particular emphasis in addressing and fostering resiliency among Mexican American students is the issue of teacher preparation with an emphasis on identifying, creating and developing positive dispositions and attitudes among teachers of Mexican American students, including validation of the students' linguistic and cultural diversity. The process of creating resilient students is enhanced if teachers possess the dispositions necessary to understand and educate Mexican American students.

---

[*] Address correspondence to: Professor Alfredo H. Benavides, Ph.D, Bilingual Education and Diversity Studies Curriculum and Instruction. College of Education, Texas Tech University Email: alfredo.benavides@ttu.edu.

INTRODUCTION

Who are Mexican Americans? This is a question that has perplexed researchers and other scholars for many years. In his 1967 epic poem "I Am Joaquín", Rodolfo "Corky" Gonzales used terms such as La Raza, Mejicano, Español, Latino and Chicano, in an attempt to help readers understand that this particular group of Mexican Americans not only possessed diversity within the group as a whole, but also the freedom to self-identify. The last line in this portion of the poem is "I refuse to be absorbed. I am Joaquín!" Note that the term *Hispanic* is not used. Simply, it had never been used to describe Mexican Americans, and thus was not part of the lexicon of the 1960's Chicano Civil Rights Movement.

Gonzales' insistence on self-identity, however, is important because in the decades that have followed, Mexican Americans have been generically grouped together and referred to as Latino or Hispanic. Therefore, for the purposes of this work we will define Mexican Americans as individuals of Mexican ancestry who are citizens or permanent residents of the United States, as well as Mexican immigrants both documented and undocumented. When the terms Latino or Hispanic appear, they are being taken from the extant literature or sources referring to these terms. These terms are also used generically where others refer to themselves specifically in this manner or when the literature uses these terms. More importantly, however, this chapter is about resiliency among Mexican Americans, and as it is applied to Mexican American students in the United States.

DEMOGRAPHICS

All measures of population growth point to the fact that Hispanics are growing in population across the country. The PEW Hispanic Center (2009) reports that there were 46,822,476 Hispanics in the U.S. in 2008. However, more recently Passel, Cohn, and Lopez (2011), report that the Hispanic population of the United States grew from 35.3 million in 2000 to 50.5 million in 2010, accounting for more than half of the nation's overall population growth during that decade. Mexican Americans account for approximately 63% of this population (Pew Research Center Publications, 2012). Of the overall Hispanic population 28,985,169 are native born and 17,837,307 are foreign born (Pew Center, 2009).

According to PEW Hispanic Center (2009), Hispanics in 2009 made up:

- 16% of the U.S. population;
- 18% of all 16-25 year-olds;
- 20% of all school-age children; and
- 25% of all newborns.

This is in sharp contrast to the 10% Hispanic population found only in the southwestern United States in the period during the Vietnam War (Rosales, 1996). Today Mexican Americans can be found living and working in all fifty states.

Mexico is by far the leading country of origin for U.S. immigrants accounting for one-third (32%) of all foreign-born residents and two-thirds (64% - 66%) of Hispanic immigrants. The U.S. is the destination point for nearly all people who leave Mexico, and about one-in-ten people born in Mexico currently lives in the United States (Passel, 2009). The United States ranks 2nd in Hispanic population (worldwide), with only Mexico having a larger population [110 million], (U.S. Census, 2008).

In 2009 the National Center for Education Statistics (NCES), reported that 20% of children ages 5-17 in the U.S. spoke a language other than English at home in 2007. About 75 % of these children spoke Spanish. Students of Mexican descent made up the largest proportion of these English language learners (ELLs). In 2008, the National Education Association (NEA) reported that about five million English language learners (ELLs) were enrolled in U.S. public schools and by 2015 the number would reach ten million. The National Clearinghouse for English Language Acquisition (NCELA, 2007) reported ELLs for the 2005-2006 school year to be 5,074,572. These numbers may seem large, however Johnson (2007) found that 34% of the Texas freshman class of 2003-2004 left school before graduating and that these numbers have actually increased in the past twenty years and are even higher for English language learners.

Carter (1970), made the point in 1970 that Mexican Americans had always been diminished by school systems because of their high dropout rate and low academic achievement. He wrote that the schools often looked at Mexican Americans as a social and educational problem needing great attention in order for the problem to be solved. He cited educators' beliefs that Mexican Americans were *culturally deprived* or *disadvantaged* and thus their home environment did not provide the skills needed to succeed in school. Flashing forward forty years, it does not appear that the problem is much different. Schools are still blaming the child and looking at his native language and culture as obstacles to be overcome and sometimes eradicated.

Other states and some U.S. senators and congressional representatives have even expressed approval for changing the 14th amendment to the U.S. Constitution, in order to deny children citizenship if they were born in the United States to parents that are here as undocumented workers (Schneider, 2010). In states such as Texas, the State Board of Education passed new social studies standards that are extremely conservative and passed only along official political party lines (McKinley, 2010). These new standards do not reflect the history of Mexican Americans prior to 1836 and fail to include accurate historical data and appropriate role models for Mexican American students. This makes validating the history, language, culture, and contributions of Mexican Americans very difficult. In Arizona, California, and Massachusetts voters passed strict laws either banning or severely restricting the use of bilingual education programs to meet the needs of Mexican American children (Crawford, 2004). How should educators and researchers view these fairly open attacks? Perhaps more importantly, how should Mexican Americans feel when they see this happening around them?

These examples serve to demonstrate how inadequate education is for many Mexican American students. Because resiliency among this population was not even a thought in 1970, it is necessary to make the point that this issue is of importance and needs to be examined judiciously by researchers and educators. The issue of resiliency among Mexican Americans needs to be brought to the attention of American educators.

Fry (2008), reported that ELLs often attend schools that have low standardized test scores. In a 2007 court ruling, U.S. Senior District Judge William Wayne Justice ruled that Texas had been complying with federal law in terms of how it educated ELLs. However, one year later, Judge Justice reversed himself ruling that secondary education programs for ELLs (in Texas) violated the federal Equal Educational Opportunities Act of 1974, and thus ordered the State of Texas to remedy the problem (Zehr, 2008). According to Sánchez (2004), the success of any student is dependent upon providing meaningful instruction that includes the integration of languages, academic development, and socio-cultural support. These are fundamental to the success of English language learners. Secondary Mexican American students in Texas are still dropping out and waiting for the remedy.

DEFINING RESILIENCY

What is resiliency? The term generally refers to those factors and processes that limit negative behaviors associated with stress and that result in adaptive outcomes even in the presence of adversity (Wolin and Wolin, 1993). It is a "process of, or capacity for, or the outcome of successful adaptation despite challenging and threatening circumstances" (Garmezy and Masten, 1991 p. 459). Resiliency is a term used to describe the set of qualities that foster a process of successful adaptation and transformation despite risk and adversity. We are all born with an innate capacity for resilience (Benard, 1995). Yet another view of resiliency is that it represents "the heightened likelihood of success in school and other life accomplishments despite environmental adversities brought about by early traits, conditions, and experiences", (Wang, Haertel, and Walberg, 1994, p. 46).

Therefore, resilient students are those who succeed in school despite the presence of adverse conditions (Waxman, Gray, and Padrón, 2003). Terms such as hardy, invulnerable, and invincible have all been used to describe resilient individuals (Wolin and Wolin, 1993).

Educational resilience is not viewed as a fixed attribute but as something that can be promoted by focusing on *alterable* factors that can impact an individual's success in school. This approach does not focus on attributes such as ability since it has not been found to be a characteristic of resilient students (Benard, 1993; Gordon and Song, 1994; Masten, Best, and Garmezy, 1990; Waxman, Gray, and Padrón, 2003). Resilience is the process of overcoming the negative effects of risk exposure, coping successfully with traumatic experiences, and avoiding the negative trajectories associated with those risks (Perez, Espinoza, Ramos, et al., 2009; Morales, 2008; Olsson, Bond, Burns, et al., 2003; Garmezy, Masten, and Tellegen, 1984; Luthar, Cicchetti, and Becker 2004; Werner and Smith 1992).

Why are some students successful in school while other students from the same socially and economically disadvantaged backgrounds and communities are not? Only a few studies have examined resiliency in schools. Most of the research has focused on comparing resilient and non-resilient students on family and individual background characteristics (Waxman, Gray, and Padrón, 2003). Morales (2008) adds that the current literature on educational resiliency is limited to the K-12 school experience and does not present models and data that stretch beyond high school to the crucial high school-to-college transitions. However, Perez, et al., (2009) studied 110 undocumented Latino high school, community college and university students. Another study by Hurtado, Saenz, Santos, and Cabrera (2008), also investigated high school, community college and university students.

Reyes and Jason (1993) examined factors that distinguished the success and failure of Latino students in an inner-city high school. Twenty-four high risk and twenty- four low risk (for dropping out of school), tenth grade participants were used in this study. They based the study on the students' ninth grade attendance rates as well as their academic achievement. The participants were interviewed on four main areas. These were family background, family support, overall school satisfaction, and gang pressures. No difference was found in the two groups with regard to socioeconomic status, parent-student involvement, or parental supervision. Low-risk students were significantly more satisfied with their school than high-risk students. High-risk students were more likely to respond that they had been invited to join a gang or had brought a weapon to school.

Gonzalez and Padilla (1997) used academic grades as criteria for resiliency. Their study utilized 133 resilient and 88 non-resilient Mexican American high school student participants. They identified resilient students as students that reported their grades as mostly A's. They identified non-resilient students as those who reported that their grades in high school were mainly D's or mostly below D's. Their findings concluded that resilient students had significantly higher perceptions of family/peer support, teacher feedback, positive ties to their school, the value placed on school, peer belonging, and familism, than non-resilient students. They also found that students' sense of belonging to school was the only significant predictor of academic resilience.

Alva (1991) used the term "academic invulnerability" for students who sustain high levels of achievement, motivation, and performance despite being at risk of dropping out. This study focused on the characteristics of a cohort of tenth grade Mexican American students from low SES backgrounds who maintained a high grade point average. Students reported higher levels of support from their teachers and friends; were more likely to "feel encouraged and prepared to attend college; enjoyed coming to school and being involved in school activities; experienced fewer conflicts and difficulties in their intergroup relations with other students; and experienced fewer family conflicts and difficulties".

Nettles, Mucherach, and Jones (2000) examined the influence of social resources such as parents, teachers, and school support. They found that access to social resources such as caring parents, participation in extracurricular activities, and supportive teachers were beneficial to student achievement. They also found that students' perceived exposure to violence had a significant impact on their mathematics achievement. However, students' perceptions of stressful life events did not have a significant effect on overall achievement.

The Center for Research on Education, Diversity, and Excellence (CREDE), sponsored several studies from 1996 to 2002 that utilized different methods to determine resiliency in students. For example, Waxman and Huang (1996) compared the motivation and learning environments of 75 resilient versus 75 non-resilient sixth, seventh, and eighth graders from an inner city middle school. Resilient students were defined as those who scored at or above the 90th percentile on standardized achievement tests over a two-year period. Non-resilient students were defined as those scoring at or below the tenth percentile on standardized achievement tests over a 2-year period. They also found that resilient students had higher perceptions of involvement, task orientation, rule clarity, satisfaction, pacing, and feedback. Resilient students also reported a higher social self-concept, achievement motivation, and academic self-concept. However, there were no significant differences between the groups on variables such as parent involvement, homework, and teacher support. A possible explanation was that both groups had low perceptions of their teacher's support and that there was a significant variability of responses within the groups.

In another CREDE study, Waxman, Huang, and Padrón (1997) compared motivation learning environments of resilient and non-resilient Latino middle school students in an urban setting. They used a stratified sample of 60 identified resilient and 60 non-resilient students. Students identified as gifted and talented and Special Education were not allowed in the sample. Students in this study were identified by test scores. They were identified as resilient if they scored above the fifty-seventh percentile and non-resilient if below the twenty-fifth percentile. They also used the four-step Problem Solving Test taken over a two-year period. Resilient students also had mostly A's and B's in math and non-resilient had mostly C's, D's, or F's in math. They found no difference on whether they spoke a language other than English before they started school. Being held back in school was deemed significant since fifty-three percent of non-resilient students had been held back one grade as compared to thirteen percent of resilient students. The researchers also found significant differences in student aspirations because:

1. Seventy-eight percent of resilient students said they would graduate high school compared to forty-three percent of non-resilient students; and
2. Ninety percent of resilient students said they would graduate college or attend graduate school, compared to only about forty-six percent of non-resilient students.

Another significant difference found in this study was that students identified as resilient spent significantly more time doing math homework than non-resilient students; and, resilient students also read more.

Waxman, Huang, and Wang (1997) asked teachers to select resilient and non-resilient students from their classrooms based on criteria provided to them by the researchers. Students then completed learning environment and learning surveys, and were observed through a shadowing experience. This study's findings were that resilient students perceived their classrooms more favorably; had higher academic self-concepts and aspirations. They also perceived their teachers as having higher expectations, providing more feedback, and more appropriate pacing than their non-resilient peers.

Padrón, Waxman, and Huang (1999) compared 250 resilient, average, and non-resilient fourth and fifth grade Hispanic students in an urban environment. Teachers were asked to select students they felt were "at-risk". Teachers were later asked to select three students from each category for observation and to complete the My Class Learning Environment Survey. The researchers found that students identified as resilient perceived a more positive learning environment and were more satisfied with their classrooms than their non-resilient peers. They also spent more time interacting with teachers as opposed to interacting with other students for social or personal purposes. Non-resilient students reported more difficulty with class work.

Read (1999) interviewed several fourth and fifth grade teachers about the concept of resiliency. Teachers reported that they had no difficulty identifying resilient and non-resilient students. They felt the resiliency framework was useful in helping them understand why some students were successful and others were not. These teachers reported that low-level or missing parental involvement, low student motivation, and low self-esteem were the major factors in the lack of success among non-resilient students. These same factors allowed resilient students to succeed. These teachers did not mention any school program or classroom factor (e.g., teaching practices) that contributed to the academic success or failure of non-resilient students. They did report that many instructional strategies worked with resilient students and only a few worked with non-resilient students. However, they did not name any.

RISK AND PROTECTIVE FACTORS

A key requirement of resilience is the presence of both risk and protective factors that either help bring about a positive outcome or reduce and avoid a negative outcome. Personality characteristics and environmental social resources are thought to moderate the negative effects of stress and promote positive outcomes despite risks. (Benard, 1995; Kirby and Fraser, 1997; Masten, 1994; Werner and Smith, 1992).

STRESSORS

Students at risk of academic failure often face problems caused by poverty as well as health and other social conditions that have made it difficult for them to succeed in school (Waxman, Gray, and Padrón, 2003). For Mexican American students we could add language proficiency in both heritage and target language, retaining the heritage culture and acculturation, immigration, legal status, migration, hours of employment, generation stage, teacher dispositions and preparation, teacher shortages, among others. Perez et al. (2009) reported that migration is one of the most radical transitions and life changes an individual or a family can endure. For immigrant children this is a dramatic experience that reshapes their lives.

Stressors related to migration include the loss of close relationships; housing problems; a sense of isolation; obtaining legal documentation; going through the acculturation process; learning the English language; negotiating ethnic identity; changing family roles; and adjusting to the schooling experience (Perez et al. 2009; Garza, Reyes, and Trueba, 2004; Portes and Rumbaut, 2001; Suarez-Orozco and Suarez-Orozco, 2001; Zhou, 1997). Acculturation stressors would include leaving relatives and friends behind when moving; feeling pressured to speak only Spanish at home; living at home with many people; and feeling that other kids make fun of the way they speak English (Perez et al. 2009; Cervantes and Castro, 1985; Padilla, 1986; Padilla, Cervantes, Maldonado, and Garcia, 1988). Stress may also be created in selecting which set of cultural norms and expectations to follow. Mexican American children and their families have to select expectations from their culture of origin or that of the mainstream culture. The differences in value of each may create pressure (Kurtines and Miranda, 1980; Perez et al. 2009).

Perez et al. (2009) also report that there are only a handful of studies on undocumented college students. De Leon's (2005) study on undocumented college students reported that these students remember: isolation, fear, and those teachers who treated them negatively. Dozier (1993) found three central emotional concerns for undocumented college students. These are fear of deportation, loneliness, and depression. Fear of deportation is very central to undocumented students. It influences every aspect of their lives. They are afraid to go to hospitals and this fear makes it impossible to obtain work authorization or they are forced to stay in bad work conditions. They are also reluctant to develop close emotional relationships with others (Dozier, 1993). All of the respondents in the study by Buriel, Perez, DeMent, Chavez, and Moran (1998) reported frustration, helplessness, shame, and fear due to their undocumented status. They also reported that language brokering was seen as a positive experience while ethnic identity formation, stereotypes about Mexicans and negotiating gender role expectations with their parents were stressors.

Garza et al. (2004) stated that for migrant children the image that has been constructed is one of a perpetuating cycle of failure. Consequently, many educators are convinced that the children of farm workers ("the ghost workers") will never be able to fly to high achieving positions. Sadly, many of these students are led to believe that they are intrinsically inferior, or that their fate is to follow the path of hopelessness that has been imposed on them for generations.

Olivarez (2006) reported that families seemed to support students' aspirations to attend college but the home environments were not always conducive to college preparation. Students had to care for younger siblings and often did their homework away from home because it was crowded in the family's small rented apartment or they secluded themselves in a corner or waited until everyone was asleep to get their work done. None of the students had a separate room in their homes where they could find a quiet space to study. Sixty percent of these students lived in crowded homes with 6 or more people and 90% lived in single studio apartments where everyone slept in the same room (Olivarez, 2006).

Some students attributed their lack of academic success to not having enough time or being too busy to complete their schoolwork to the best of their ability and others held jobs that sometimes left them too tired to focus on school. Again, 60% reported working after school or on the weekends between 16 and 40 hours per week and 60% also participated on athletic teams (Olivarez, 2006). High school employment was considered a risk factor if students worked more than 20 hours per week (Perez et. al 2009; Steinberg and Cauffman, 1995; Steinberg and Dornbusch, 1991; Steinberg, Fegley, and Dornbusch, 1993).

In a report by the Pew Center, Lopez (2009), states that the main reasons given by 16-25 year-old Latinos for dropping out of school were economic (74%), poor English skills (40%), and a general dislike of school (40%). These types of statistics and reasons for low achievement have perplexed educators for decades. Latino schooling in the U.S. has long been characterized by high dropout rates and low college completion rates. Both problems have moderated over time, but a persistent educational attainment gap remains between Hispanics and whites (Lopez, 2009). Length of time in the US also seemed to play a role in academic success. Those who had spent 10 years or more in the U.S. had lower GPAs than those who had been in the U.S. from 3 to 8 years (Olivarez, 2006). Does this mean that the longer students attend U.S. schools, the less learning is taking place among these students? What factors and conditions are responsible for these dropout rates? How can they be addressed by the educational system?

Latino education in the U.S. has been normally characterized by high dropout rates and this is especially true among foreign-born Latino students (34%). Foreign-born Latino students also suffer low college completion rates (Chapman, Laird, Ifill, and KewalRamani, 2011). Hadaway, Vardell and Young (2004), point out that native-born and foreign-born Latino students have major differences in their lives and that these impact their schooling. For example:

1) Students born in the U.S. may have a weak first language model at home while foreign-born students generally have a strong first language model in their homes. Strong first

language skills help to reinforce language concepts and structures and therefore can serve as a bridge to learning another language. 2) U.S.-born students may also experience difficulty in acquiring another language due to the inconsistent modeling in one or both home languages. 3) Because U.S.-born Latinos inhabit two worlds, they are often at odds with fitting into either or both. This may lead to confusion and perhaps marginalization (Hadaway, Vardell and Young, 2004). According to Hadaway, Vardell and Young (2004), there are many other factors that make life difficult for U.S. or foreign-born Latinos in the United States. Many of these factors have to do with poverty, poor health, limited resources, discrimination, and low teacher expectations among others.

Parental education was considered a risk factor if the parental education was less than a high school education (Perez, 2009). Research reveals that Latino educators seem likely to welcome parents and families to schools, and capitalize on their cultural and Spanish language knowledge (Gomez, Rodriguez and Agosto, 2008). In preparing for a parent/teacher conference, teachers need knowledge of parent, student history and culture awareness. Family size was considered another risk factor among Latino students if there were three or more siblings (Perez et al., 2009; Grissmer, Kirby, Berends, and Williamson, 1994; Sameroff, Seifer, Baldwin, and Baldwin, 1993; Seifer, Sameroff, Baldwin, and Baldwin, 1992).

ENVIRONMENTAL RISKS

Abrego (2006) reports that both documented and undocumented students in her study encountered various incidents of violence near their homes and schools, and attended poorly funded schools with four-year college attendance rates of less than ten percent. Social forces such as prejudice, economic inequality, and attitudes toward violence in mainstream American culture interact with the influences of early childhood to foster the expression of violence (National Center for Mental Health Promotion and Youth Violence Prevention, 2009). Familismo or placing family needs above individual needs may keep Latino youth from being unduly influenced by delinquent youth groups, such as gangs, however it may also serve as a risk factor that draws them to gangs. In families where there is instability or dysfunction, gangs and delinquent groups can serve as surrogate families (National Center for Mental Health Promotion and Youth Violence Prevention, 2009; Soriano, 1995). Risk factors include being a minority student attending an inner-city school or coming from a low income home where English is not the primary language (Dauber, Alexander and Entwisle, 1996).

PROTECTIVE FACTORS

Resiliency theory identifies protective factors present in the families, schools, and communities of successful youth that are often missing in the lives of troubled youth (Krovetz, 1999). Benard (1993) found four personal characteristics that resilient children typically display: social competence; problem-solving skills; autonomy; and a sense of purpose. Social competence includes qualities such as responsiveness, especially the ability to elicit positive responses from others; flexibility, including the ability to move between cultures, empathy; communication skills; and a sense of humor. Problem-solving skills encompass the ability to plan; to be resourceful in seeking help from others; and, to think critically, creatively, and reflectively (Benard, 1995).

Critical consciousness, a previously omitted protective factor, is the development of a reflective awareness of the structures of oppression (be it from an alcoholic parent, an insensitive school, or a racist society), and creating strategies for overcoming them has been important (Benard, 1995). Autonomy is having a sense of one's own identity and an ability to act independently and to exert some control over one's environment, including a sense of task mastery, internal locus of control, and self-efficacy. The development of resistance (refusing to accept negative messages about oneself) and of detachment (distancing oneself from dysfunction) serves as a powerful protector of autonomy (Benard, 1995).

According to Benard (1995), resiliency manifests itself as a sense of purpose and a belief in a bright future, including goal direction, educational aspirations, achievement motivation, persistence, hopefulness, optimism, and spiritual connectedness. Students who do well in the classroom show a positive self-evaluation of their academic status at school (Wylie, 1979) and a sense of control over their academic success and failure. (Dweck and Licht, 1980; Dweck and Wortman, 1982; Stipek and Weisz, 1981; Willig, Harnisch, Hill, and Maehr, 1983). Gordon (1996) found that a strong belief in their own cognitive skills was one of the main differences between resilient and non-resilient Latino students in an urban school environment. The high academic achievers excelled because they believed in their own capabilities to achieve. Also, being identified as gifted was considered a personal protective factor.

Students who reported understanding, speaking, reading, and writing both English and Spanish "very well" were considered as having the protective factor of being highly bilingual (Perez et al., 2009). The valuing of school by parents, friends and self were also considered to be personal protective factors in addition to participating in volunteer and extracurricular activities (Perez et al., 2009).

Caring relationships are also very important. Benard (1995) states that the presence of at least one caring person is very important to students who are resilient. This person must convey an attitude of compassion and understanding. This understanding and caring provides support for healthy development and learning. The most frequently- mentioned positive role model in the lives of resilient children outside the family was a favorite teacher who was not just an instructor for academic skills for the children but was also a confidant and positive model for personal identification (Werner and Smith, 1989).

Contrast this to the relationship that Midobuche (1999) developed with her fifth-grade teacher. Midobuche writes:

> This lack of respect was rampant when I was in elementary school. It became so bad that I had nightmares, stomach cramps, and difficulty sleeping. My mother met with my teacher to explain what was happening. (My real problem was my fear of the teacher and what she was doing to all of us.) Because my mother spoke no English, she had to find an interpreter. She explained to the teacher that I was having sleeping problems because I was not comfortable in school. After my mother left, the teacher called me to the front of the classroom. She asked the class to point to me and call me "baby." She told the students that I was not mature enough to be in her class, that I was afraid of her, and that that I was such a baby that my mother had to speak to her. I never again said anything to my mother. I even pretended to sleep through the night. I actually thanked God in my prayers when I got the chicken pox that year. Why

not? It kept me out of school for two weeks. To this day, when I smell the perfume this teacher wore, my stomach gets butterflies. (p. 80-81)

According to Noddings (1988), teachers need to have the motivation for wanting to succeed in establishing caring relationships with students and their families. Children will work harder for people they love and trust. Caring relationships need to be established beyond student and teacher, and include teacher to teacher as well as teacher to parent. Caring relationships are a means of relating to youth, their families, and each other that conveys compassion, understanding respect, and interest. According to Midobuche (1999) these types of relationships were rare in her schooling experience.

However, Midobuche (2011) also recounts her experience with a high school biology teacher who inspired her to higher levels of achievement. Midobuche writes:

> One such teacher was my high school biology teacher, who always encouraged all of his students. I recall him repeatedly meeting with my parents and though he was non-Hispanic, speaking to them in Spanish in order to answer the questions that they might have about considering whether or not to send me away to a four-year university. The respect that this man demonstrated through his use of my native language as well as his understanding of how difficult this decision was for Mexican parents, was, in one word, inspiring. Here was a human being who although different from my culture, understood my parents and me so well. He went out of his way to understand. However, the truly beautiful part of his understanding was that it didn't make you feel indebted to him. He was understanding of me and my family because somewhere he had learned that this was part of being a good teacher. (p. 87)

High expectations and support often result in high rates of academic success. Academic success will in-turn lower rates of behavior such as dropping out, drug abuse, teen pregnancy, delinquency, etc. (Rutter et al., 1979). Also, high expectations for students occur at several levels. Most obvious and powerful is the relationship level where teachers and other school staff communicate the message that the student has everything needed to be successful. Tracy Kidder (1990) states: "For children who are used to thinking of themselves as stupid or not worth talking to… a good teacher can provide an astonishing revelation. A good teacher can give a child at least a chance to feel." The child then responds by feeling that if the teacher thinks I am worth something, maybe I am.

Relationships need to convey high expectations. Students learn to believe in themselves and their future as well as develop critical resiliency traits of self-esteem, self-efficacy, autonomy, and optimism. Schools also communicate expectations in a structured and organized way with curriculum that supports, respects, and validates their language and culture. There should also be opportunities for participation by the student. According to Sarason, (1990) and Benard, (1995) this participation should include meaningful involvement; caring and respect for fundamental human needs; asking questions that encourage critical thinking and dialogue; making learning more hands on; and cooperative approaches.

When schools ignore the basic needs of both students and teachers, schools become alienating places (Sarason, 1990). When schools are places where the basic human needs for support, respect, and belonging are met, motivation for learning is fostered. However, how are schools to become these places when there is a shortage of teachers who educate Mexican American children—especially those who are English language learners?

SHORTAGE OF TEACHERS

Most Mexican American children are taught by teachers who do not know their language or culture and are unfamiliar with them and their backgrounds. Many of these teachers also bring negative attitudes toward Ells because they believe that these students bring too many deficits to the learning experience and are not capable of learning the subjects required of them and thus the teacher feels that they cannot overcome these deficits (Walker, Shafer, and Iiams, 2004). For example, 48 % of K-12 students in Texas are Hispanic, while only 22% of all teachers are Hispanic. Meanwhile, White students make up 34% of all Texas students, yet 67% of all teachers are White (Texas Education Agency [TEA], 2009). This shortage of Mexican American teachers as well as bilingual educators has remained critical since the early 1980's. Gold (1992) referred to this shortage as "the single greatest barrier to the improvement of instructional programs for limited English proficient (LEP) students" (p. 223). The lack of a bilingual teacher supply is supported in studies by: Gándara (1986); Macías (1989); Quezada (1991); Torres-Guzman and Goodwin (1995); Crawford (1997); Menken and Holmes (2000); and Menken and Antunez (2001); and Abdelrahim (2005). The lack of a supply of teachers that understand the students they teach is also a negative factor for Mexican American students (Midobuche and Benavides, 2011).

Abdelrahim (2005), points out that schools will need to hire as many as two million new teachers in the coming decade and suggests that hiring teachers from abroad might alleviate the critical teacher shortage in bilingual education. The National Clearinghouse for English Language Acquisition (NCELA 2007) noted that bilingual and ESL education would be particularly crucial in this great teacher shortage. The convergence of this shortage and other factors has created a need to carefully examine what bilingual education, ESL, and mainstream teachers need to know about meeting the needs of ELLs. These needs will affect how best practices are incorporated into everyday classrooms across our educational landscape as well as affect the development of resiliency among Mexican American students.

The U.S. Department of Education National Center for Education Statistics (NCES 2002) provides statistics showing that while many teachers have ELLs in their classrooms, the number of educators to complete at least 8 hours of training in the past three years on teaching ELLs was exceedingly low. The following table provides selected examples from the National Center for Education Statistics Report (2002).

State	% of Teachers Who Taught ELLs	% with 8 or more hours of formal preparation
Arizona	67.8%	23.2%
Colorado	53.2%	13.2%
Georgia	35.2%	6.2%
Illinois	37.1%	7.1%
Indiana	29.0%	1.9%
New Mexico	64.7%	33.2%
California	75.2%	49.2%
Nevada	67.5%	18.6%
Arkansas	29.9%	12.5%
Louisiana	16.4%	3.1%
Oklahoma	32.9%	5.2%
Texas	57.7%	17.9%

QUALIFIED TEACHERS

The No Child Left Behind Act mandates that all children should have highly qualified teachers. To be deemed highly qualified teachers must have: 1) a bachelor's degree, 2) full state certification or licensure, and 3) prove that they know each subject they teach. However, there is no mention of how to determine teacher dispositions for promoting resiliency or working with Mexican American children. Yet, principals are sometimes pressured by higher administration to hire teachers in order to fill shortages, regardless of preparation. Principals sometimes feel that they have to play the "waiting game" where they can not hire new faculty until the faculty (sometimes inefficient) from within the district surplus list are reassigned first. Principals feel that they have to wait until they can get new faculty to their campus or hire the "lesser of all evils" (Levin, Mulhern, and Schunck, 2006). Mainstream teachers often take the required certification exams needed for bilingual and ESL education without any formal preparation in teaching ELLs. These teachers often take teaching positions in school districts without the proper teacher preparation or experience in ESL or Bilingual Education. They are faced with the tremendous pressure of having one year to pass their certification exams and of trying to get their students ready to pass assessment exams such as the State of Texas Assessments of Academic Readiness (STAAR), in a language that they are themselves not fluent in (Texas Education Agency, 2012). Even College of Education advisors have inconsiderately recommended that mainstream teachers challenge the ESL exams without the proper courses needed in preparing them to teach Ells.

TEACHER DISPOSITIONS

Whether teachers are produced by a university preparation program or through some form of alternative certification, it is not a guarantee that the critical caring dispositions needed to promote resiliency in students will be present in their classrooms. Well beyond the three R's and even strong pedagogical preparation, well prepared teachers who are ready to meet the needs of an increasingly diverse population must not only possess the skills and knowledge necessary to do so, but also the dispositions needed to accomplish this goal (Thornton and Eisenman, 2008). Definitions of dispositions are inconsistent within the literature and across teacher preparation programs. There has been a proliferation of terminology and perspectives ranging from tendencies, values, habits of mind, attitudes, and behaviors, thus making them difficult to define (Richhart, 2001). According to the National Council for Accreditation of Teacher Education (NCATE, 2006), dispositions are defined as:

> The values, commitments, and professional ethics that influence behaviors toward students, families, colleagues, and communities and affect student learning, motivation, and development as well as the educator's own professional growth. Dispositions are guided by beliefs and attitudes related to values such as caring, fairness, honesty, responsibility, and social justice. For example, they might include a belief that all students can learn, a vision of high and challenging standards, or a commitment to a safe and supportive learning environment. (p.30)

Thornton (2006) stated that dispositions remain a neglected part of teacher education. Yero (2002) and Talbert-Johnson (2006) also report that while it is easy to measure teachers' content knowledge and pedagogical skills, the assessment of dispositions is much more involved and difficult. However, dispositions, attitudes, and perceptions of others play a vital role in determining success in the world of teaching (Cline and Necochea, 2006).

When candidates enter a teacher preparation program they come with their own set of beliefs, values, and dispositions. In a teacher preparation program students examine these attitudes, beliefs, values, and dispositions. They are expected to expand their horizons and open new ways of thinking, seeing, and behaving. A philosophical mismatch may occur when a professor asks students to reconsider their prejudices and misconceptions, and become more critical and reflective. When this happens students could possibly exhibit rudeness, defensiveness, and uncooperativeness. This could be because of poor self-esteem, inadequate academic preparation, or they could simply be out of their element and want to simply use the field of bilingual education or ESL education in order to be considered more marketable (Major and Brock, 2003).

What teachers and candidates alike should be striving for is true authenticity in their values, attitudes, and dispositions. We need to observe our students closely in order to avoid political correctness in their speaking and writing. This could have implications for online instruction due to issues in evaluating teaching effectiveness. It is also problematic to admit teacher candidates whose dispositions are troubling, and yet they continue through the program unchecked (Talbert-Johnson, 2006). Why is this allowed to happen? Changing beliefs and dispositions is a difficult proposition that takes time and must involve thoughtfully designed curricular experiences. If the dispositions go unchecked and no one intervenes and teacher candidates become licensed to teach, many high risk Mexican American children could receive less than effective instruction with no protective factors. Unfortunately, there is limited literature that addresses the dispositions that would pertain specifically to teachers working with ELLs (Cline and Necochea, 2006).

DISPOSITIONS AND TEACHER PREPARATION

Unfortunately, the skills and techniques that teachers learn and practice in college classrooms are not always maintained over time, nor do they necessarily transfer to actual classrooms with children (Scheeler, 2007). In order to address issues that arise from changing demographics that often impact values, attitudes, beliefs, and dispositions it is important for all institutions to periodically conduct critical self-examinations.

In a 2008 study at Texas Tech University (TTU), Burley, Agnello, Borrego, and Ramirez, surveyed 896 freshmen students about their attitudes toward several issues within multicultural education and diversity themes in general. The following five questions were asked as part of the survey.

1. TTU should be committed to the creation of a multicultural community.
2. TTU should be committed to the creation of a campus, which is supportive of diversity in various forms (gender, political orientation, etc.).

3. TTU should be actively seeking qualified minority candidates for faculty and staff positions.
4. TTU should actively recruit minority students.
5. TTU should strive for its student population to be reflective of the ethnic composition of the region and state.

The responses to these questions were somewhat disheartening. To Question #1, 68% of these freshmen students responded with 'Disagree or Strongly Disagree'. To Question #2, the students responded with 76% indicating 'Disagree or Strongly Disagree'. Questions 3 and 4 both received responses that indicated a 40% 'Disagree or Strongly Disagree' response. Question #5 also drew a 42% 'Disagree or Strongly Disagree' response from the students.

While there may be many reasons for these responses, more troubling are the implications for those who decide to become teachers. Undoubtedly, some of these freshmen students will choose education as their field of study. Educators should be concerned if they bring the survey attitudes with them. How can these dispositions be changed in any meaningful way? Would students with these dispositions be able to appreciate the language, cultural, and socioeconomic differences that might exist between them and many potential students? Would these future teachers be able to produce the resiliency that is needed by the children that they most certainly will teach?

In attempting to create higher levels of resiliency among Mexican American students, and in developing the proper and positive dispositions for working with them, it is important for these future teachers to understand the student's language and cultural heritage. In order to promote and develop resiliency in Mexican American children, teachers must demonstrate a genuine interest in the student as well as allow the student to feel a sense of self-worth. Many students with these types of teachers won't have a chance. Teacher candidates are often raised to believe in the old stereotypical expectations of low achievement and non-resilience among Mexican American students—when we as educators should know better. Carter (1970) wrote that even Mexican American teachers often held the same negative attitudes and dispositions towards the Mexican American students that they taught. Perhaps this could be attributed to the prevailing attitudes of the era and how difficult it was then for Mexican Americans to become teachers or even finish college. Regardless, there should be no excuses today. Today, we know far more about educating all students than we could have ever hoped for in 1970 or before.

SUMMARY

We believe that the keys to teaching Mexican American children are the dispositions that a teacher brings to the educational experience. Yet there are very few courses in Colleges of Education that specifically address the language and culture of Mexican Americans. Usually this is left to bilingual or multicultural education courses that tend to generalize a great deal and homogenize all groups into the *'Hispanic'* label. While it is important to recognize these ethnic differences for everyone's edification, it is extremely important to recognize particular segments of the school population, especially when that population comprises a large majority of the student body.

Mexican Americans students in states such as Texas and Arizona are today facing school boards and even state laws that limit their education as it concerns their ethnic group and in many ways their identity as well. In Texas, the State Board of Education dropped many references to Mexican Americans in their social studies curriculum, thus continuing the exclusion of Mexican Americans in the history of Texas (McKinley, 2010). In Arizona, the state legislature passed a law banning ethnic studies in state schools. This gave the Tucson Unified School District the impetus to close the Mexican American Studies Program at Tucson High School. This law was applied only to the Mexican American Studies Program and not the African American, Pan-Asian, or American Indian programs (Sleeter, 2012). This seems to be a concerted attempt to prevent these students from learning about themselves and gaining the self-esteem that we all know is so valuable to any student.

It appears that the mis-education that was occurring among Mexican American students in the last century is continuing today in much of the country. Bilingual education has been attacked for many years and state legislatures are not squeamish about passing anti-immigrant laws. Arizona even passed a law banning teachers with accents from teaching (Jordan, 2010). How do these policies align with the notion that all students deserve a fair and equitable education? More specifically, how are Mexican American students being identified as resilient or non-resilient? Is attendance a good measure? Are high or low grades a good measure? Mexican American students often face many obstacles to achievement such as working to help support the family, language barriers in English, poverty at home, constant moving to different apartments or housing arrangements, no help or support from parents who are also stressed from multiple jobs and low wages. Do these students have a level playing field in the classroom? Do they have teachers who understand these backgrounds and can go beyond mere teaching to support these students?

We believe that the answer lies in teachers who understand their students and are not afraid to teach them what they need to know in order to survive in our society. Better prepared teachers with the dispositions to reach out to and teach these students can and will make the difference in lifting their educational status and creating the resiliency that these students need to succeed in school and life. By creating more resilient students these teachers will also be able to contribute in significant ways to our nation and society. If resiliency is the key to promoting achievement in Mexican American students, then positive dispositions are indispensible. We need to research more specifically how to identify these dispositions in students at different levels. Teacher candidates will then be better prepared to enter the teaching profession and to in turn produce more resilient graduates.

REFERENCES

Abdelrahim, S. (2005) NCELA FAQ No. 24, Q: How can I become a teacher? OELA's national Clearinghouse for English Language Acquisition and Language Instruction Educational Programs. Retrieved from http://www.ncela.gwu.edu/expert/faq/24teacher.htm

Abrego, L. (2006). "I can't go to college because I don't have papers": Incorporation patterns of Latino undocumented youth. *Latino Studies*, 4, 212-231.

Alva, S. A. (1991). Academic invulnerability among Mexican-American students: The importance of protective resources and appraisals. *Hispanic Journal of Behavioral Sciences*, 13, 18-34.

Benard, B. (1993). Fostering resiliency in kids. *Educational Leadership*, 51, 44-48.

Benard, B. (1995). Fostering resiliency in kids: Protective factors in the family, school and community. San Francisco: West Ed Regional Educational Laboratory.

Benavides, A., Midobuche, E., and Carlson, P., (Eds.) (2011). Hispanics in the southwest: issues of immigration, education, health, and public policy, Bilingual Press, Arizona State University, Tempe, AZ, (Book on CD).

Buriel, R., Perez, W., De Ment, T., Chavez, D., and Moran, V. (1998). The relationship of language brokering to academic performance, biculturalism, and self-efficacy among Latino adolescents. *Hispanic Journal of Behavioral Sciences,* 20, 283-287.

Burley, H., Agnello, M.F., Borrego, J., and Ramirez, L. (2008) Multicultural Core Requirement Summary Report, Texas Tech University.

Carter, T. P. (1970). Mexican Americans in school: A history of educational neglect. New York: College Entrance Examination Board.

Cervantes, R. C., and Castro, F. G. (1985). Stress, coping and Mexican American mental health: A systematic review. *Hispanic Journal of Behavioral Sciences*, 1, 1-73.

Chapman, C., Laird, J., Ifill, N., and KewalRamani, A. (2011). Trends in High School Dropout and Completion Rates in the United States: 1972–2009 (NCES 2012-006). U.S. Department of Education. Washington, DC: National Center for Education Statistics. Retrieved April 5, 2012 from http://nces.ed.gov/pubsearch

Cline, Z. and Necochea, J. (2006). Teacher dispositions for effective education in the borderlands. *The Education Forum, 70*, 268-281.

Crawford, J. (2004). Educating English learners: language diversity in the classroom, Bilingual Educational Services, Los Angeles, CA, 5th Edition.

Crawford, J. (1997). *Best evidence: Research foundations of the bilingual education act.* Washington, D.C.: National Clearinghouse for Bilingual Education. [Online]. Available: http://www.ncbe.gwu.edu/ncbepubs/ reports/bestevidence/index.htm [1999, January].

Dauber, S. L., Alexander, K. L., and Entwisle, D. R. (1996). Tracking and transitions through the middle grades: Channeling educational trajectories. Sociology of Education, 69, 290-307.

De Leon, S. (2005). Assimilation and ambiguous experience of the resilient male Mexican immigrants that successfully navigate American higher education. Austin: Unpublished doctoral dissertation, University of Texas.

Dozier, S. B. (1993). Emotional concerns of undocumented and out-of-status foreign students. *Community Review*, 13, 29-33.

Dweck, C.S. and Licht, B.G. (1980). Learned helplessness and academic achievement. In J. Gerber and m. Seligman (Eds.), *Human helplessness: Theory and application* (pp. 197-221). New York, NY: Academic Press.

Dweck, C.S., and Wortman, C. (1982) Learned helplessness, anxiety, and achievement motivation: Neglected parallels in cognitive, affective, and coping responses. In H.W. Krohne and L. Laux (Eds.), Achievement, stress, and anxiety. Washington, DC: Hemisphere.

Fry R. (2008). The role of schools in the English Language Learner achievement gap. Pew Hispanic Center: Washington DC. http://justspanish4u.com/yahoo_site_admin/assets/docs/Pew-Hispanic_Center.23880753.pdf

Gandara, P. (1986). Bilingual education: Learning English in California. Sacramento, CA: Assembly Office of Research.

Garmezy, N., and Masten, A. (1991). The protective role of competence indicators in children at risk. In E. M. Cummings, A. L. Greene, and K. H. Karraker, Life-span developmental psychology: Perspectives on stress and coping (pp. 151-174). Mahwah, NJ: Lawrence Erlbaum.

Garmezy, N., Masten, A. S., and Tellegen, A. (1984). The study of stress and competence in children: A building block of developmental psychopathology. *Child Development*, 55, 97-111.

Garza, E., Reyes, P., and Trueba, E. (2004). Resiliency and success: Migrant children in the United States. Boulder, CO: Paradigm.

Gold, N.C. (2009). Solving the shortage of bilingual teachers: policy implications of California's staffing initiative for LEP students. Retrieved from http://www.ncela.gwu.edu/files/rcd/BE019299/Solving_The_ Shortage.pdf

Gordan, K.A. (1996). Resilient Hispanic youths' self-concept and motivational patterns. *Hispanic Journal of Behavioral Sciences, 18*, 63-73.

Gordon, E. W., and Song, L. D. (1994). Variations in the experience of resilience. In M. C. Wang and E. W. Gordon (Eds.), Educational resilience in inner-city America: Challenges and prospects (pp. 27-43). Hillsdale, NJ: Erlbaum.

Gómez, M. L., Rodriguez, T. L., and Agosto, V. (2008). Who are Latino prospective teachers and what do they bring to US schools. *Race, Ethnicity, and Education, 11*(3), 267-283.

Gonzales, R. (1967). *I am Joaquin*, La Causa Publications, Santa Barbara, California. Retrieved from http://www.latinamericanstudies.org/latinos/ joaquin.htm

Gonzales, R., and Padilla, A. M. (1997). The academic resilience of Mexican American high school students. *Hispanic Journal of Behavioral Sciences*, 19, 301-317.

Gordon, E. W., and Song, L. D. (1994). Variations in the experience of resilience. In M. C. Wang, and E. W. Gordon, Educational resilience in inner-city America (pp. 27-43). Mahwah, NJ: Lawrence Erlbaum.

Gordon, K. (1996). Resilient Hispanic youths' self-concept and motivational patterns. Hispanic Journal of Behavioral Sciences, 18, 63-73.

Grissmer, D. W., Kirby, S. N., Berends, M., and Williamson, S. (1994). Student achievement and the changing American family. Santa Monica, CA: RAND.

Hadaway, N.L., Vardell, S.M., and Young, T.A. (2004). *What every teacher should know about English learners.* Boston: Person Allyn and Bacon.

Hurtado, S. H., Saenz, V. B., Santos, J. L., and Cabrera, N. L. (2008). Advancing in higher education: A portrait of Latina/o college freshmen at four year institution, 1975-2006. Los Angeles, CA: UCLA.

IES, U.S. Department of Education, National Center for Education Statistics (2008). The Condition of Education 2008. Participation in education: Elementary/secondary education, Language Minority School-Age Children Indicator 7.

Johnson, R. L. (October 2007). Texas School Attrition Study 2006-07, Texas school holding power worse than two decades ago. Retrieved on July 31, 2008 from http://www.idra.org/

IDRA_Newsletter/October_2007_School_Holding_Power/Texas_Public_School_Attrition_Study_2006_07/

Jordan, M. (2010). Arizona Grades Teachers on Fluency: State Pushes School Districts to Reassign Instructors With Heavy Accents or Other Shortcomings in Their English, *The Wall Street Journal*. Retrieved from http://online.wsj.com/article/SB10001424052748703572504575213883276427528.html#printMode.

Kidder, T. (1990). *Among schoolchildren*. New York: Avon Books.

Kirby, L. D., and Fraser, M. W. (1997). Risk and resilience in childhood. In M. D. Fraser, Risk and resilience in childhood: An ecological perspective (pp. 10-33). Washington, D. C.: NASW.

Krovetz, M. L. (1999). Fostering resiliency: expecting all students to use their minds and hearts well. Thousand Oaks, CA: Corwin.

Kurtines, W., and Miranda, M. (1980) Differences in self and family role perceptions among acculturating Cuban American college students. *International Journal of Intercultural Relations*, 4, 167-184.

Levin, J., Mulhern, J., and Schunck, J. (2006, June). Unintended Consequences: The Case for Reforming the Staffing Rules in Urban Teachers' Union Contracts. *Primary Sources*, pp. 1-2.

Luthar S.S. (1991). Vulnerability and resilience: A study of high-risk adolescents. *Child Development, 62*, 600-616.

Luthar, S.S., Cicchetti, D., and Becker, B. (2000). The construct of resilience: a critical evaluation and guidelines for future work. *Child Development, 71*, 543-562.

Lopez, M. H. (2009, Octoaber 07). *Latinos and education: Explaining the attainment gap*. Retrieved June 28, 2010, from PEW Hispanic Center: http://pewhispanic.org/reports/report.phb?ReportID=115

Macias, R. (1989). The national need for bilingual teachers. Claremont, CA: Tomas Rivera Center.

Major, E. M. and Brock, C. H. (2003). Fostering positive dispositions toward diversity: Dialogical explorations of a moral dilemma. *Teacher Education Quarterly*, 30(4), 7-26.

Masten, A. S. (1994). Resilience in individual development: Successful adaptation despite risk and adversity. In M. C. Wang, and E. W. Gordon, Educational resilience in inner-city America: Challenges and prospects (pp. 3-25). Hillsdale, NJ: Lawrence Erlbaum.

Masten, A. S., Best, K. M., and Garmezy, N. (1990). Resilience and development: Contributions from the study of children who overcome adversity. *Development and Psychopathology, 2*, 425-444.

McKinley, J. (2010). Texas conservatives win curriculum change. *The New York Times*. Retrieved March 25, 2010, from http://www.nytimes.com/2o10/03/ 13education/ 13texas.html.

Menken, K., and Antunez, B. (2001). An overview of the preparation and certification of teachers working with limited English proficient students. Washington, DC: National Clearinghouse of Bilingual Education. Retrieved July 28, 2003, from http://www.ericsp.org/pages/ digests/ncbe.pdf.

Menken, K. and Holmes, P. (2000). Ensuring English language learners' success: Balancing teacher quantity with quality. Washington, DC: NCBE.

Midobuche, E. (1999). Respect in the Classroom. *Educational Leadership, 56,* 80-82.

Midobuche, E. (2011). "Becoming a dream catcher for English language learners: Implications for teachers, students, and self", in *Hispanics in the Southwest: Issues of Immigration, Education, Health, and Public Policy,* in Benavides, A. Midobuche, E. and Carlson, P. (Eds.), Bilingual Press, Arizona State University, Tempe, AZ, (E-book on CD).

Midobuche, E. and Benavides, A., (2011) *ESL and Mexican American Students: Learning in a Climate of Politics, Standards, Immigration Reform, and Fear.* Paper presentation at the 9th *Annual Hawaii International Conference on Education* (HICE), January 4 -7, 2011, Honolulu, Hawaii.

Morales, E. E. (2008). Academic resilience in retrospect following up a decade later. *Journal of Hispanic Higher Education, 7,* 228-248.

National Education Association, (2008). English language learners face unique challenges, NEA Education Policy and Practice Department, Retrieved on April 9, 2012 from http://www.weac.org/Libraries/PDF/ELL.sflb.ashx.

National Clearinghouse for English Language Acquisition (NCELA) (2007), The growing numbers of limited English proficient students, Retrieved on July 29, 2008 from http://www.ncela.gwu.edu/policy/states/reports/ statedata/2005LEP/GrowingLEP_0506.pdf.

National Center for Education Statistics (2009). *Dropout rate in the United States: 2009.* Retrieved from http://nces.ed/gov/fastfacts/display.

National Center for Mental Health Promotion and Youth Violence Prevention, Education Development Center, Meeting the Needs of Latino Youth: Part I: Risk, Retrieved from**:** http://www.promoteprevent.org/publications/ prevention-briefs/meeting-needs-latino-youth-part-i-r.

National Council for Accreditation of Teacher Education. (2006). NCATE News: A statement from NCATE on professional dispositions, Retrieved fromhttp://www.ncate.org/public/ 0616_MessageAWise.asp?ch=150.

Nettles, S. M., Mucherach, W., and Jones, D. S. (2000). Understanding resilience: The role of social resources. Journal of Education for Students Placed at Risk, 5, 47-60.

Noddings, N. (1988). An ethic of caring and its implication of instructional arrangements. American Journal of Education, 96, 215-230.

Olivarez, P. M. (2006). Ready but restricted: An examination of the challenges of college access and financial aid for college-ready undocumented students in the U. S. Unpublished doctoral dissertation, University of Southern California.

Olsson, C. A., Bond, L., Burns, J. M., Vella-Brodrick, D. A., and Sawyer, S. M. (2003). Adolescent resilience: A concept analysis. Journal of Adolescence, 26, 1-11.

Padilla, A. M. (1986). Acculturation and stress among immigrants and later generation individuals. In D. Frick, H. Hoefert, H. Legewie, R. Mackerson, and R. K. Silbereisen, The quality of urban life: Social, psychological, and physical conditions (pp. 100-120). Berlin, Germany: de Gruyter.

Padilla, A. M., Cervantes, R. C., Maldonado, M., and Garcia, R. E. (1988). Coping responses to psychosocial stressors in Mexican and Central American immigrants. Journal of Community Psychology, 16, 418-427.

Padrón, Y. N., Waxman, H. C., and Huang, S. L. (1999). Classroom and instructional learning: Environment differences between resilient and nonresilient elementary school students. *Journal of Education for Students Placed at Risk,* 4, 63-81.

Passel, JS; Pew Research Center (2006). The size and characteristics of the unauthorized migrant population in the U.S. estimates based on the March 2005 Current Population Survey, March 7, 2006. Retrieved from http://pewhispanic.org/files/reports/61.pdf.

Passel, J. S., Cohn D., Lopez, M.H. (2011). Census 2010: 50 Million Latinos Hispanics account for more than half of nation's growth in past decade. Pew Hispanic Center: Washington DC. http://www.pewhispanic.org/ files/reports/140.pdf.

Perez, W. (2009). We are Americans: undocumented students pursuing the American dream, Sterling, VA: Stylus Publishing.

Perez, W., Espinoza, R., Ramos, K., Coronado, H., and Cortes, R. (2009). Academic resilience among undocumented Latino students. *Hispanic Journal of Behavioral Sciences,* 31, 149-181.

Pew Hispanic Center. (2009). *Between two worlds: How young latinos come of age in america.* Washington, DC: Author. Retrieved from http://pewhispanic.org/files/reports/117.pdf.

Pew Research Center (July 2011). The mexican american boom: births overtake immigration, Retrieved from: http://pewresearch.org/pubs/2058/-immigration-mexican-immigrants-mexican-american-birth-rate.

Portes, A., and Rumbaut, R. G. (2001). Legacies: The story of the immigrant second generation. Berkeley, CA: University of California Press.

Quezada, M. District remedies to eliminate the shortage of qualified teachers of Limited English Proficient students in California. Doctoral dissertation, University of Southern California, 1991.

Read, L. (1999). Teachers' perceptions of effective instructional strategies for resilient and nonresilient students. Teaching and Change, 7, 33-52.

Reyes, O., and Jason, L. A. (1993). Pilot study examining factors associated with academic success for Hispanic high school students. Journal of Youth and Adolescence, 22, 57-71.

Ritchhart, R. (2001). From IQ to IC: A dispositional view of intelligence. *Roeper Review,* 23, 143-150.

Rosales, F. Arturo. (1996). Chicano! The History of the Mexican American Civil Rights Movement. Houston, Tex.: Arte Público Press.

Rutter, M. et al (1979). Fifteen thousand hours. London: Open Books.

Sameroff, A. J., Seifer, R., Baldwin, A., and Baldwin, C. P. (1993). Stability of intelligence from preschool to adolescence: The influence of social and family risk factors. *Child Development,* 64, 80-97.

Sánchez, H. (2004). *Improving your child's education: A guide for Latino parents.* Washington. The Education Trust.

Sarason, S. B. (1990). The predictable failure of educational reform: Can we change course before it's too late? San Francisco: Jossey Bass.

Scheeler, M.C. (2007). Generalizing effective teaching skills: The missing link in teacher preparation. *Journal of Behavioral Education, 17*(2): 145-159.

Schneider, B. (2010). *Politics Daily,* Illegal Immigration Foes Focus on 14th Amendment 'Citizenship Clause', HuffPost Politics, Retrieved from: http://www.politicsdaily.com/bloggers/brian-schneider/

Seifer, R., Sameroff, A. J., Baldwin, C. P., and Baldwin, A. (1992). Child and family factors that ameliorate risk between 4 and 13 years of age. *Journal of American Academy of Child and Adolescent Psychiatry,* 31, 893-903.

Sleeter, C. (2012). Ethnic studies and the struggle in Tucson, Education Week, Retrieved from http://www.edweek.org/ew/articles/2012/02/15/ 21sleeter.h31.html?tkn=QVXFtyhi F8vDM9WJO3yD%2BYpAHQgQslK9nTIqandcmp=ENL-CM-VIEWS1.

Soriano, F. I. (1995). *Conducting needs assessments: A multidisciplinary approach.* Thousand Oaks, CA: Sage Publications.

Steinberg, L. D., Fegley, S., and Dornbusch, S. M. (1993). Negative impact of part-time work on adolescent adjustment: Evidence from a longitudinal study. *Developmental Psychology*, 29, 171-180.

Steinberg, L., and Cauffman, E. (1995). The impact of employment on adolescent development. *Annals of Child Development*, 131-166.

Steinberg, L., and Dornbusch, S. (1991). Negative correlates of part-time employment during adolescence: Replication and elaboration. *Developmental Psychology*, 304-313.

Stipek, D., and Weisz, J. (1981). Perceived personal control and academic achievement. *Review of Educational Research*, 51, 101-137.

Suarez, J. A. (1983). The Mesoamerican Indian Languages. Melbourne, Australia: Cambridge University Press.

Suarez Orozco, C. and Suarez Orozco, M.M. (2001). *Children of Immigration*. Cambridge, MA: Harvard University Press.

Talbert-Johnson, Carolyn. 2006. "Preparing Highly Qualified Teacher Candidates for Urban Schools: The Importance of Dispositions." *Education and Urban Society* 39: 147–161.

Taylor, P. et al., (2009, December 11). Between two worlds: How young Latinos come of age in America. Retrieved June 22, 2010, from Pew Hispanic Center: http://pewhispanic.org/reports/report.php?ReportID=117

Texas Education Agency, (2012) STAAR Resources, retrieved from http://www.tea.state.tx.us/student.assessment/staar/

Thornton, H. (2006). Dispositions in action: Do dispositions make a difference in practice? *Teacher Education Quality*, 53-68.

Thornton, H. and Eisenman, G. (2008). Reaching students and keeping teachers: Studying and assessing quality teacher dispositions and classroom management. Paper presented at the annual meeting of the American Association of Colleges for Teacher Education. Retrieved from http://www.allacademic.com/meta/p35753_index.html

Torres-Guzmán, M. E. and Goodwin, A. L. (1995) Mentoring Bilingual Teachers. Focus. Washington, D.C.: NCBE.

Torres-Guzmán, M. E. and Goodwin, A. L. (1995). Urban Bilingual Teachers and Mentoring for the Future. Education and Urban Society. 28(1): 48-66.

U.S. Census Bureau (2008). Population Projections, Retrieved October 10, 2010 from http://www.census.gov/population/www/projections/ 2008projections.html

U.S. Department of Education, National Center for Education Statistics (2002*). Schools and staffing survey, 199-2000: Overview of the data for public, private, public charter, and bureau of Indian Affairs elementary and secondary schools, Washington, DC: Author. Table 1.19. pp. 43-44.* Retrieved from http://nces.ed.gov/pubsearch/pubsinfo.asp?pubid=2002313 and from http://nces.ed.gov/pubs2002/2002313.pdf

Wang, M. C., Haertel, G. D., and Walberg, H. J. (1994). Educational resilience in inner cities. In M. C. Wang, and E. W. Gordon, Educational resilience in inner-city America (pp. 45-72). Mahwah, NJ: Lawrence Erlbaum.

Waxman, H. C., and Huang, S. L. (1996). Motivation and learning environment differences between resilient and nonresilient inner-city middle school students. *Journal of Educational Research,* 90, 93-102.

Waxman, H. C., Gray, J. P., and Padrón, Y. N. (2003). *Review on research on educational resilience.* LA: Center for Research on Education, Diversity and Excellence.

Waxman, H. C., Huang, S. L., and Padrón, Y. N. (1997). Motivation and learning environment differences between resilient and non-resilient Latino middle school students. *Hispanic Journal of Behavioral Sciences,* 19, 137-55.

Waxman, H. C., Huang, S. L., and Wang, M. C. (1997). Investigating the multilevel classroom learning environment of resilient and nonresilient students from inner-city elementary schools. International Journal of Educational Research, 27, 343-53.

Werner, E. E., and Smith, R. S. (1992). Overcoming the odds: High-risk children from birth to adulthood. New York: Cornell University Press.

Werner, E. E. 1993. "Risk, Resilience, and Recovery: Perspectives from The Kauai Longitudinal Study." *Development and Psychopathology.* 2, pp. 225-444.

Werner, E. E. and Smith R.S. (1992). *Overcoming the Odds: High Risk Children from Birth to Adulthood.* Ithaca: Cornell University Press.

Werner, E., and Smith, R. (1989). Vulnerable but invincible: A longitudinal study of resilient children and youth. New York: Adams, Bannister and Cox.

Willig, A. C., Harnisch, D. L., Hill, K. J., and Maehr, M. L. (1983). Sociocultural and educational correlates of success-failure attributions and evaluation anxiety in the school setting for Black, Hispanic, and Anglo children. American Educational Research Journal, 20, 385-410.

Wolin, S. J., and Wolin, S. (1993). The resilient self: How survivors of troubled families rise above adversity. New York: Villard.

Wylie, R.C. (1979). The self-concept (Vol. 1). Lincoln, NE: University of Nebraska Press.

Yero, J, L, (2002) *Teaching in mind: how teacher thinking shapes education.* Retrieved from http://www,teachersmind,coni/leaming,htm

Zehr, M. (2008). States struggle to meet achievement standards for ELLs. Education Week, 27, 12.

Zhou, M. (1997). Growing up American: The challenge of immigrant children and children of immigrants. *Annual Review of Sociology*, 23, 63-95.

Section 4. Social Policy and Institutional Support

In: Youth: Practices, Perspectives and Challenges
Editor: Elizabeth Trejos-Castillo

ISBN: 978-1-62618-067-3
© 2013 Nova Science Publishers, Inc.

Chapter 15

YOUTH PARTICIPATION AND PROTECTION: FROM THEORY TO PRACTICE

Maria Manuela Calheiros[*,1], *Joana Patrício*[1]
and Sónia Bernardes[1]
[1]CIS - ISCTE-IUL, Lisbon University Institute, Portugal

ABSTRACT

The right of children and youth to participation is one of the key principles of the UN Convention on the Rights of the Child (UNCRC, 1989). Participation is a means for young people to express their needs and claim their rights, and studies that consider the perspective of young people have recently increased (Holland, 2009). However, several recent studies reveal that: a) there are few studies investigating the perspectives and experiences of children and youth at risk (e.g. Southwelland Fraser, 2010); b) the lack of participation and of influence on decisions are perceived by the youth as a major fault in the social systems (e.g. Mares, 2010); and c) young people's viewpoint is seldom used to change the services (e.g. Strolin-Goltzman, Kollar, andTrinkle, 2010). Therefore, the voice of children and youth remains under-represented in the research and practice domains. Consequently, this chapter aims to cover and illustrate some developments in the concept and practices of youth participation. In the first part, different perspectives, models and practices to promote youth participation are described. In the second part, two studies undertaken within the health-care and youth protection systems are presented. These studies illustrate how the right of youth to participation can be promoted through participatory research, namely through needs assessment and youth involvement in social and health services design. Both studies used qualitative methods to assess the needs of young people and promote their participation in residential and health-care services design (i.e., a residential care facility for transition to independent living and a health care facility for youth, respectively). The first study was conducted with 21 adolescents aged 15 to 18 years, in a residential care setting. The second was conducted with 346 youngsters aged 11 to 25 years old in community support institutions. Finally, some challenges to the integration of young people's participation in the services evaluation and design in the common social policies and practices are discussed.

---

[*] CIS-ISCTE-IUL. Corresponding author e-mail address: maria.calheiros@iscte.pt.

INTRODUCTION

Studies and practices on youth participation have intensified in recent decades (e.g. Holland, 2009) since the declaration of youth's right to participation in the UN Convention on the Rights of the Child (UNCRC, 1989), which states that: "1) states Parties shall assure to the child who is capable of forming his or her own views the right to express those views freely in all matters affecting the child (...), 2) for this purpose, the child shall in particular be provided the opportunity to be heard in any judicial and administrative proceedings affecting the child" (p. 4). As such, according to this convention, all young people have the right to participate and adults are responsible for facilitating their participation and ensuring that their opinions are taken into account (Horwath, Hodgkiss, Kalyva, andSpyrou, 2011).

However, we are still far from achieving the goal of youth participation at an acceptable level (Horwath et al., 2011). Their voices continue to be excluded and undervalued, and the right to participation is not being implemented consistently at a political, legislative and practical level (Lloyd-Smith andTarr, 2000; Hill, Davis, Prout, andTisdall, 2004) in the areas of social care, education and health care (Morgan, Gibbs, Maxwell, and Britten, 2002). In addition, there are still very few studies that have investigated young people's perspectives and experiences in the protection system for children and youth at risk (e.g. Fox andBerrick, 2007; Southwelland Fraser, 2010).

Young people have expressed the lack of participation and influence in decision-making as one of the main failures of the systems they belong to (e.g. Mares, 2010; SouthwellandFraser, 2010) and their opinions are rarely used to change these systems (Strolin-Goltzman, Kollar, andTrinkle, 2010). In this way, the voice of young people remains underrepresented in research, practice and policies.

Faced with this overview, the purpose of this chapter is to help bridge this gap by highlighting not only the predominant theoretical perspectives on participation, but above all by illustrating how it can be promoted in research.

PART I - PERSPECTIVES, MODELS AND PRACTICES TO PROMOTE YOUTH PARTICIPATION

In this part, we will begin with a brief synopsis of the main conceptual models on participation, highlighting its benefits for individuals, organizations and society. We will then describe several fundamental practices for promoting youth participation, namely those involving the identification and selection of participants, facilitators and participation methods. Finally, we will underscore the particular importance of participation in the context of research, by describing the characteristics and benefits of participatory research.

Perspectives, Theoretical Models and Benefits of Participation

Although there exists no single consensual definition of participation, it is understood as: a) a process which entails the involvement, sharing of responsibilities, influence and inclusion of youth in decisions affecting their life; b) a vehicle of change, and of ensuring that the interests, opinions and perspectives of youth are respected; and c) an opportunity to develop the autonomy, independence, social skills and resilience of youth (Gesellschaft für Technische Zusammenarbeit [GTZ], 2010; Horwath et al., 2011; Mattheus, Limb, and Taylor, 1999).

The study of participation results in at least five theoretical models that facilitate this concept's conceptualization and operationalization, as indicated by the review of Horwath et al. (2011), namely the models of Hart (1992), Huskins (1996), Treseder (1997), Shier (2001) and Kirby, Lanyon, Cronin and Sinclair (2003). Despite their distinctions, all of these models conceptualize the concept in different categories reflecting different degrees and forms of participation and involvement, from a more basic participation, where the young person is involved in the process, interacts with the adult and is heard, to more in-depth participation, where the young person may initiate the process, make decisions and share power and responsibilities with adults. In fact, has shown in Table 1, these theories indicate that youth involvement can take place at different levels through which youth acquire increasingly more autonomy and responsibility in the participatory and decision-making process.

When analysing these models, it should be noted that only the levels of involvement described in the last five columns of Table 1 are part of the perspective of participation. In fact, the first three categories mentioned by Hart (1992) are manipulative forms of participation, since the involvement of youth does not have effective results; they do not know the reason for their participation or do not receive any feedback from it. Along these same lines, the first three levels of involvement referred to by Huskins (1996) are steps prior to participation, in that the young person is involved in the process, but does not have a proactive role until later.

It should also be noted that these levels are not all hierarchical, i.e. categories involving more in-depth youth participation are not necessarily superior or better than those involving more basic participation. In this way, these categories may be conceptualized in a horizontal non-hierarchical relationship where they are all at the same level, or in a vertical hierarchical relationship where the categories of more basic participation are seen as below those of more in-depth participation.

In fact, while the model of Hart (1992) is hierarchical, the model of Treseder (1997), based on the first, is non-hierarchical, arguing that the most suitable level of participation depends on the purpose of participation and the choice of young people.

Although we have no knowledge of evidence linking these different models and levels of participation to different benefits for the participants, especially for youth, a number of studies have shown that participation in general has numerous advantages at the individual, organizational and societal levels.

With regard to the benefits of participation for youth, studies stress the positive consequences of youth participation in activities, initiatives and projects, in their daily living contexts (e.g., school, residential care settings) or in contexts where they can speak for themselves, be heard and advocate for their rights.

These types of participation, where youth are supported and taken into account when expressing their views, promotes citizenship and social inclusion by encouraging, from early on, their involvement in public and community life, and by promoting the communication of children and young people from different socioeconomic and cultural backgrounds (Kirby, Lanyon, Cronin, and Sinclair, 2003). Participation also results in personal and social education and development, helping to develop more confident and resilient youth with diverse skill sets (e.g. communication, teamwork) and greater self-esteem (Checkoway and Richards-Schuster, 2004; GTZ, 2010; Kirby et al., 2003; Sekulovic, 2007). Moreover, there may be an increased sense of power and coping skills among youth involved in the participatory process (GTZ, 2010; Niekerk, 2007). Benefits have also been seen in terms of knowledge acquisition and building, improved relationships with adults and peers, an increased sense of belonging, efficiency, responsibility and autonomy, and in the comprehension of the individual's situation and sense of ownership (Checkoway and Richards-Schuster, 2004; GTZ, 2010; Horwath et al., 2011).

Table 1. Models of participation

Model	Categories/Levels of participation						
Hart (1992)	Manipulation	Decoration	Tokenism	Assigned but informed	Consulted and informed	Adult-initiated shared decisions with children	Child-initiated and directed	Child-initiated shared decisions with adults
Huskins (1996)	First contact	Familiarizing	Socializing	Taking part	Being involved	Organizing	Leading	Peer coaching
Treseder (1997)				Assigned but informed	Consulted and informed	Adult-initiated shared decisions with young people	Young people-initiated and directed	Young people-initiated shared decisions with adults
Shier (2001)				Children are listened	Children are supported in expressing their views	Children's views are taken into account	Children are involved in decision-making processes	Children share power and responsibilities for decision-making
Kirby, Lanyon, Cronin, and Sinclair (2003)					Children's and young people views are taken into account	Children and young people are involved in decision-making in an active and direct way	Children and young people share power and responsibility for decision-making	Children and young people make autonomous decisions

Youth participation also has benefits for projects, organizations and services, particularly for improvement of services (Oldfield and Fowler, 2004). In fact, youth participation in developing, implementing and evaluating services makes them more effective, appropriate, relevant and sustainable (Feinstein, Karkara, and Laws, 2004; GTZ, 2010). Participation also increases the commitment, access to and use of services on the part of youth, which maximizes resources (Kirby et al., 2003; Sekulovic, 2007).

With regard to the benefits for society, adults have reconsidered their views by acknowledging the value and fostering the participation of youth (Welsh Assembly Government, 2007). On a more global scale, participation encourages citizenship and democracy (Horwath et al., 2011), and is beneficial for informed policymaking leading to changes in: practices, services and organizational structures, developing and designing strategies, decision-making, practices involving the recruitment and selection of human resources, as well as in the production of material and information resources (Checkowayand Richards-Schuster, 2004; Horwath et al., 2011). In summary, participation not only promotes individual empowerment, but also interpersonal, organizational and community empowerment, together with ownership and capacity building for all of those involved (Viswanathan et al., 2004).

Participation Practices

Participation can be promoted in various contexts of young people's lives, from more informal (e.g. family and peer group) to more formal settings (e.g. participation in the community, schools, public policy decision-making and society) (GTZ, 2010). In fact, young people should have various venues and means of involvement, as well as time to develop the skills needed for effective participation, with education and support to this end over the course of the participation process (O'Donoghue, Kirshner, andMclaughlin, 2002).As such, in order to adopt participatory practices – above all in formal contexts – different factors must first be considered, such as identifying and selecting participants, facilitators and participation methods.

With regard to participant selection, it is important to consider inclusion and representativity. In fact, it is difficult to ensure that the youth participating are representative of a group, above all when they are selected by the organizations themselves; clear and specific information must thus be given on the project's nature and the characteristics of the youth to be included (Horwath et al., 2011). In this process of identifying and selecting participants, one must take into account the ages, understanding and experience of participation, the group's size, the available resources and methods, past experiences, and the diversity, ethnicity, religion and culture of the participants to tailor the activities to them (Horwath et al., 2011). Moreover, in an initial youth participation phase, the participation's goals should be clearly defined and monitored, mutual expectations should be clarified, informed consent with clear confidentiality boundaries should be established, together with agreed rules and the identification of an appropriate participatory context (GTZ, 2010; Horwath et al., 2011).

With regard to the facilitators, the adults' training is particularly important. In fact, in order to adapt and be able to promote youth participation, the adults must change the way they perceive and understand youth, and learn how to be allies of the participation (O'Donoghue et al., 2002). As facilitators, the adults play a key role in guiding and connecting the youth to the resources and information needed for participation, and should help familiarize them with the contextual norms where it will occur (O'Donoghue et al., 2002). The facilitator is responsible for ensuring that the youth understand the goals of the participation, for establishing a safe and friendly environment, and for guaranteeing that all of the youth have the time and support needed to express their opinions (Horwath et al., 2011). The facilitator is also responsible for initiating the participation process, and should monitor the discussion's progress, cope with participants' emotions, manage conflicts and misunderstandings, recap key points and receive feedback from the session, assuming more of a leadership or management role in the processdepending on the goal and type of activity (Horwath et al., 2011).

With regards to participation methods, these should be chosen according to the goals of the participation and the participants' needs and characteristics. According to the review of Horwath et al. (2011), there exist more formal participation methods (e.g. consultations, meetings and suggestion boxes) as well as more informal ones (e.g. dialogues and spontaneous remarks), as well as individual or group methods. These are further broken down into written methods (e.g. questionnaires, checklists, arrangements and completion of sentences), oral methods (e.g. storytelling), exhibition and disseminated methods (e.g. campaigns and presentations), technological, visual and artistic methods (e.g. production of images, books, video and photo diaries, websites, social networking and virtual group platforms), and dramatization methods (e.g. drama and role-playing), among others.

In summary, to ensure inclusive, representative, effective, meaningful, and beneficial participation for youth and institutions alike, youth participation must be promoted in a wide range of contexts and through different practices, adapting them not only to the processes' goals but also to the participants themselves. Moreover, in addition to the care in choosing participants and forms of participation, the participation must be facilitated by adults who are competent to this end, which requires a global effort in building the resources, structures, practices and cultures supporting these participatory processes (O'Donoghue et al., 2002).

Participatory Research

Besides the participation of youth in their daily lives formal and informal contexts (e.g., family, school), it is important that they also participate are involved in the research/academic context, in order to provide a more in-depth understanding of their own realities and perspectives. In this regard, participatory research is of particular importance. It is characterized by principles of inclusion, and acknowledging the importance of involving the beneficiaries, users and stakeholders tied to the research's purpose (Cargo and Mercer, 2008). It is also distinguished by being action-driven, since it focuses on the transfer of knowledge into practice, bridging the gap between theory and practice that exists in public services (Glasgow and Emmons, 2007). Participatory research entails a partnership providing a balance between goals of scientific excellence and social and cultural relevance, resulting in for benefits for everyone involved. In fact, with participation, the evidence collected in a research process has more validity (external, social and cultural), more credibility, and more widespread applicability (Cargo and Mercer, 2008), since knowledge is produced based on the population's needs. Moreover, involving the different stakeholders gives insight into various perspectives on problems and priorities, thereby enriching the understanding of the issues under analysis (Holland, 2009). This facilitates the transformation of knowledge into action, through change, not only in individual behaviour and practices, but also in political and organizational systems (Cargo and Mercer, 2008). In addition, it allows more comprehensive and coordinated responses, giving decision-makers the knowledge needed on how to improve the development, implementation and provision of programs and services (Cargo and Mercer, 2008). In research projects, it is important to involve young people throughout the entire process, including the analysis and interpretation of data, where they can verify the validity of analytical conclusions and interpretations and help to develop key messages, making them feel that their participation is proactive and meaningful (Mainey, 2008). Youth participation in participatory research is thus essential, particularly in systems where they are the end beneficiaries and users (e.g., residential care, school/educational or health-care systems), and should occur in two core situations: 1) needs assessment; and 2) designing services. With regard to needs assessment, not only is it important for young people to have the right to participate in decisions affecting them, but their needs are much better served when they participate in such decisions (Horwath et al., 2011). In fact, young people are the true "experts" in terms of their own lives, and have a one-of-a-kind ability to impart their experiences and perspectives (Clark and Moss, 2001). With regard to designing services, it should be emphasized that scientific knowledge produced through youth participation can be used to improve existing programs or to create new programs, practices, services and policies (Teufel-Shone, Siyuja, Watahomigie, and Irwin, 2006). Thus, by integrating young people's perspectives, the appropriate services can be developed to meet the needs of the system and its end-users (Viswanathan et al., 2004), while also ensuring their greater effectiveness, suitability, relevance, and sustainability (Feinstein et al., 2004). In summary, participatory research is a means of promoting and safeguarding young people's right to participation, as well as leveraging its benefits for youth, institutions and society at large. However, as previously mentioned, youth participation in research still falls short of the ideal, and is seldom used to change services. The next part aims at illustrating how this might be accomplished.

PART II - STUDIES THAT PROMOTE YOUTH PARTICIPATION WITHIN THE HEALTH-CARE AND YOUTH PROTECTION SYSTEMS

In this part, we present two research projects promoting youth participation by involving them in assessing needs and designing services in the area of residential care (Autonomy Development and Integration Project/Calheiros, Graça, Patrício, andLouceiro, 2009) and health care services (Project for the Assessment of Risk/Protection Factors and Institutional Social Support in Health Care, Calheiros/Bernardes, Paulino, and Pereira, 2005). These projects are examples of best practices in promoting youth participation in research and practice, simultaneously contributing to young people's well-being, promoting their skill building, protecting their rights and improving services.

Autonomy Development and Integration Project

Context and Goals

The Autonomy Development and Integration Project (Calheiros, Graça, Patrício, and Louceiro, 2009) arose from the need to promote transition programs between residential care and independent living, aimed at facilitating and encouraging the social integration of youth in residential care. This project was developed in Portugal, through a protocol between a residential care institution in Lisbon and the Social Research and Intervention Center (CIS-IUL). In fact, young people's departure from residential care has been a topic of major concern since, most often, they leave the institutions without the resources, support and life skills needed for self-sufficiency (Colca and Colca, 1996), and without a support network allowing a gradual, sustained transition to independent living (Geenenand Powers, 2007). A number of studies have consolidated this idea, showing that adolescents in prolonged care face greater challenges during this transition process, with their failure leading to poor academic performance, housing difficulties, financial and job seeking difficulties, physical and mental health problems, substance abuse, and other psychosocial adjustment difficulties (e.g. Barth, 1990; McMillenand Tucker, 1999).

These were the grounds for extending independent living support services to those groups of youth still lacking a specific response in this regard. This project, thus, entails the initial phase of putting together this new service, aimed at identifying the young people's needs and designing a service to support this transition to independent living.

Methodology

A qualitative methodology was used in this project. More specifically, four focus groups were held including a total of N= 21 young people in residential care aged 15 to 18 years (M=16; SD=1.07; 52% female). To ensure the heterogeneity and representativity of the sample, the participants came from 20 residences of care in Lisbon, coordinated by the same institution, and were chosen according to the following criteria: a) minimum age of 15 years; b) participants of both sexes; c) participants with and without recorded behavioral problems; and d) with at least three years of care. Participants were contacted directly and asked about their availability to participate.

The focus groups were conducted by three researchers who had no connections with the institutions, two as moderators and one as an outside observer. The focus groups lasted from one to two hours, with the number of participants in each session ranging from four to six. In all of the sessions, the same introductory instructions were given, and the questions were asked in the same order. In addition, the participants were ensured that all data collected would be kept confidential and anonymous and gave us their informed consent to participate. The participants were also asked for their consent to record the focus groups, which were then transcribed and analyzed.

The focus groups were conducted using a semi-structured script covering: 1) questions and discussion topics involving five areas common to various needs assessment approaches available in the literature – housing situation, family and social relationships, physical and psychological health, behaviours and skills, and education and employment; and 2) questions on the design of a new support service for autonomy development and integration, covering different areas such as housing conditions, operating rules, location and relationships between residents, technicians and outside people.

The data gathered from the focus groups underwent a mixed content analysis, i.e. with categories defined both a priori and a posteriori (Vala, 2003). The reliability of this category system was checked by determining inter-rater agreement (Cohen Kappa = 0.968), followed by a structural analysis, valence analysis and occurrence analysis of the category system. This analysis is presented in two different points: I) Identification of the needs of youth in residential care; and II) Participatory design of a support service for the transition to independent living.

Results

Identification of the Needs of Youth in Residential Care

The categories resulting from the identification of the needs of youth in residential care (total of 834 units of analysis) show that young people place particular importance on a set of factors comprising seven areas, described in descending order of importance in the discourses:

1. Life context (405; 48.6%) includes young people's perceptions, feelings and positions on their life context in residential care. Of particular note in this area is the perception of educators (24%), where the young people pointed out several negative aspects such as improper behaviour, turnover and lack of motivation, although they also expressed admiration for them. After this came physical space (22.5%), where they expressed some dissatisfaction with the space's décor and physical conditions, together with ambivalent perspectives involving satisfaction with the space's capacity; the social image of residential care (17.3%), which was negative and unstructured overall; and services (12.3%), where they expressed some dissatisfaction with regard to food. Dissatisfaction with residential care rules (8.6%) and climate of insecurity due to theft (6.7%) had less weight. Finally came changes and stability in their care plan (5%) and desire to leave residential care (3.7%).
2. Social and family relationships (216; 25.9%) correspond to relationships both within and outside the institution. Here, the most frequently mentioned areas were interactions with educators (48.2%), where the young people pointed out the quality of the relationship and the support provided by educators, but also the lack of empathy, trust and friendliness in their relationship with them, and with the peer group (37.5%), where they pointed out distrust between residents, but also the support and the quality of the relationship between them. The relationships with technicians, i.e. psychologists and social workers (8.3%), based on a positive and supporting relationship, and with the family (6%), where they were reluctant to speak (only mentioning positive aspects), had less weight.
3. Education (88; 10.6%) includes a number of school-related questions involving the educational context (56.8%), characterized by conflicts and difficulties in school integration, together with moderate levels of academic satisfaction and motivation (21.6%) and a high frequency of changes of schools (21.6%).
4. Skills and behaviour (58; 6.9%) involve the young people's verbalizations revolving around their conduct in residential care. In this area, they expressed some difficulties in self-management skills for autonomy (84.5%), as well as some behavioural problems (8.6%) and some cases of isolation and refusal of support (6.9%).
5. Factors for psychological health (28; 3.4%) include the youth's perspectives on factors promoting/threatening their degrees of well-being and psychological health, underscoring several extrinsic factors (53.6%), such as their life context in residential care, and intrinsic factors (46.4%), such as resilience.
6. Employment (22; 2.6%) includes the young people's references to positive and negative aspects of the professional context. Here, they identified the perception of work as a personal development opportunity (50%), positive contacts and experiences from work (22.8%) and the functional aspects of work (13.6%), such as

the salary, as positive aspects of employment, and the difficulties experienced at work (13.6%), such as strict work schedules, as negative aspects.
7. Factors for physical health (17; 2%) include the young people's perspective on factors promoting physical health, such as healthy practices (70.6%) like regular sleep, a balanced diet and athletic activity, and the use of health care services (29.4%).

Participatory Design of a Supportive Service for Independent Living Transitioning

The categories identified for the participatory design of a supportive service for independent living transitioning (total of 358 units of analysis) show that young people place particular importance on a set of factors comprising four areas, described in descending order of importance in the discourses:

1. Physical space (132; 36.9%) corresponds to the housing conditions and structure of the residence supporting independent living. This includes aspects such as location (43.2%), which should be central with good access, community resources, leisure facilities and refuge from social problems, type (30.5%), which refers to apartments with structures and facilities that are comparable to those found in most housing, limited capacity (15.2%), where the young people underscored the importance of moderate levels of housing density, generally from three to five inhabitants, and décor (14.4%), involving their ability to be part of planning and, above all, personalizing the space.
2. Rules and functioning (126; 35.2%) correspond to the residence's rules, routines and management principles. It is comprised of autonomous decision-making (19.8%), with the young people pointing out the need for more freedom and independence in the new setting; conflict resolution (19.8%), affirming their ability to resolve conflicts between themselves as a group of residents; financial management (14.3%), emphasizing that this should be oriented according to the residence's maintenance expenses; length of stay (13.5%), with most suggesting a maximum length of stay at the residence of two to three years; task organization (8.7%), where they reaffirmed their ability to self-govern themselves as a group responsible for organizing, planning and completing domestic tasks in rotation; and visitation rules (8.7%), where they stressed the importance of consent among the residents with regard to visitors. A sense of security at the residence (7.1%), participation in establishing internal house rules (4%) and understanding/participating in house admission criteria (4%) had less weight.
3. Educators (61; 18.7%) include the young people's verbalizations revolving around educators' role in the new service, namely educator characteristics (54.1%) – not controlling, moderately demanding, understanding, experienced, trustworthy, friendly and not too old – and their functions (45.9%) – support/monitoring, being informed and accessible, and conflict resolution/mediation. Thus, they seem to view educators as individuals that can be a source of social support, in addition to their role of control and supervision, being physically present but more "backup" in nature.
4. In the relationship between residents (39; 10.9%) the most commonly cited aspect was trust (33.3%), with the unanimous belief that a relationship based on mutual trust

was essential from the very outset. This was followed by understanding and flexibility (12.9%), respect (17.9%), privacy (17.9%) and the possibility of conflicts (7.7%).

Conclusion

This project explored residential care system's youth perspectives in regards to their needs and the development of a transitioning service into independent living.

With regard to young people's needs, we found that these primarily revolved around the relationship with educators and with the peer group, as well as the structural (e.g. suitability of the physical space) and functional life context (e.g. suitability/comprehension of rules). The aspects arising from this study are consistent with those found in prior studies, such as the importance of relationships and normalization of the care, among others (e.g. Geenen and Powers, 2007; Strolin-Goltzman, Kollar, andTrinkle, 2010).

With regard to the design of the ideal autonomous residence, the young people stressed that it should have a central location in a non-problematic zone, normative structures, and personalized décor and three to five residents. In terms of rules and functioning, of particular interest was self-governance through references to the importance of autonomous decision-making, conflict resolution and task organization, although the need for support in financial management was also mentioned. According to the young people, in this context, educators should primarily provide social support and monitoring, in addition to control and supervision. In the relationship with residents, they emphasized the importance of trust.

This data reinforces the importance placed by young people on structural and functional aspects of their life contexts; the ideas put forward for the new residence are precisely aimed at solving some of the shortcomings identified by youth in the current service (e.g. décor/furnishings, self-governance, trust, etc.).

Despite the project's limitations (e.g., small size of the sample group, and the fact that all of the participants belonged to the same institution), the results obtained provide a better understanding of this population, identify strong and weak points in the residential care system, and help to develop justified, specific policies and practices focused on the final beneficiaries: the young people themselves.

Project for the Assessment of Risk/Protection Factors and Institutional Social Support in Health Care

Context and Goals

The Project for the Assessment of Risk/Protection Factors and Institutional Social Support in Health Care (Calheiros, Bernardes, Paulino, and Pereira, 2005) was developed in 2005, in Portugal, through a protocol between a community support institution (with healthcare services) and the Social Research and Intervention Center (CIS-IUL). This project arose primarily due to the fact that adolescence is a critical time for the adoption of key health-related behaviour (Jessor, Turbin, and Costa, 1998). This development phase is considered crucial in terms of health and illness, since many positive health habits are established during adolescence, as well as many high-risk behaviours. The patterns from this phase of life will most likely persist for the remaining lifetime (Maggs et al., 1993, cited by Jessor et al., 1998), thus having long-lasting results on the individual's health and well-being.

Moreover, adolescents have the lowest levels of health care service use (Ryan, Millstein, Greene, and Irwin, 1996). They show high resistance to approaching health care institutions, while these have difficulties in attracting the adolescents that seek them (Muza and Costa, 2002). In this way, attracting young people to these services may be a strategy for promoting health and preventing illness during adolescence. In this way, one of the purposes of this project was to identify the needs of young people using health facilities, thereby helping to understand their concept of ideal health care centre, in order to layout guidelines to develop a health care service for this population.

Methodology

Similarly to the previous project, qualitative methodologies were used; one extensive in nature (open-ended questionnaire) and another intensive in nature (focus groups). In the first, N= 346 youth, aged 11 to 25 years old (M=16.58; SD=2.0; 56.6% male) attending community support institutions for youth at risk responded in writing to two open-ended questions on their perspectives on the ideal health care centre ("In your opinion, what would the ideal health care centre be like? Compared to the existing one, what should it have?"; "In your opinion, what could a health care centre have to make people of your age want to go there?") In the second, N= 21 young people were selected from these N= 346, aged 13 to 21 years (61.9% male) to take part in three focus groups. These were conducted using a semi-structured script including questions on the use of health care services, taking into account youth in general and their own experience. (e.g. "Why do young people avoid going to health care services?"). In the end, the topic of the ideal health care centre was introduced through the question "In your opinion, what would an ideal health care centre for youth be like?".

The data from the open-ended questionnaire and focus groups underwent a content analysis, carried out similarly to the one described in the previous project. This analysis is presented in two different points: I) Identification of young people's needs and perspectives on the use of health care services; and II) Design of the ideal health care centre for youth.

Results

Identification of Young People's Needs and Perspectives on Health Care Services Use

The identification of young people's needs and perspectives on the use of health care services includes the results from the first part of the focus groups, where questions were asked on the use of health care services and the factors influencing this. In this analysis, a total of 205 units of analysis were identified, divided into two main areas: use and non-use.

1. The area of "use" (104; 53.33%) includes the reasons that bring young people to health care services (76.92%), primarily involving the type of need of these youth (56.25%), who may use the services for needs involving prevention or care for an illness/symptom. There are also socio-demographic factors tied to use (23.75%), such as age and gender, with the young people saying that girls use health care services more often, mainly for reasons involving family-planning; and factors of

family context (20%), with references to the importance of family support for the use of health care services. The types of services that the young people use (23.08%), namely the hospital, emergency room and gynaecology/obstetrician, were also mentioned.

2. In the area of "non-use" (91; 46.67%), there was greater detail in specifying the underlying reasons (87.91%), which involved aspects of the technicians, services and youth. Reasons involving technicians (45%) included the difficulty of the technician/youth relationship (66.67%) (e.g. distrust, embarrassment), the antipathy of administrative technicians (22.22%) and the lack of competence and involvement of health care technicians (11.11%). Reasons for non-use involving services (27.5%) included the lack of accessibility (81.82%), comprising waiting time, distance of the service and difficulty scheduling appointments, and the cost of appointments (18.18%). Reasons involving the youth (27.5%) included the lack of prevention values (81.82%), absence of family support (9.1%) and existence of a self-healing perspective (9.1%). The type of services least used by youth was also mentioned (12.09%), with some references again to hospitals, and with references to health care centres.

Design of the Ideal Health Care Centre for Youth

In order to understand youth's representation of the ideal health care centre, both the data collected by the focus groups and the open-ended questionnaires were analysed. In this analysis, a total of 488 units of analysis were identified, organized into the following areas, described in descending order of importance in the discourses:

1. Integrated services (133; 27.4%) -The ideal health care centre should offer a series of integrated services, namely community intervention programs (49.6%), focused primarily on topics of substance abuse and sexuality, using strategies based on fun/informal activities. There should also exist health support services (17.3%) such as family planning, nursing and pharmacies, together with psychological consultations (16.5%), specialized medical consultations (10.5%) and emergency services (6.0%).
2. Promotion of services (122; 25.1%) - Strategies were proposed for the ideal health care centre to promote its services, such as leisure and entertainment activities (46.7%) (e.g. games, television), computers with Internet access (16.4%), cultural activities (12.3%) (e.g. theatre groups), athletic activities (6.6%) (e.g. yoga) and background music (6.6%).
3. Characteristics of technicians (81; 16.67%) -The technicians who work at the ideal health care centre should be young (23.5%), nice (16.1%), competent (13.6%), trained in the area of adolescence (12.4%) and understanding (12.4%).
4. Functioning (53; 10.91%) –The health care centre's functioning should discourage bureaucracy in services by computerizing the management of its users and flexible scheduling processes (32%), in order to provide faster service (18.9%). The articulation between technicians and multidisciplinary expertise (18.9%) were a desirable characteristic of operation. Costs should be tailored to users' available resources (13.2%).

5. Technician/adolescent relationship (44; 9.1%) - A relationship of trust (25%), involvement (25%), confidentiality (20.5%) and support (15.9%) was considered important.
6. Physical space (42; 8.64%) - The structural features of the building were emphasized (26.2%), particularly with regard to the space's amplitude. However, more than the building's structure, its interior features were important (73.81%). The ideal health care centre should be well decorated and comfortable, with an informal, relaxed environment.
7. Location (11; 2.26%) – Some said that psychology and counselling services should be located outside of the neighbourhood, while general clinical services should be located within it, due to issues of confidentiality and anonymity.

Conclusion

This project explored young people's perspectives on their current health care service needs, and the development of an ideal youth health care service. The identification of young people's needs and perspectives vis-à-vis health care services was illustrated by the reasons for their use and non-use. The reasons for their use included those that bring young people to health care services, and involving prevention and the identification of illnesses or symptoms. However, greater details were provided regarding reasons for no service use, involving aspects of the technicians (technician/youth relationship, antipathy of administrative technicians and the lack of competence and involvement of health care technicians), the services (accessibility, difficulty scheduling appointments and financial factors) and the youth themselves (lack of prevention values, absence of family support and existence of a self-healing perspective). These results are consistent with other empirical evidence demonstrating that the demand for services is not only determined by the perception of a health problem, but also by factors involving the health care system. Examples of such factors are the relationship with health care professionals, the guarantee of confidentiality, respect for the patient, sociability, anonymity, appointments without the need for prior scheduling, financial accessibility and the existence of a regular health care service, among others (Pommier et al, 2001).

With regards to designing the ideal health care centre for youth, participants emphasized that it should offer a series of integrated services and strategies to promote its services. Technicians working at the centre should be young, nice, competent, trained in the area of adolescence and understanding. The technician/adolescent relationship is also emphasized, placing importance on a relationship of trust, involvement, confidentiality and support. Aspects involving the health care centre's operation are also mentioned (non-bureaucratic services, scheduling processes, prompt service, articulation between technicians and multidisciplinary expertise, costs matching users' available resources), the physical space (the space's amplitude, décor, comfort, informality and relaxed environment) and the location of the services (within or outside the neighbourhood). Once again, these results are consistent with prior evidence showing the importance of the space's characteristics and the competence of the health care service's technicians (Pommier et al., 2001).

In general, it can be concluded that the results obtained provide a better understanding of young people's perspectives on current health care centres and the factors involved in their use or non-use; they also help to develop policies and practices in the health care system based on aspects that are critical to this population.

Discussion - Contributions of Participatory Research

The projects discussed here exemplify the combination of research and action through an approach of participatory research to ensure youth participation and influence on improving social and health care services. From these projects, specific concerns and priorities of youth can be identified to help improve and develop services that are tailored to the specific characteristics and needs of youth, thereby increasing their potential effectiveness (Axford, Little, Morphet, andWeyts, 2005). The results obtained in these projects can also beused to assist in making decisions, solving problems in a timely manner, correcting or discontinuing negatively assessed services, and developing new services based on the input gathered that better address young people's needs.

In fact, in the area of residential care services, the results obtained can define a variety of guidelines to improve existing services and build a new one to support the transition from residential care to independent living, such as: a) quality of interpersonal relationships; b) investment in the selection, training and goal management of educators; c) stability; d) institutional image management; e) physical space (community resources, normalization, personalization and regulation of personal spaces); f) participation in planning routines and norms to manage each residential unit; g) strong support and incentives for the training and qualification of practitioners; h) skill building (personal/interpersonal and self-care); i) response designed according to the needs and characteristics of a given target group; j) normalization; and, k) awareness and engagement of technicians and educators.

Also in the area of health care, the results obtained can help define a variety of guidelines to improve youth health care services to bring them ever closer to the image of the ideal health care centre defined by them, such as: a) health care practitioners with ongoing and specialized training in the area of adolescence; b) technician/adolescent relationship based on confidentiality; c) implementation of integrated services at strategic locations in terms of accessibility; d) informal, comfortable interior space, with cultural and leisure facilities; e) integrated operation and exchange between different health care technicians, with other community services, families and schools f) services involving sex education/health education; and g) reinforced medical care services, with a greater variety of specialized consultations.

Furthermore, besides promoting youth participation, these projects built knowledge on how to improve and develop more effective services. However, despite its potential and benefits, this participation still falls short of the ideal, prompting reflection on its obstacles and challenges, which will be presented in part three of this chapter.

PART III - CHALLENGES TO YOUTH PARTICIPATION IN THE SERVICES EVALUATION AND DESIGN

The declaration of young people's right to participation is a fundamental step in acknowledging youth as active citizens, as individual people with their own ideas who are capable of speaking for themselves; however, as we have already asserted, this does not mean that their participation actually occurs. In order for it to occur, there must be a joint effort between research, policy and practice to safeguard and promote young people's right to participation.

The projects and review of literature presented in this chapter show that it is possible – and advisable – to integrate the participation of youth in assessing and designing services in common social practices and policies. In fact, youth participation builds knowledge for action, underscoring critical aspects to refine and develop new services, and promoting better public policies, stronger organizations, more relevant services and healthier communities (Ginwrightand James, 2002). However, the right to participation is not being consistently implemented in political, legislative and practical terms (Lloyd-Smith andTarr, 2000, Hill et al., 2004). Therefore, in this part of the chapter, we will reflect on some of the obstacles to participation, as well as recommendations for practice and research.

Obstacles to Participation

Despite the benefits of participation for youth, services, organizations, and societies in general, as presented over the course of this chapter, there also exist various obstacles to participation, such as: the lack of definition and confusion revolving around the concept of participation, cultural barriers to youth participation, adults' resistance to participation and unwillingness to share power, the persistence of social biases that impede adults from seeing youth as social and political agents, and adults' inability and inexperience in facilitating and promoting participation (AICAFMHA, 2008; IAWGC, 2008).

Among youth, there is also the lack of confidence, information, time, skills, power and resources, location and lack of transportation, low socio-economic status, and ambiguity with regards to roles and responsibilities (AICAFMHA, 2008). Moreover, among adults and organizations, there are obstacles such as: organizational mind-sets, which generally do not acknowledge youth participation, organizational disagreement on the right forms and types of participation, community resistance, believing that young people's opinions and abilities are inferior to those of adults, and the different abilities and skills of youth and adults (AICAFMHA, 2008).

In fact, there is a lack of formal methods to promote youth involvement (Horwath et al., 2011), as well as structures and public desire to involving youth in the decision-making processes (GTZ, 2010). In addition, the quality of the participation must be considered, since poor practices give youth a sense of lost confidence and time, thereby harming future attempts at public involvement (Together We Can, 2005).

Furthermore, political support for youth participation is primarily a product of demagogy since, in practice, youth participation is limited in various contexts, namely: in voting, elections and political activities; at school, where students are rarely entitled to influence how the school is managed, and do not participate in decisions that affect them; and in legal systems, where young people are often excluded and not consulted (Bessant, 2004). In fact, in most places, a culture of non-participation predominates, where young people have few opportunities to participate in discussions on their future or express their preferences; this culture is enhanced by doubts and uncertainties on young people's abilities, and the on suitability, benefits and forms of their involvement (Mattheus, Limb, and Taylor, 1999). Participation is even more difficult to achieve in cultures favouring hierarchical relationships and with specific groups of youth, such as youth from rural zones, minorities, institutions, living alone, isolated and with disadvantaged socio-economic circumstances (AICAFMHA, 2008; GTZ, 2010).

Also participation is limited by a lack of financial resources, human resources and time demanding effective and inclusive participation, and by the youth themselves, who often times do not see themselves as a group that should participate or that, when they want to participate, do not know how to proceed and do not have the resources (Checkoway and Richards-Schuster, 2004). As such, the development, implementation and maintenance of youth participation strategies is restricted and hampered by a series of barriers among youth, organizations and communities (AICAFMHA, 2008).

Ethically, youth participation also requires that a number of aspects be considered. Among these is the importance of considering that the participants may not benefit directly from the changes derived from their participation. As such, young people must be informed, before they participate, that they may not benefit directly from the changes, but that policies and practices enhancing the experiences and lives of youth in general may change if the results are properly used and disseminated. These limitations are further minimized if we consider the benefits for youth arising from their participation (Kendrick, Steckley, andLerpiniere, 2008). It should be further clarified that the information gathered will not be used to the detriment of the participants, and that it is confidential and anonymous; it is important that confidentiality boundaries be clearly laid out (Horwath et al., 2011). In addition, care should be taken not to create unrealistic expectations among young people, and – to avoid exclusion and discrimination – adults should ensure that all social groups have the chance to participate in accordance with their emotional and cognitive skills (Horwath et al., 2011).

Recommendations for Practice

For participation to be effective and meaningful we must help institutions and adults create an environment where participation is facilitated and change is encouraged in social structures, policies, and attitudes (GTZ, 2010). We must involve youth in democracy, projects, programs and institutions, give them the space to express themselves, learn to respect and listen to their perspectives, see them as capable and competent social agents who can participate meaningfully in decision-making processes, take their opinions into account and be willing to invest the financial and human resources needed to allow and facilitate high-quality participation (GTZ, 2010; Horwath et al., 2011).

Some countries already have youth organizations, government departments and non-governmental organizations addressing this issue and promoting youth involvement. However, policies and structures are needed to develop youth participation and support this process of representation, consulting and co-management, fostering a culture of participation in which youth involvement from early on is seen as something natural and responsible (Mattheus, Limb, and Taylor, 1999). It is also important to empower youth organizations to participate in designing policies and action plans (GTZ, 2010).

Some participation promotion strategies include: political participation on a local and national scale; developing abilities that strengthen youth and youth organizations; youth participation in local development initiatives; increased awareness of the potential and right of youth to participate through media or public debates; promoting the right to vote and political participation; promotion of proactive youth participation in research, in policy analysis, in policy and program design, in implementing, monitoring and evaluating programs, and in campaigns; developing dissemination skills; and organizing and holding conferences (GTZ, 2010).

In summary, the following are necessary: a) strengthening youth participation, making it systematic, sustained and integrated (Hart, 2007); b) viewing young people as drivers of change and proactive citizens who speak for themselves; c) consulting with young people to learn how they would like to be involved and supported (Sekulovic, 2007); and d) utilizing inclusive practices allowing young people to share their experiences, while also being an opportunity to improve their life circumstances (Fox andBerrick, 2007).

Recommendations for Future Research

It is important to sustain lines of scholarship providing a more in-depth and detailed understanding of the conditions needed to foster effective youth participation and its benefits (Bessant, 2004; O'Donoghue et al., 2002). Moreover, the evolution of this concept would benefit from empirical studies with more complex models and quasi-experimental and multilevel designs, allowing us to identify which factors empower effective participation and its benefits at various levels.

Along the same lines, as stated by O'Donoghue et al. (2002), questions of power must also be studied to understand whether adults are willing to involve youth in a meaningful manner, and whether young people are willing and prepared to take on the role of decision makers and public agents.

General Conclusion

Since participation is a right to which young people are entitled, and since it has benefits at a number of levels, the purpose of this chapter was to systematize the evolution of this concept in theoretical and practical terms, the benefits of (and obstacles to) effective participation, and the best practices for promoting participation. In this regard, we exemplified the use of participatory research partnerships as a potential effective means of initiating this process, as they promote youth participation, build knowledge for action, and simultaneously promote the capacity building of services and ownership of methods, cultures and policies for participation's continuity. In the end, this chapter is aimed at clearly establishing the importance of promoting systematic, effective youth participation by adopting policies, structures and cultures that hold it in high regard.

REFERENCES

AICAFMHA (2008). *National youth participation strategy scoping project report*. Stepney: Australian Infant, Child, Adolescent and Family Mental Health Association.

Axford, N., Little, M., Morpeth, L., andWeyts, A. (2005). Evaluating children's services: Recent conceptual and methodological developments. *British Journal of Social Work, 35*, 73-88.

Barth, R. (1990). On their own: The experiences of youth after foster care. *Child and Adolescent Social Work Journal, 7*, 419-440.

Bessant, J. (2004). Mixed messages: Youth participation and democratic practice. *Australian Journal of Political Science, 39*, 387-404.

Calheiros, M., Bernardes, S., Paulino, P., and Pereira, J. (2005). Projeto Avaliação dos Factores de Risco/Protecção e do Suporte Social Institucional na Área da Saúde. Relatório final não publicado, CIS-IUL, ISCTE - Instituto Universitário de Lisboa.

Calheiros, M., Graça, J., Patrício, J., and Louceiro, A. (2009). Projeto de Integração e Desenvolvimento da Autonomia. Relatório final não publicado, CIS-IUL, ISCTE - Instituto Universitário de Lisboa.

Calheiros, M., Lopes, D., and Patrício, J. (2011). Assessment of the needs of youth in residential care: Development and validation of an instrument. *Children and Youth Services Review, 33*, 1930-1938.

Cargo, M., and Mercer, S. (2008). The value and challenges of Participatory Research: Strengthening its practice. *Annual Review of Public Health, 29*, 325-350.

Checkoway, B., and Richards-Schuster, K. (2004). Youth participation in evaluation and research as a way of lifting new voices. *Children, Youth and Environments, 14*, 84-98.

Clark, A., and Moss, P. (2001). *Listening to young children: The Mosaic approach*. London: National Children's Bureau.

Colca, L., andColca, C. (1996). Transitional independent living foster homes: A step towards independence. *Children Today, 24*, 7-11.

Feinstein, C., Karkara, R., and Laws, S. (2004). A workshop report on child participation in the UN study on violence against children. London: Save the children alliance.

Fox, A., andBerrick, J. (2007). A response to no one ever asked us: A review of children's experiences in out-of-home care. *Child and Adolescent Social Work Journal, 24*, 23-51.

Geenen, S., and Powers, L.E. (2007). "Tomorrow is another problem" The experiences of youth in foster care during their transition into adulthood. *Children and Youth Services Review, 29*, 1085-1101.

Gesellschaft für Technische Zusammenarbeit (2010). *Toolkit "Get youth on board!". Youth participation*. Eschborn: Deutsche Gesellschaft für Technische Zusammenarbeit.

Ginwright, S., and James, T. (2002). From assets to agents of change: Social justice, organizing and youth development. *New Directions for Youth Development, 96*, 27-46.

Glasgow, R., and Emmons, K. (2007). How can we increase translation of research into practice? Types of evidence needed. *Annual Review of Public Health, 28*, 413–433.

Hart, R. (1992). *Children's participation: From tokenism to citizenship*. Florence: UNICEF International Child Development Centre.

Hart, S. (2007). Child participation and child protection. *The International Society for Prevention of Child Abuse and Neglect Special Report, 1*.

Hill, M., Davis, J., Prout, A., andTisdall, K. (2004). Moving the participation agenda forward. *Children and Society, 18*, 77–96.

Holland, S. (2009). Listening to children in care: A review of methodological and theoretical approaches to understanding looked after children's perspectives. *Children and Society, 23*, 226-235.

Horwath, J., Hodgkiss, D., Kalyva, E., andSpyrou, S. (2011). *You respond. Promoting effective project participation by young people who have experienced violence. A guide to good practice through training and development*. Retirado de http://www.you-respond.eu/files/you-respond-practical-guide-english.pdf

Huskins, J. (1996). *Quality work with young people: Developing social skills and diversion from risk*. London: Youth Clubs UK.

IAWGCP (2008). *Children as active citizens: A policy and programme guide*. Bangkok: Inter-Agency Working Group on Children's Participation (IAWGCP).

Jessor, R., Turbin, M. S., and Costa, F. M. (1998). Protective factors in adolescent health behavior. *Journal of Personality and Social Psychology, 75*, 788-800.

Kendrick, A., Steckley, L., andLerpiniere, J. (2008). Ethical issues, research and vulnerability: Gaining the views of children and young people in residential care. *Children's Geographies, 6*, 79-93.

Kirby, P., Lanyon, C., Cronin, K., and Sinclair, R. (2003). *Building a culture of participation: Involving children and young people in policy, service planning, delivery and evaluation*. Nottingham: Department for Education and Skills Publications.

Lansdown, G. (2005). *The evolving capacities of children: Implications for the exercise for rights*. Florence: UNICEF, Innocenti Research Centre.

Lloyd-Smith, M., andTarr, J. (2000). Researching children's perspectives: A sociological dimension. In A. Lewis and G. Lindsay (Eds.), *Researching Children's Perspectives* (pp 59-70). Buckingham: Open University Press.

Mainey, A. (2008). *Evaluating participation work: The toolkit*. London: National Children's Bureau.

Mares, A. (2010). An assessment of independent living needs among emancipating foster youth. *Child and Adolescent Social Work Journal, 27*, 79-96.

Mattheus, H., Limb, M., and Taylor, M. (1999). Young people's participation and representation in society. *Geoforum, 30*, 135-144.

McMillen, C., and Tucker, J. (1999). The status of older adolescents at exit from out-of-home care. *Child Welfare, 78*, 339–360.

Morgan, M., Gibbs, S., Maxwell, K., and Britten, N. (2002). Hearing children voices: Methodological issues in conducting focus groups with children aged 7-11 years. *Qualitative Research, 2*, 5-20.

Muza, G., and Costa, M. (2002). Elementos para a elaboração de um projecto de promoção à saúde e desenvolvimento dos adolescentes – O olhar dos adolescentes. *Cadernos de Saúde Pública, 18*, 321-328.

Niekerk, J. (2007). Child participation: The challenges for child protection workers. *The International Society for Prevention of Child Abuse and Neglect Special Report*, 10-11.

O'Donoghue, J., Kirshner, B., andMclaughlin, M. (2002). Introduction: Moving youth participation forward. *New Directions for Youth Development, 96*, 15-26.

Oldfield, C., and Fowler, C. (2004). *Mapping children and young people's participation in England*. London: DfES.

Pommier, J., Mouchtouris, A., Billot, L., Romero, M., Zubarew, T., andDeschamps, J. (2001). Self-reported determinants of health service use by French adolescents. *International Journal of Adolescent Medicine and Health, 13*, 115-130.

Ryan, S., Millstein, S., Greene, B., and Irwin, C. (1996). Utilization of ambulatory health services by urban adolescents. *Journal of Adolescent Health, 18*, 192-202.

Sekulovic, R. (2007). Involving children in advocacy: What does it mean? *The International Society for Prevention of Child Abuse and Neglect Special Report, 2-3.*

Shier, H. (2001). Pathways to participation: Openings, opportunities and obligations. A new model for enhancing children's participation in decision-making, in line with article 13.1 of the UNCRC. *Children and Society, 15,* 107-117.

Southwell, J., and Fraser, E. (2010). Young people's satisfaction with residential care: Identifying strengths and weaknesses in service delivery. *Child Welfare, 89,* 209-228.

Strolin-Goltzman, J., Kollar, S., andTrinkle, J. (2010). Listening to voices of children in foster care: Youths speak out about child welfare workforce turnover and selection. *Social Work, 55,* 47-53.

Teufel-Shone, N. I., Siyuja, T., Watahomigie, H. J., and Irwin, S. (2006). Community-based Participatory Research: Conducting a formative assessment of factors that influence youth wellness in the Hualapai community. *American Journal of Public Health, 96,* 1623-1628.

Together We Can (2005). *People and participation: How to put citizens in the heart of decision-making.* London: Involve.

Treseder, P. (1997). *Empowering children and young people: Promoting involvement in decision making.* London: Children´s Rights Office and Save the Children.

UNCRC, (1989). *United Nations convention on the rights of the child.* Retirado de http://www2.ohchr.org/english/law/pdf/crc.pdf

Vala, J. (2003). Análise de conteúdo. In A. Silva and J. Pinto (Eds.), *Metodologia das Ciências Sociais* (pp. 101-128). Porto: Edições Afrontamento.

Viswanathan, M., Ammerman, A., Eng, E., Gartlehner, G., Lohr, K., Griffith, D., Rhodes, S., Samuel-Hodge, C., Maty, S., Lux, L., Webb, L., Sutton, S., Swinson, T., Jackman, A., and Whitener, L. (2004).Community-based Participatory Research: Assessing the evidence. *Evidence Report/ Technology Assessment, 99.* (Prepared by RTI–University of North Carolina Evidence-based Practice Center under Contract No. 290-02-0016). AHRQ Publication 04-E022-2. Rockville, MD: Agency for Healthcare Research and Quality.

Welsh Assembly Government (2007). *Conwy children and young people's partnership. Participation strategy.* Retirado de http://www.conwy.gov.uk/upload/public/attachments/360/Conwy_CYPP _ Participation_Strategy_NEW.pdf.

In: Youth: Practices, Perspectives and Challenges
Editor: Elizabeth Trejos-Castillo

ISBN: 978-1-62618-067-3
© 2013 Nova Science Publishers, Inc.

Chapter 16

REFORMING JUVENILE JUSTICE: CASE STUDIES IN REINVESTMENT AND REALIGNMENT

Douglas N. Evans[*,1] *and Lisa Marie Vasquez*[2]

[1]Indiana University, Bloomington, IN, US
[2]Rutgers University, NJ, US

ABSTRACT

As crime rates continue to decline in the United States, some state juvenile justice systems have developed reforms to limit the number of juveniles that are placed in secure facilities. Because incarceration rates are not always related to crime rates, these reforms may only be a temporary response to the crime drop. However, certain reforms have proved to be long lasting and unresponsive to fluctuations in juvenile crime rates. This chapter discusses two different strategies for juvenile justice reform. The first, reinvestment strategies, promote the creation of financial incentives that encourage county governments to limit the number of juvenile offenders they send to secure state facilities. The state rewards counties for reduced youth incarceration by allocating funds to counties for the development of community-based supervision and treatment programs that enable juveniles to be rehabilitated close to their homes. The second method, realignment, is the shifting of management and responsibility, typically from the state to the county level. This model requires counties to take control of juvenile justice operations and severely limits their ability to place juveniles in secure state facilities. Both models enable states to save on juvenile justice expenditures and to promote youth rehabilitation and community safety, but they do so to varying degrees. State representatives can scale back on reinvestment initiatives if juvenile crime rates start to increase. Realignment has shown to be the more durable reform strategy because it involves a complete shift in control. Compared to state governments, counties are in the optimal position to supervise and provide for adjudicated and at-risk juveniles locally and in the most cost-effective way. This chapter also compares several states that have employed reinvestment and realignment models.

---

[*] Address Correspondence to: Douglas N. Evans, Indiana University Email: dnevans@indiana.edu.

INTRODUCTION

State governments are responsible for managing juvenile justice systems. There is no federal system that governs juvenile justice and therefore there is no unified set of laws, regulations or policies that guide juvenile justice in the United States. State and local officials make determinations regarding youth policy and state and county courts generally decide dispositional outcomes for juvenile delinquents. This arrangement results in considerable differences in the ways that states process juvenile offenders, pay for the costs of juvenile facilities and services, and manage and oversee juvenile justice operations.

States vary in the extent to which they incarcerate juvenile offenders. Although many people believe that the amount of crime determines the correctional population, oftentimes the size of the juvenile correctional population is unrelated to the crime rate. Incarceration is a policy decision. Some state policymakers pass legislation and make funding decisions that encourage the use of confinement. Other states favor the use of community-based supervision and treatment programs and reserve confinement for the most violent and serious juvenile offenders. The decision to fund secure confinement facilities is crucial because the costs associated with youth confinement are considerable. States that invest heavily in juvenile confinement facilities risk depleting the resources that would enable them to create a balanced juvenile justice system (Butts and Evans, 2011).

The cost of confinement is a sizeable expense for state governments. It costs around $100,000 annually to confine one juvenile, and in New York the costs have reached $266,000 (New York Juvenile Justice Advisory Group, 2010). Because more than 80,000 juveniles spent time in a secure state facility in 2008, youth confinement creates significant expenditures for states nationwide (Sickmund, 2010). The traditional financial arrangement in juvenile justice absolves local governments from financial accountability for youth confinement. Because local governments are generally responsible for the costs of community-based supervision and treatment, cities and counties are willing to send more adjudicated youth to secure facilities in order to conserve financial resources.

Several states experienced two key consequences that resulted from an overreliance on youth incarceration: the high costs and a lack of rehabilitative success associated with confinement. Annually, states expend $5.7 billion to confine juvenile offenders, many of which are non-violent and low-level offenders. Juveniles who are incarcerated have higher recidivism rates when compared to juveniles who are treated in their own communities (Petteruti, Walsh and Velazquez, 2009). The root of the problem lies within the financial arrangement between states and local governments. Community-based programs rarely receive the necessary state funding and political support to achieve maximum success and because state governments are typically responsible for the costs of confinement, counties that send juvenile offenders to secure state facilities evade financial accountability.

Clearly, juvenile justice systems need some access to confinement facilities, but first there has to be a decision on how states should balance confinement and community-based interventions for juvenile delinquents. Some states have explored structural reform modifications that enable juvenile justice systems to reduce their reliance on expensive confinement that is no more effective than probation at reducing recidivism (Mulvey, Steinberg, Piquero, Besana, Fagan, Schubert and Cauffman, 2010). There are a number of states pursuing reform strategies for reducing youth confinement. This chapter focuses on two such strategies: reinvestment and realignment, and discusses states and jurisdictions that have implemented these reforms. The remainder of this chapter explores these strategies and discusses states that have implemented them to reform juvenile justice policy and practice. Reinvestment and realignment initiatives have enabled local jurisdictions to keep more youth close to home and have shifted funding from costly confinement facilities toward community-based programs that demonstrate better outcomes for youth (Tyler, Ziedenberg and Lotke 2006). This chapter builds on juvenile justice reform literature by providing an overview of the development of reinvestment and realignment and analyzing states that have implemented these reforms.

REINVESTMENT

Reinvestment involves financial incentives that encourage state and local governments to reduce expenditures on confinement and reallocate resources toward community-based supervision and treatment programs. Reinvestment strategies alter the financial obligations between states and counties by holding counties accountable for the costs of youth confinement and requiring state governments to fund community-based programs for youth (Butts and Evans, 2011). The financial reorganization includes monetary rewards for counties that keep youth confinement numbers down and penalties for jurisdictions that exceed a predetermined limit of state-confined youth. A popular technique was for state governments to charge counties for youth confinement on a sliding scale. The lower the severity of a juvenile's offense, the more money the county was responsible for paying to confine a juvenile. Several states launched reinvestment initiatives as early as the 1960s (Hartney, Krisberg, Vuong and Marchionna, 2010). Reinvestment has helped several jurisdictions to reduce youth confinement and budgetary expenditures. The following sections provide an overview of states that have implemented reinvestment initiatives.

California

California was the first state to implement a reinvestment strategy. In the early 1960s, probation[1] was a standard sentence for non-violent and first time offenders. As probation caseloads grew and staff size remained constant, probation officers were required to manage caseloads as high as three times the recommended number. Probation services became ineffective and meaningful supervision was unrealistic because much of a probation officer's daily work was spent on quick check-ins and routine paperwork. Probation officers responded to this burden by referring more offenders to state correctional facilities. From 1952 to 1968, the number of beds in juvenile facilities increased from 2,500 to 6,421 (Breed, 1974). As the population of persons in state confinement increased, taxpayer money spent on state corrections grew to some of the highest in the nation.

To reestablish the importance of community supervision and reduce confinement, the California legislature passed the Probation Subsidy Act of 1965. Although the act targeted juveniles and adults, California laid the groundwork for later reform in the juvenile system

---

[1] A sentence in which an offender forgoes confinement but remains under court supervision

specifically. The legislation offered financial incentives to counties willing to use probation rather than state corrections. State officials believed that probation was the most effective and cost-efficient method for handling at least one-fourth of the offenders that would have been sent to state correctional facilities. The Probation Subsidy Act granted county probation departments between $2,000 and $4,000 for each offender not committed to a state facility (Smith, 1972).

The Probation Subsidy Act improved many aspects of the California justice system. From 1965 to 1969, the percent of convicted offenders sent to state correctional facilities decreased from 23 percent to 10 percent (Smith, 1972). Between 1970 and 1971, 44 participating counties reduced their combined institutional commitments by 4,495 and as a result received more than $18 million in state subsidies (Breed, 1974). County probation departments hired more officers, supervisors, and support staff. The Subsidy Act ultimately enabled counties to divert of more than 45,000 offenders from state custody (Smith, 1972). Although it was successful on many levels, probation became increasingly expensive as more offenders entered the system, mostly for drug-related crimes. Because the state never raised the $4,000 subsidy and proposed treatment programs never materialized at the county level, California discontinued the Probation Subsidy Act in 1978 and replaced it with a program that offered grants for counties seeking to improve community-based youth programming (Nieto, 1996).

County participation in the grant program gradually waned because it was cheaper for counties to send juvenile offenders to state facilities than to supervise and treat them locally. Counties were accountable for only $25 a month per juvenile for state confinement and the state paid the remainder (Hartney et al., 2010). The minimal costs for confinement created an unintended incentive to incarcerate juvenile offenders. The population of juveniles in state confinement increased considerably through the 1980s and 1990s until it peaked at 10,122 in 1996 (Dawood, 2009). In addition to the spike in youth confinement, the costs of incarceration grew as high as $225,000 a year per juvenile (Ferriss, 2010). In 2008, California spent $200 million more to incarcerate juvenile offenders than it did in 1996 when the institutional youth population was five times as large (Little Hoover Commission, 2008). There were other issues that were more salient to the public. Institutional overcrowding became a problem in some facilities, and reports of severe institutional abuse and youth inmate suicide appeared in the media (Hartney et al., 2010). In response to escalating criticisms, California passed Senate Bill 681 in 1996.

Senate Bill 681 created a "sliding scale" fee for counties that placed juveniles in state facilities. The legislation required counties to pay little to nothing to incarcerate a violent juvenile offender, but the cost of confinement increased as the severity of offense decreased. The sliding scale fee led to a considerable reduction in the youth custodial population. By 2010, there were only 1,118 juveniles in state facilities, which is an 89 percent decrease from the 1996 youth custodial population (Juvenile Research Branch, 2010).

Pennsylvania

Pennsylvania was the next state to implement a reinvestment strategy in its juvenile justice system. In the 1960s, there were no incentives for counties to develop community-based supervision or treatment programs for juvenile offenders. The state paid the costs of youth incarceration, so counties could send juvenile offenders to state facilities at no cost

(Tyler et al., 2006). County courts sent many juveniles to the State Correctional Institution at Camp Hill, which was an adult facility not far from Harrisburg. In 1975, a court ruling outlawed the incarceration of juveniles at Camp Hill and became the spark for juvenile justice reform (Youth Advocate Programs, 2011).

The Pennsylvania legislature passed Act 148 in 1976 to reduce youth incarceration and stimulate the development of community-based programs for juveniles. Prior to the legislation, most Pennsylvania counties lacked the resources to create local alternatives to confinement for juvenile offenders. Act 148 offered counties financial incentives to create community-based programs for at-risk youth and compelled courts to put them to use by requiring courts to use the least restrictive disposition for juvenile offenders. The state government reimbursed counties for 80 percent of the cost of community-based youth programming but only covered 40 percent of the costs of youth confinement (Petteruti et al., 2009).

Act 148 demonstrated successes within a short time after its enactment. From 1981 to 1984, state subsidies to counties for community-based alternatives increased from $65 million to $114 million. Counties sent 24 percent fewer juveniles to state facilities compared to previous years. The number of juveniles enrolled in community-based programs increased 20 percent and there was a 52 percent increase in juveniles entering day treatment (Arnya, Lotke, Ryan, Schindler, Shoenberg and Soler, 2005). Counties used state reimbursements to develop programming for at-risk youth, improve youth counseling services, and expand community-monitoring services.

The financial structure of Act 148, however, concerned state and local governments. The state worried that county expenditures would far exceed budget estimations while counties did not want to be locked into a fixed budget and risk depleting state funds before the end of the fiscal year. An amendment in the early 1990s created a system of needs based planning and budgeting to allow for a more flexible use of state funds. The amendment called for counties to submit a proposed budget for intended services, and it provided the state with more detailed information and budgetary oversight.

The achievements of Act 148 have been long lasting. In 2003, only five percent of adjudicated youth removed from their homes were confined in a state facility (Arnya et al., 2005). The reductions in youth confinement have generated considerable savings that Pennsylvania has funneled into the counties. Counties have used most of the money to fund private service providers that develop and manage many of the community-based youth services. Act 148 built on the reinvestment mechanisms of the California Probation Subsidy Act and provided a framework for subsequent states seeking to reduce juvenile justice costs and improve youth rehabilitation programs.

Wisconsin

Wisconsin introduced the Youth Aids program in 1981. Previously, the state was financially responsible for youth confinement and counties had to pay for local alternatives to confinement. Most counties lacked the available funding to create and sustain community-based programs so the primary destination for a majority of juvenile offenders was state confinement facilities. Youth Aids halted this trend by reversing the financial mechanisms that supported youth confinement.

The central objective of Youth Aids was to decentralize the financial structure of the Wisconsin juvenile justice system and enable counties to fund and manage smaller, local-based juvenile justice systems. To achieve this objective, counties had to limit the number of juvenile offenders they sent to state facilities and instead, supervise and treat them locally. Because confinement may be necessary for some juveniles, Youth Aids sought to reduce the duration of time they spent in state facilities (Stuiber, Flood, Chrisman, Monroe, Morris and Sommerfeld, 1999).

Youth Aids legislation specified a formula for state disbursements to counties. The state government allocated funds to each county based on three statistics: the juvenile population per county, the number of juvenile arrests per county, and the number of juveniles from each county sent to a state facility (Tyler et al., 2006).

Counties use the funds, which are a combination of federal and state money, to pay for the costs of juvenile justice placements. Youth Aids encourages counties to supervise and treat as many youth as possible in their communities because community-based services are far more cost-efficient than youth confinement. Counties are required to pay for the cost of youth confinement before they pay for community-based services, so counties that over-confine youth risk exhausting their Youth Aids funds quickly. There are some exceptions to the county's financial obligations. If a court judge determines that a juvenile is a serious offender or if a judge waives a juvenile to adult court and he or she subsequently serves time in a juvenile facility, the state covers the cost of placement (Carmichael, 2007).

Wisconsin's youth institutional population has steadily declined since Youth Aid's enactment. Between 1997 and 2006, the number of juveniles in state facilities decreased by 33 percent (Sickmund, Sladky and Kang, 2008). In Milwaukee County, the largest county in the state, there was a 75 percent decline in the population of juveniles in confinement facilities from 1995 to 2005 (Tyler et al., 2006).

Youth Aids is not solely responsible for the reduction in youth confinement, however, because the recent crime drop also has lessened the state's use of confinement. From 1997 to 2006, youth drug offenses decreased 52 percent, youth property crime decreased 46 percent, and the number of juvenile arrests dropped 25 percent even though the juvenile population grew slightly during that time (Carmichael, 2007). It remains to be seen whether youth confinement rates will remain low if juvenile crime rebounds.

The Youth Aids program has experienced many funding issues during its 30-year existence. The cost to counties for in-home youth services to continue to rise while state allocations have remained constant and even decreased in some years. In 1992, Youth Aids funds covered nearly 65 percent of the costs of local alternative programming for youth. By 1997, Youth Aids covered only 45 percent of the $181 million cost to counties for community-based services. Because of the funding deficit, only 18 counties had enough resources to pay for local youth services, whereas 42 counties had the available funds to cover these costs in 1992 (Stuiber et al., 1999).

Despite freezes in state allocations to counties and the rising cost of services, Youth Aids continues to provide resources for counties to treat eligible juvenile offenders close to home.

Ohio

Several factors affected increases in the number of confined youth in Ohio through the 1980s. Juvenile court judges had minimal dispositional outcomes available for adjudicated youth so their options were limited to incarceration or releasing a juvenile to the custody of his or her parents. Determinate youth sentencing practices established a minimum duration of confinement and limited judicial authority for setting the length of time that juveniles could spend in custody (Moon, Applegate and Latessa, 1997). The result was a considerable growth in the youth institutional population in Ohio to the point that some juvenile facilities experienced overcrowding. In 1991, four of the 20 most overcrowded juvenile facilities in the nation were in Ohio (Austin, Krisberg, DeComo, Rudenstine, and Del Rosario, 1995). By 1992, the number of youth in state confinement was nearly twice the size of its designed capacity (National Criminal Justice Association).

To expand judicial dispositions for juvenile offenders, reverse the incentives for incarcerating juveniles, and reduce the Department of Youth Services (DYS) institutional population, Ohio initiated Reasoned and Equitable Community and Local Alternatives to the Incarceration of Minors (RECLAIM Ohio) in 1994. RECLAIM established state funding allocations for counties to pay for DYS placements and community-based youth services. The specific amount of funds depends on the average number of youth felony adjudications over a four-year span. As an incentive, counties can earn extra funds in subsequent years for reducing their number of DYS placements. A built-in disincentive requires counties to pay 75 percent of the costs of DYS confinement (Tyler et al., 2006). There are exceptions to this requirement. Counties are not responsible for any confinement costs in the event that a juvenile commits murder or rape (Moon et al., 1997). The costs of youth confinement are considerable. Ohio spends $123,370 annually to confine one youth in a DYS facility. It costs only $8,539 to place a juvenile in a community-based RECLAIM program. For every dollar that counties spend on RECLAIM programs, the state saves between $11 and $45 on the cost of confinement (Lowenkamp and Latessa, 2005a).

RECLAIM started as a pilot program in nine Ohio counties. Pilot counties used state funds to develop community-based programs that enabled them to reduce DYS commitments by 42 percent in one year. During that year, non-pilot counties sent 23 percent more youth to DYS facilities than in the previous year (Moon et al., 1997). There was little change in the number of felony diversions pre- and post-pilot RECLAIM, but pilot counties sent significantly fewer low-level youth offenders to DYS facilities in the first year of RECLAIM compared to non-pilot counties (Lowenkamp and Latessa, 2005b). Based on its initial successes, Ohio launched RECLAIM statewide in 1995.

RECLAIM grew quickly, serving 6,945 juveniles through community-based diversion programs in 1995 (Latessa, Turner, Moon and Applegate, 1998). However, early funding deficits threatened the effectiveness of RECLAIM. In 1995, the Ohio legislature proposed allocating $71 million for counties to use in support of RECLAIM, but the counties received only $17.6 million (Latessa et al., 1998). State funding gradually increased and by August of 2011, Ohio made $252 million in RECLAIM funds available to the counties (Ohio Department of Youth Services, 2011).

RECLAIM Ohio has reduced the DYS population and increased the availability of local alternatives to confinement. The DYS population decreased each year between 2000 and 2009. There were 2,453 youth in state custody in 2001 and by 2009 there were 1,228 youth in custody. In 2009, Ohio counties admitted 130,000 juveniles to more than 650 RECLAIM programs across the state (Ohio Department of Youth Services). There were 736 juveniles in DYS facilities as of March 2011. Because of the declining DYS population, Ohio shut down three youth facilities and plans to shut down at least one more (Johnson, 2011). The reductions in state confinement suggest that RECLAIM has achieved success. However, it remains to be seen how county judges will respond if or when youth crime increases.

Illinois

Illinois modeled its reinvestment program after RECLAIM Ohio. The initial basis for reform was the high cost for youth confinement and the number of juveniles in Illinois Department of Juvenile Justice (IDJJ) facilities, which lingered around 1,800 from 2000 to 2004. At an annual cost of more than $70,000 per youth, Illinois spent over $100 million per year on youth confinement (Illinois Department of Human Services, 2008a). The root of the problem was the financial arrangement that held the state, not the counties, accountable for the costs of IDJJ placement.

IDJJ placement became a common destination for juvenile offenders, regardless of their offense. Through the 1990s, 40 percent of youth sent to IDJJ facilities had violated parole and another 30 percent was sent for mental health evaluations (Illinois Department of Human Services, 2010). In 2004, one-third of the youth placed in IDJJ facilities were sent for a court-ordered mental health evaluation and nearly one-half were sent for a property offense (Tyler et al., 2006). This indicates that less than 20 percent of IDJJ commitments committed a serious or violent offense in 2004. Equally as concerning as the overuse of confinement for low-risk youth, IDJJ placement demonstrated minimal rehabilitative effects. The three-year recidivism rate for youth released from IDJJ facilities remained around 50 percent from the early 1990s through 2005 (Illinois Department of Human Services, 2008b; Illinois Department of Human Services, 2010). The extent of youth confinement combined with the costs and negative impacts prompted policymakers to pursue reforms.

The Illinois General Assembly enacted Redeploy Illinois in 2004. To participate in the Redeploy program, counties must commit to reducing their IDJJ commitments by 25 percent of the average of the prior three years by the end of the first year of participation (Tyler et al., 2006). The state then reimburses participating counties that handle juvenile offenders through community-based alternatives. If a county exceeds its target number of IDJJ commitments, it is required to pay $4,000 per excess commitment (Illinois Department of Human Services, 2008).

Similar to RECLAIM Ohio, Redeploy Illinois started as a pilot program. The four pilot counties initially shared $2 million of state money to develop a variety of community-based programs including aggression replacement training, functional family therapy, cognitive education and treatment, life skills training, substance abuse and mental health treatment, home detention, psychological assessments, and community service programs (Illinois Department of Human Services, 2007). Counties are free to fund their own unique programming as long as it adheres to the mission of reducing youth confinement and strengthening rehabilitation.

Redeploy programs are less costly than IDJJ confinement. The annual cost of one IDJJ placement is more than $70,000 while the cost of placing a juvenile in a Redeploy program for one year is between $3,000 and $10,000 (Illinois Department of Human Services, 2010). For every $1 million spent on community-based Redeploy programs, the state avoids spending more than $3.5 million on IDJJ confinement. Within three years, Redeploy helped to divert 382 juveniles from IDJJ placement and generated nearly $19 million in cost savings to the state (Illinois Department of Human Services, 2008b).

Participation in Redeploy is a difficult task for some counties. Cook County, the most populated county in Illinois, was forced to suspend its participation in Redeploy because it was unable to reduce its IDJJ commitments by 25 percent within the first year (Illinois Department of Human Services, 2008b). Kankakee County applied to participate in Redeploy but did not receive adequate state funding and was forced to terminate its community-based youth programs (Kankakee County Board, 2010).

Redeploy operated in 27 of 102 Illinois counties and diverted nearly 800 juveniles from IDJJ placement as of 2011 (Illinois Government News Network, 2011). In 2009, the governor signed legislation to extend Redeploy Illinois to every county in the state (Redeploy Illinois, 2010). Redeploy has been so successful that the state is considering applying the financial incentives to the adult system.

Additional State Reinvestment Programs

Several other states have adopted similar reinvestment strategies to reduce youth confinement, conserve financial resources, and develop local alternative programs that are more conducive to rehabilitation. North Carolina reformed its juvenile justice system with the passage of the Juvenile Justice Reform Act (JJRA) in 1998. The JJRA sets aside state funds for counties that appoint a Juvenile Crime Prevention Council (JCPC) to manage juvenile justice locally. JCPCs consist of 25 community members and are responsible for submitting annual proposals, securing state funding, and evaluating youth rehabilitation programs (Mason, 1999). Counties must match between 10 percent and 30 percent of the state contributions to JCPCs (Durham County Juvenile Crime Prevention Council, 2011). Five years after the JJRA, the number of youth in state custody in North Carolina declined 65 percent (North Carolina Department of Juvenile Justice and Delinquency Prevention, 2011). State budget cuts and the rising costs of confinement threaten future juvenile justice developments across the state.

Deschutes County, Oregon introduced the Community Youth Investment Project (CYIP) in 2001. The CYIP made Deschutes County financially autonomous and obligated the county government to pay for youth placed out their homes. Incentives enabled the county to receive a full state refund for each youth diversion. The refund was equal to the annual cost of one youth placement. Deschutes allocated approximately 70 percent of the state reimbursements toward rehabilitation programs and reinvests the remaining funds in prevention programs, parenting training, home visits, tutoring, and after school activities (Maloney and Holcomb, 2001).

Florida started the Redirection Program in 2004 to divert low-level youth offenders from secure facilities and lessen its juvenile justice expenses. Redirection consists of two primary diversion programs: Multi-Systemic Therapy and Functional Family Therapy. The programs spread quickly across the state. By 2008, Redirection operated in 41 of 67 Florida counties. By the end of 2009, Redirection programs served 3,956 juveniles, and 2,821 (71 percent) successfully completed the program. As of 2010, Redirection generated more than $51 million in savings (Office of Program Policy Analysis and Government Accountability, 2010). Youth who completed the program were less likely to be re-arrested, especially for a violent offense.

Lastly, Texas initiated a juvenile justice reinvestment strategy after its youth confinement population grew considerably in the late 1980s. From 1988 to 1992, Texas experienced a 285 percent increase in youth confined for a violent offense (Texas Youth Commission, 2010). However, by 2000 half of the 5,646 youth confined in Texas were non-violent offenders. At a cost of more than $130,000 per commitment and few rehabilitation programs in facilities, the Texas budget suffered and the youth re-arrest rate grew to more than 50 percent (Texas Youth Commission, 2011). Instead of spending billions on new prisons and juvenile facilities, Texas reinvested less than $250 million on treatment programs and passed the Commitment Reduction Program (CRP) to create incentives for counties to reduce youth confinement. The CRP requires counties to pay for youth confinement that exceeds an established threshold. A year after the CRP began youth confined decreased 40 percent (Levin, 2010).

REALIGNMENT

Realignment generally includes aspects of reinvestment, but realignment is much different in that it involves structural shifts rather than just financial alterations. Realignment is a reconfiguration of justice system management in which the state transfers responsibility and oversight to local governments and reduces or removes its own control (Butts and Evans, 2011). The primary line of reasoning underlying realignment strategies is that localities are in the optimal position to provide extensive and cost-effective supervision and treatment services to youth offenders.

A few jurisdictions in the U.S. have explored realignment approaches, but California is the only state that has enacted juvenile justice realignment statewide (Little Hoover Commission, 2008). Texas has realigned a portion of its juvenile justice population by giving counties the authority to handle juvenile misdemeanants. Wayne County, Michigan has fully realigned its juvenile justice system and privatized its youth services. Realignment may be the most effective mechanism of juvenile justice reform because it withstands fluctuations in youth crime. When state facilities are no longer available for youth confinement, counties are forced to handle youth using the most cost-efficient means. Locally managed juvenile justice appears to minimize the impact of increases in youth crime on incarceration rates.

Wayne County

Wayne County, home of Detroit and more juveniles than every other Michigan county, had few options for youth offenders up until the turn of the century. Juvenile judges could order probation or confinement. There were no intermediary options so confinement became a common albeit expensive option in for Wayne County youth. From the early 1980s through the 1990s, Wayne County spent $150 million annually to confine youth offenders (Latona, Smith and Chaney, 2006). County juvenile facilities were in bad shape; some were overcrowded and showed signs of deterioration. Staff was overworked and youth supervision suffered as a result. Approximately two-thirds of juveniles released from confinement returned to the system within six months of their release. The county needed major change.

The initial impetus for reform was the threat of federal takeover of Wayne County's juvenile intake and detention centers due to overcrowding. To avoid losing control of its facilities, Wayne County officials agreed to a compromise in which many juveniles in detainment would be sent home and monitored electronically. The courts reduced delays between arrest and pre-trial hearings to no more than five days. These changes reduced the juvenile detention population by 35 percent and negated the threat of federal takeover (Latona et al., 2006).

In the mid 1990s, the former director of the Michigan Department of Human Services offered counties grant money if they agreed to assume control for court-ordered juvenile placements. Wayne County was the only county to accept this responsibility. In 2000, Wayne County implemented realignment and took control of its juvenile justice system. During the transition, county officials co-opted private service providers to manage a network of community-based youth programs and services. The arrangement became known as the Juvenile Assessment Center/Care Management Organization (JAC/CMO) system. The JAC, an independent, non-profit agency, is the entry point for youth diversions. JAC personnel assess youth and refer them to one of five CMOs that are dispersed by zip code across Wayne County. Each CMO oversees 300 to 500 youth and is charged with implementing individualized service plans for every youth (Kresnak, 2002). CMOs utilize community-based services if youth are responsive to them, but in the instance that a youth requires a more restrictive intervention, CMOs are responsible for the costs of confinement.

Wayne County has an agreement with the state to split the costs of juvenile justice services. As long as the county submits an annual budget and plan of services, it can bill the state for up to a 50 percent reimbursement for services such as assessments, academic support, substance abuse treatment, mental health counseling, and family services (Wayne County Children and Family Services, 2010a). Realignment has generated considerable savings for the county. In 1999, youth confinement cost the state and Wayne County $113 million. Ten years later, Wayne County spent $73 million on youth confinement (New York State Juvenile Justice Advisory Group, 2010). The JAC/CMO has become more financially efficient and its costs have lessened each year. In 2008, the five CMOs spent $115 million on youth services. Two years later the CMOs spent $87 million (Wayne County Children and Family Services, 2010b).

Realignment reduced county and state expenditures and youth confinement. The average daily population of confined youth in Wayne County was 906 in 1996. By 2003, there were 40 Wayne County youth in confinement (Kresnak, 2002). By 2010, there were only two youth in a secure facility (Wayne County Children and Family Services, 2010a). The recidivism rate has fallen as well. More than 70 percent of the 4,000 youth in CMOs from 2009 to 2010 fulfilled their court-order conditions satisfactorily (Wayne County Children and Family Services, 2010b). A quasi-experimental evaluation study compared 1,900 CMO-served youth with a similar group of youth released from confinement prior to the realignment. The recidivism rate for CMO-served youth was less than five percent while the recidivism rate for youth released from confinement was more than 50 percent (Plante and Moran, 2006). The success of realignment and the JAC/CMO system has saved the state and county millions on expenses and nearly eliminated the need for juvenile facilities in Wayne County.

Texas

Along with its reinvestment endeavors, Texas passed Senate Bill 103 in 2007 to partly realign its juvenile justice system and prohibit counties from incarcerating juvenile misdemeanor offenders. The legislation transferred authority for youth misdemeanants from the state to the counties. The purpose was to reduce youth confinement and to compel counties to devise alternative methods for handling low-level youth offenders.

Counties were no longer able to confine youth misdemeanor offenders in state facilities so they needed alternatives. Texas allocated financial resources to counties to support the development of local programs and services for at-risk youth. For each youth diverted from state confinement, the state contributes more than $51,000 to local juvenile probation departments to subsidize the costs of supervision and treatment (Texas Juvenile Probation Commission, 2010). The State Legislature provides additional funding for county programs.

The realignment had an immediate impact on youth confinement. In 2007, there were 4,709 youth in state confinement and less than two years after the realignment there were 2,259 youth confined in Texas (Levin, 2010). Because of the reduction in confinement, state representatives proposed closing several juvenile facilities across the state and abolishing the Texas Youth Commission and the Texas Juvenile Probation Commission, which collectively oversee juvenile justice in Texas. The Texas Juvenile Justice Department (JDD) will replace the two agencies. The central mission of the JDD will be the establishment of a continuum of youth and family-focused rehabilitation services that will maximize positive youth outcomes and minimize the likelihood of youth confinement.

California

The sliding scale fee helped to reduce youth confinement in California, but problems within the state juvenile justice system persisted. Juvenile facilities were in falling apart, conditions inside facilities were poor, and there were reports of abuse of youth wards (Hartney et al., 2010). To address these issues, Governor Schwarzenegger signed Senate Bill 81 in 2007. Referred to as the "Juvenile Justice Realignment" Bill, the legislation limited confinement to sexual, violent, and serious youth offenders and realigned responsibility for the majority of youth offenders from the state to the counties (California Department of Corrections and Rehabilitation, 2010).

Senate Bill 81 set up a grant program to support county-level juvenile justice. The state distributes an average of $117,000 per juvenile delinquent to county probation departments to support community-based programs and services for youth (Brown, 2011). Precise allocations are determined by a formula: the $117,000 amount is multiplied by the number of realignment-eligible youth in California and the aggregate amount is then divided up based on each county's juvenile population and felony adjudication rate (Ramadas, 2008).

Realignment has contributed to substantial reform in the California juvenile justice system. The population of youth in state confinement declined 80 percent between 2000 and

2010, which allowed the state to close five juvenile facilities (Hartney et al, 2010). However, realignment also has generated some concerns at the county and state-level. The state enacted the realignment within a week after passing Senate Bill 81. The quick turnaround led to delays in funding and left county probation departments little time to create alternatives for influx of youth who were no longer eligible for state confinement. Senate Bill 81 did not delineate a method for state oversight so counties lacked guidelines for best practices and had minimal accountability financially (Dawood, 2009). Counties are not mandated to recount their expenditures and they are not required to disseminate reports on meeting proposed outcomes so it is difficult to ascertain the extent to which counties are succeeding in their efforts to supervise and rehabilitate youth offenders (Little Hoover Commission, 2008). Another concern is that the youth's current offense is the sole determining factor of whether or not they are eligible for community-based placement. Judges do not have to consider prior offenses so former violent or repeat youth offenders with a current low-level offense could avoid confinement (Hartney et al., 2010).

As counties adjust to realignment, the shift will save money for county and state governments and increase rehabilitative options for at-risk youth. Considering the recent budget crises that California has endured, the state needs to conserve as many resources as possible. State budget officials estimate that when the realignment transition is complete, California will save approximately $250 million per year (Brown, 2011). The governor hopes that realignment will enable the staff to eliminate the Department of Juvenile Facilities by June of 2014.

A key legal ruling will impact the future of incarceration in California and possibly the entire country. In May 2011, the Supreme Court declared prison overcrowding to be unconstitutional when state prisons were filled to twice their capacity (Biskupic, 2011). The ruling required California to reduce its prison population by 33,000 within two years. In response, the state passed the Criminal Justice Realignment Bill (A.B. 109), which mandated that counties assume responsibility for all offenders that have not committed a violent, sexual, or serious offense. It also proscribes counties from sending parole violators to state prison (Luhrs, 2011). Some counties are preparing for these changes by increasing their bed space in local jails.

CONCLUSION

Confinement is not simply a reaction to crime. It is the collective decision of policymakers, juvenile justice practitioners, and budget specialists. The rate of youth confinement may be correlated to the youth crime rate at times, but at other times the two may diverge completely. Of all the dispositional options available to juvenile courts for youth offenders, confinement is the most costly and has the most enduring impact on youth. Other than waivers to adult to court, youth confinement is the most prominent issue facing juvenile justice systems.

Community-based supervision and treatment programs have become viable alternatives to confinement. The advantage to community-based youth programs is that they are more cost-effective, more rehabilitative, and less invasive than confinement. However, funding for community-based programs is inevitably tied to expenditures on youth confinement (Miller,

1991). The more budgetary resources that state governments allocate toward confinement, the less funds that are available for alternative programs.

Several jurisdictions across the country have explored strategies to limit the use of state confinement. Even when confinement is needed, youth do not have to be sent to state facilities that are hundreds of miles from their homes. They can be supervised in their communities, and if confinement is warranted, small, locally based facilities managed by city or county officials could fill the void left by the phasing out of state-level confinement.

When cities and counties consider juvenile justice reforms, it is necessary to consider the size of the jurisdiction and the availability of resources. Larger communities may have the resources to manage a local juvenile justice system and out-of-home placement options. However, smaller communities may lack the resources to offer an array of programs, services, and out-of-home placement options for youth. If this is the case, small jurisdictions may require state support to run an effective juvenile justice system. Realignment may be the most effective strategy for large cities that have the budgetary resources to implement a range of interventions for at-risk youth. For smaller counties, reinvestment initiatives may work best because they give counties incentives to reduce confinement and also ensure that county governments have access to state resources.

The prison population in the United States currently is the largest in the world. Institutional overcrowding, poor conditions inside some facilities, and occasional reports of abusive staff practices have drawn attention to problems associated with confinement. But as long as jails, prisons, and secure facilities exist, criminal and juvenile justice systems will continue to use incarceration as a punishment for certain offenders. The available space inside secure facilities determines the size of institutional populations to some extent. Just as building more prisons will increase the prison population, closing secure facilities will ultimately reduce the institutional population.

Jurisdictions that are considering the reforms discussed in this chapter should learn from the efforts of other states and communities that have implemented these reforms. Each community needs to find the appropriate balance between community-based youth programs and confinement given its availability of resources and prevalence of juvenile delinquency. Realignment strategies are longer lasting than reinvestment strategies because their impact is more durable. Reinvestment strategies can be scaled back as crime rates increase but realignment is a structural shift that is difficult to reverse. Whatever strategy best fits, state policymakers should pursue reforms transparently and collaboratively with city and county officials and ensure continual oversight and evaluation of the results.

This chapter has important implications for the fields of social work and other youth-focused organizations. When jurisdictions effectively implement reinvestment and realignment, the result is less youth confinement. Without confinement, alternative forms of supervision and treatment become critical. It is important for social workers and youth organizations to develop programs that address the wide range of needs of at-risk and justice-involved youth. Reinvestment and realignment strategies compel state and local governments to collaborative in the establishment of a variety of programs and services that improve youth outcomes.

The application of reinvestment and realignment strategies to juvenile justice systems appears to be limited to the United States. However, international jurisdictions have utilized other mechanisms to reduce youth confinement. The British government has passed several pieces of legislation to reduce the duration of youth confinement and shift from policies that favor confinement toward community supervision sentences (Allen, 2002). Germany, France, and Spain also have passed legislation to increase the usage of alternative and community sanctions for youth (Dunkel, 2006; Castaignede and Pignoux, 2010; Alberola and Molina, 2003). Legislation does not alter the funding streams or the structural arrangements of juvenile justice systems as reinvestment and realignment do, but it is does persuade judges to consider alternative sentences in lieu of confinement.

Future research should explore state realignment and reinvestment strategies to learn the best methods for implementing the reforms. Many jurisdictions have been successful in their efforts but some locales have experienced setbacks that have hindered their attempts at reform. Justice reforms, especially those implicating confinement, are comprehensive and often involve a network of decision makers and stakeholders. Research can suggest how these individuals and processes work together to achieve effective and long lasting reform.

Additional research should consider the impact of community-based supervision and treatment programs on offenders diverted from confinement. Programs are only effective to the extent that they meet the particular needs of the individuals they serve. Research must evaluate the various aspects of alternatives to incarceration programs including youth assessment, matching juveniles with the appropriate programs, the nature of each program, and the consistency between program goals and outcomes. This line of research could provide support for community-based programs and increase their political viability. Mass incarceration is not sustainable in the long-term because it depletes state and county resources and does little to improve the lives of offenders. Community-based programs offer effective alternatives, and realignment and reinvestment are two mechanisms for enhancing their usage.

REFERENCES

Alberola, C. R. and Molina, E. F. (2003). Juvenile justice in Spain: Past and present. *Journal of Contemporary Criminal Justice, 19*(4), 384-412.

Allen, Rob (2002). *Juvenile justice reform in England and Wales*. Paper presented at the United Nations Asia and Far East Institute For the Prevention of Crime and the Treatment of Offenders, 118th International Training Course, Tokyo, JP. Retrieved from www.unafei.or.jp/english/pdf/PDF_rms/no59/ch09a.pdf.

Aryna, N., Lotke, E., Ryan, L., Schindler, M., Shoenberg, D. and Soler, M. (2005). *Keystones for reform: Promising juvenile justice policies and practices in Pennsylvania*. San Francisco, CA: Youth Law Center. Retrieved from *www.jlc.org/mfc/ keystonesforreform.pdf.*

Austin, J., Krisberg, B., DeComo, R., Rudenstine, S. and Del Rosario, D. (2005). *Juveniles taken into custody: Fiscal year 1993*. Washington, DC: Office of Juvenile Justice and Delinquency Prevention. Retrieved from http://www.ncjrs.gov/pdffiles/154022.pdf

Biskupic, Joan (2011). Supreme Court stands firm on prison crowding. *USA Today*, May 24, 2011. Retrieved from http://www.usatoday.com/news/ washington/judicial/2011-05-24-Supreme-court-prisons_n.htm.

Breed, A. F. (1974). California Youth Authority. In Bremner, Robert H. (Ed.) *Children and youth in America: A documentary history* (pp. 1062-1068). Washington, DC: The American Public Health Association.

Brown, E. G. (2011). *2011-12 Governor's budget summary*. Sacramento, CA: California Department of Finance. Retrieved from http://tinyurl.com/88ulmhu.

Butts, J. A. and Evans, D. N. (2011). *Resolution, reinvestment and realignment: Three strategies for changing juvenile justice*. New York, NY: Research and Evaluation Center, John Jay College of Criminal Justice.

California Department of Corrections and Rehabilitation (2010). *2010 juvenile justice outcome evaluation report: Youth released from the Division of Juvenile Justice in fiscal year 2004-05*. Sacramento, CA: Author. Retrieved from http://tinyurl.com/3dkegut.

Carmichael, C. D. (2007). Juvenile justice in Wisconsin. In Bogenschneider, Karen and Heidi Normandin (Eds.) *Cost-effective approaches in juvenile and adult corrections: What works? What doesn't?* Madison, WI: Wisconsin Family Impact Seminars.

Castaignede, Jocelyn and Nathalie Pignoux (2010). France. In Dunkel, Frider, Joanna Grzywa, Philip Horsfield and Ineke Pruin (Eds). *Juvenile justice systems in Europe: Current situation and reform developments vol.1* (pp. 483-546). Monchengladbach, DE: Forum Verlag Godesberg GmbH.

Dawood, N. (2009). *Juvenile justice at a crossroads: The future of senate bill 81 in California*. Berkeley, CA: Prison Law Office. Retrieved from http://tinyurl.com/8494kz9.

Dunkel, Frieder (2006). Juvenile justice in Germany: Between welfare and justice. In Junger-Tas, Josine and Scott H. Decker (Eds.) *International Handbook of Juvenile Justice* (pp. 225-262). New York, NY: Springer.

Durhman County Juvenile Crime Prevention Council (2011). *Request for proposals: DJJDP continuation funding 2011-2012*. Durham, NC: Author. Retrieved from http://tinyurl.com/8a4pl6u.

Ferriss, S. (2010). Steinberg calls for social services shift to California counties. *Sacramento Bee*, May 30, 2010. Retrieved from http://bitly.com/ferriss2010.

Hartney, C., Krisberg, B., Vuong, L., and Marchionna, S. (2010). *A new era in California juvenile justice: Downsizing the state youth corrections system*. Berkeley, CA: Berkeley Center for Criminal Justice. Retrieved from http://tinyurl.com/7q27zyb

Illinois Department of Human Services (2007). *Redeploy Illinois annual report 2007: Implementation and impact*. Springfield, IL: Author. Retrieved from http://www.dhs.state.il.us/page.aspx?item=33334.

Illinois Department of Human Services (2008a). *Request for proposals for pilot sites to implement Redeploy Illinois*. Springfield, IL: Author. Retrieved from http://tinyurl.com/7bh73ed.

Illinois Department of Human Services (2008b). *Redeploy Illinois annual report 2008: Implementation and impact*. Springfield, IL: Author. Retrieved from www.dhs.state.il.us/page.aspx?item=41157.

Illinois Department of Human Services (2010). *Redeploy Illinois annual report to the governor and general assembly*. Springfield, IL: Author. Retrieved from http://tinyurl.com/82n6dc8.

Illinois Government News Network (2011). *Illinois Department of Human Services Redeploy Illinois initiative saves state millions: Statistics reveal significant reductions in juvenile incarceration rates*. IL: Author. Retrieved from http://tinyurl.com/73jv9pa.

Johnson, A. (2011). State to close 4th juvenile prison, end local program. *The Columbus Dispatch*, Mar. 22, 2011. Retrieved from http://tinyurl.com/7glwlkj.

Juvenile Research Branch (2010). *Division of juvenile justice population overview as of December 31, 2010*. Sacramento, CA: California Department of Corrections and Rehabilitation. Retrieved from http://tinyurl.com/7zqgk98.

Kankakee County Board (2010). *Redeploy Illinois program cut due to lack of funding*. Kankakee, IL: Author. Retrieved from http://tinyurl.com/72toc5p.

Kresnak, J. (2002). Juvenile treatment improves: Wayne County helps more, for less per teen. *Detroit Free Press*, Aug. 13, 2002. Retrieved from http://tinyurl.com/7c6t4gu.

Latessa, E. J., Turner, M. G., Moon, M. M. and Applegate, B. K. (1998). *A statewide evaluation of the RECLAIM Ohio initiative*. Washington, DC: Bureau of Justice Assistance. Retrieved from *www.uc.edu/ccjr/Reports/ProjectReports/Reclaim.PDF*.

Latona, C. J., Smith, C. J. and Chaney, D. L. (2006). *Advocating success: A groundbreaking approach to juvenile justice*. Detroit, MI: The Juvenile Assessment Center.

Levin, M. (2010). *Juvenile justice*. Austin, TX: Texas Public Policy Foundation. Retrieved from http://www.texaspolicy.com/pdf/2011-JuvenileJustice-CEJ-ml.pdf.

Little Hoover Commission (2008). *Juvenile justice reform: Realigning responsibilities*. Sacramento, CA: Author. Retrieved from http://bitly.com/LittleHoover.

Lowenkamp, C. T. and Latessa, E. J. (2005a). *Evaluation of Ohio's Reclaim funded programs, community correctional facilities, and DYS facilities: Cost-benefit analysis supplemental report*. Washington, DC: Office of Juvenile Justice and Delinquency Prevention. Retrieved from http://tinyurl.com/43kgdbq.

Lowenkamp, C. T. and Latessa, E. J. (2005b). *Evaluation of Ohio's Reclaim funded programs, community corrections facilities, and DYS facilities: Executive summary*. Washington, DC: Office of Juvenile Justice and Delinquency Prevention. Retrieved from http://tinyurl.com/7k6adgx.

Luhrs, Emily (2011). *San Francisco leading the way in criminal justice realignment*. San Francisco, CA: Center on Juvenile and Criminal Justice. Retrieved from http://tinyurl.com/7jfltev.

Maloney, Dennis and Deevy Holcomb (2001). In pursuit of community justice: Deschutes County, Oregon. *Youth and Society, 33*(2), 296-313.

Mason, J. (1999). *Reform act*. Raleigh, NC: The North Carolina Department of Juvenile Justice and Delinquency Prevention. Retrieved from http://tinyurl.com/7bv6r8e.

Miller, J. G. (1991). *Last one over the wall: The Massachusetts experiment in closing reform schools*. Columbus, OH: Ohio State University Press.

Moon, M. M., Applegate, B. and Latessa, E. J. (1997). RECLAIM Ohio: A politically viable alternative to treating youthful felony offenders. *Crime and Delinquency, 43*(4), 438-456.

Mulvey, E. P., Steinberg, L., Piquero, A. R., Besana, M., Fagan, J., Schubert, C. and Cauffman, E. (2010). Trajectories of desistance and continuity in antisocial behavior following court adjudication among serious adolescent offenders. *Development and Psychopathology, 22*(2): 453-475.

National Criminal Justice Association (n.d). *Juvenile justice reform initiatives in the states: 1994-1996*. Washington, DC: Office of Juvenile Justice and Delinquency Prevention. Retrieved from http://www.ojjdp.gov/pubs/ reform/ch3_d.html.

New York State Juvenile Justice Advisory Group (2010). *Tough on crime: Promoting public safety by doing what works.* New York, NY: Author. Retrieved from http://bitly.com/NYSJJAG

Nieto, M. (1996). *The changing role of probation in California's criminal justice system.* Sacramento, CA: California Research Bureau. Retrieved from http://1.usa.gov/Nieto1996

North Carolina Department of Juvenile Justice and Delinquency Prevention (2011). *2010 annual report.* Raleigh, NC: Author. Retrieved from http://bitly.com/NC2010

Office of Program Policy Analysis and Government Accountability (2010). *Redirections saves $51.2 million and continues to reduce recidivism.* Tallahassee, FL: Author. Retrieved from www.oppaga.state.fl.us/MonitorDocs/Reports/pdf/1038rpt.pdf.

Ohio Department of Youth Services (n.d.). *RECLAIM Ohio statistics.* Columbus, OH: Author. Retrieved from http://tinyurl.com/7lk9gfg.

Ohio Department of Youth Services (2011). *DYS fact sheet: August 2011.* Columbus, OH: Author. Retrieved from http://tinyurl.com/74xcegj.

Petteruti, A., Walsh, N. and Velasquez, T. (2009). *Costs of confinement: Why good juvenile justice policies make good fiscal sense.* Washington, DC: Justice Policy Institute. Retrieved from http://tinyurl.com/7bz934k.

Plante and Moran (2006). *Operational review of the juvenile justice and abuse and neglect programs of the Children and Family Services Department: County of Wayne.* Ann Arbor, MI: Author. Retrieved from http://tinyurl.com/3z2j2rm.

Ramadas, S. (2008). California youth and criminal law: 2007 juvenile justice reform and gang prevention initiatives. *Berkeley Journal of Criminal Law, 13*(1), 145-174.

Redeploy Illinois Program, Pub. Act No. 095-1050 §730 ILCS 110/16.1 (2010). Retrieved from http://www.ilga.gov/legislation/publicacts/fulltext.asp?Name=095-1050andGA=95.

Sickmund, M., Sladky, T. J. and Kang, W. (2008). *Census of juveniles in residential placement databook.* Washington, DC: Office of Juvenile Justice and Delinquency Prevention. Retrieved from http://www.ojjdp.gov/ojstatbb/ezacjrp/.

Sickmund, M. (2010). *Juveniles in residential placement: 1997-2008.* Washington, DC: Office of Juvenile Justice and Delinquency Prevention. Retrieved from http://tinyurl.com/842mjpo.

Smith, R. L. (1972). *A quiet revolution: Probation subsidy.* Washington, D.C.: Office of Juvenile Delinquency and Youth Development. Retrieved from http://1.usa.gov/Smith1972.

Stuiber, P., Flood, V., Chrisman, J., Monroe, K., Morris, D. and Sommerfeld, R. (1999). *Youth Aids: An evaluation.* Madison, WI: Legislative Audit Bureau. Retrieved from http://bitly.com/WI1999.

Texas Juvenile Probation Commission (2010). *Board meeting minutes.* Austin, TX: Author. Retrieved from www.tjpc.state.tx.us/events/MeetingMinutes/100917.pdf.

Texas Youth Commission (2011). *Average TYC cost per day per youth.* Austin, TX: Author. Retrieved from http://www.tyc.state.tx.us/research/cost_per_day.html.

Tyler, J. L., Ziedenberg, J. and Lotke, E. (2006). *Cost-effective youth corrections: Rationalizing the fiscal architecture of juvenile justice systems.* Washington, D.C.: Justice Policy Institute. Retrieved from http://tinyurl.com/3kdu8ns.

Wayne County Children and Family Services (2010a). *Key performance measures and outcomes: Juvenile justice services through FY 2010*. Detroit, MI: Author. Retrieved from http://bitly.com/Wayne2010b.

Wayne County Children and Family Services (2010a). *Comprehensive statistical report through fiscal year 2010: Juvenile justice services, Wayne County care management system*. Detroit, MI: Author. Retrieved from http://bitly.com/Wayne2010a.

Youth Advocate Programs, Inc. (2011). *About YAP*. Harrisburg, PA: Author. Retrieved from http://www.yapinc.org/about-yap/.

In: Youth: Practices, Perspectives and Challenges
Editor: Elizabeth Trejos-Castillo

ISBN: 978-1-62618-067-3
© 2013 Nova Science Publishers, Inc.

Chapter 17

SYSTEM MATURATION: LEVERAGING CHANGE AND REDUCING DISPROPORTIONATE CONTACT THROUGH RISK ASSESSMENT

Eyitayo Onifade[*]
Florida State University, Tallahassee, FL, US

ABSTRACT

In so much as risk assessments are valid predictors of recidivism with diverse populations, risk assessments by their very nature can reduce system contribution to disparities in adjudication rates through squeezing out the biases found at the early stages of the justice process. Theoretically, these instruments should do a better job than informal assessments at identifying youth likely to offend repeatedly, regardless of race or gender. Thus low risk members of marginal groups with disproportionate representation in juvenile justice systems can be diverted from extensive system contact. For these groups, this in turn results in "narrowing of the net", the reduction of disproportionate marginal group contact with law enforcement. This chapter will detail the challenges and successes of a juvenile justice system in the mid-west that attempted to reduce disproportionate minority contact using the risk assessment approach.

INTRODUCTION

In so much as delinquency is a by-product of the interaction between youth and the social expectations of society; disparities in contact with the United States' justice system are as much a result of the behavior of justice system as they are the behavior of the youth. This is not to say delinquency is merely a social construct, but is to say that delinquency models of adolescent development that fail to account for person-environment fit are incomplete. This incomplete picture disadvantages practitioners tasked with creating interventions based on

---

[*] Address Correspondence to: Eyitayo Onifade, Assistant Professor, Social Policy and Administration, College of Social Work, Florida State University, Email: eonifade@fsu.edu.

these theories of development. Note, most programs aimed at reducing disproportionate contact of members of marginalized groups like African Americans or adolescent girls with the justice system target youth themselves for intervention. The presumption being that delinquency as indicated by common metrics like arrests, petitions, convictions and offense level reflect disparities in misconduct perpetuated by these groups of individuals. The extent to which this is true has been the subject of much debate, conjecture and finally research; as evidenced in the plethora of DMC studies conducted over the past two decades. What those studies have discerned is that whatever contribution individual behavior makes to the disparities, system factors also play significant part in DMC; therefore, interventions that focus exclusively on youth have a self-imposed limit on their overall efficacy. Since 1988, the Juvenile Justice and Delinquency Prevention Act has required that states that receive block grant funding must both document the extent to which DMC exists and devise strategies for the reduction of DMC. Although most states have devoted considerable resources to assessing disparities in contact with juvenile justice, few states have successfully devised comprehensive strategies to reduce that contact. In the most recent review of existing strategies, systems have generally adopted four practices: 1) mapping out decision points, 2) cultural competence training of system actors, 3) community based programming, 4) removing subjectivity during decision-making through risk assessment. What follows is a brief treatise on the attempts of a courageous juvenile justice system in the Mid-west to implement innovative changes in its system behavior to reduce disproportionate minority contact using risk assessment. The county had over 277,000 residents, 61,000 of which youth under the ages of 18. African Americans represented 11% of the population but nearly 40% of the juvenile offender probation case-load. That amounted to a DMC risk index of 4[1]. In the sections that follow, I provide a brief background on the underlying conceptual framework of reducing DMC through risk assessment, as well as share the experiences of the county juvenile justice system attempting to implement the strategy over a nearly decade long period.

CONCEPTUAL FRAMEWORK OF DMC REDUCTION THROUGH RISK ASSESSMENT

Delinquent as Different

If one thinks of crime as undesirable social behavior so egregious that informal sanction, mores, and traditions are incapable of providing a sufficient response, then the juvenile justice system is a formalized system of social control by society. Society has mechanisms in place that compel children and adolescents to conform to its expectations and norms through punishment, deterrence, or rehabilitation and criminalization of those respective behaviors (Kraska, 2006). Actors in systems of justice response are faced with a tough question whose simple wording belies our collective difficulty in responding to it. Why do some youth commit crimes, while others do not?

---

[1] DMC Index is calculated by dividing the percent representation in the offender population by the percent representation of the group in the over-all population. Thus, the closer the risk index is to 1, the lower the disparity in representation for that group.

The common denominator in most of these perspectives is that those that commit crimes are different in their person or context; in turn, the juvenile justice response has always hinged on the identification of individuals with those differences and addressing the criminogenic (crime causing) factors that comprise those differences between delinquents and law-abiding youth. In identifying criminogenic differences, society has tried everything from phrenology to profiling to standardized risk assessments. Each of these presupposes delinquents have identifiable differences that can be relied upon to separate out individuals that society can target with juvenile justice resources. The differences between these methods depend on the theory from which they originate. With the wide cross-section of theories explaining delinquency, the resulting system is an amalgamation of delinquency reduction models with often counter-intuitive and conflicting means that either widen or narrow the adjudication net depending on any number of factors including but not limited to age, race, class, gender, community, and policing philosophy (Pope and Feyerham, 1992). Specifically, these disparate methods of crime control occur in three ways:

- through emphasizing law enforcement in particular communities
- the criminalization of undesirable behavior associated with certain groups
- the decision making of criminal justice practitioners at various junctions of the adjudication process (Schrantz and McElroy, 2000).

Disparate Methods of Crime Control

First, with regards to over-emphasis of law enforcement in certain communities, communities vary in the degree to which they use the juvenile justice system to respond to undesirable and maladaptive behavior (Stucky, 2005). Socioeconomic conditions like adequate education and employment opportunities, access to health care, and treatment programs can reduce problem solving to the overuse of the criminal justice system (Loftin and McDowall, 1982; Maguire, 2001; Stucky, 2005). Moreover, policing levels are also associated with the perceived threat from the marginalized group (Stucky, 2005). Thus, local government systems that are more susceptible to political pressure from the power group are more likely to increase policing resources in marginal communities (Stucky, 2005; Wilson, 1968). The difference in communities' willingness to use the criminal justice system is also dependent upon the availability of alternative systems that can appropriately address the respective undesirable and maladaptive behaviors of individuals in that community. Due to economic restraints, huge gaps in allocations of social support services remain intractable for low income communities, making the criminal justice system the first and primary responder to a broad array of social problems (Weisman, Lamberti, and Price, 2004). This is further demonstrated by the within community variance in the adoption of zero- tolerance practices by pillar institutions that primarily serve minors like schools; this ultimately affects the ratio of reported and unreported delinquency (Mauer, 1999). Consequently, some communities will have a higher rate of "crime" than their counterparts whether the prevalence of the underlying undesirable behavior is similar or not.

Second, communities can selectively enforce laws based on group membership (Taxman, Byrne, and Pattavinia, 2005). For instance, African Americans are more likely than Whites to be arrested for drug offenses, yet Whites have comparable drug usage rates according to public health sources (Freudenberg, 2002). Selective criminalization of marginal groups can occur through targeting certain neighborhoods and areas with justice resources and policies (Eck and Weisburd, 2004). Curfews are often passed that make it a violation for youth of a certain age to be out after a certain time at night, yet those ordinances are differentially enforced at a neighborhood level. In an effort to fight the proliferation of gangs in certain communities, ordinances have been passed that prohibit individuals that "look like" gang-members from loitering or aggregating in a particular area for extended periods of time. The Supreme Court struck down a city ordinance that used just such language in prohibiting said behavior, but recommended the law be re-drafted to specify such loitering cannot be done with the purpose of facilitating "criminal conduct." With greater surveillance of these communities, the contributions of criminals to the larger cultural trends of the community they belong to can also become a source of selective criminalization. The State of Florida has passed laws prohibiting "sagging", a fashion trend that originated in prisons but matriculated into the larger youth culture over time and is now commonly associated with African American males. Opponents of the code contend this law unfairly targets African American youth while allowing other popular fashion trends such as low ride cut jeans and tank tops that are popular amongst other groups.

Finally, disparities in contact can occur through the basic decision-making of justice officials. Prosecutors, for instance, often have wide latitude as to plea negotiations. These decisions can be swayed by prevailing public opinions at the time of those decisions. Despite sentencing guidelines, prosecutor discretion allows for significant departures from these guidelines based on the decisions of the prosecution which are not reviewable under the law (Kerstetter, 1990). Furthermore, police have some degree of choice in whether to warn and let go, or arrest and detain, with that decision affected by many factors including their appraisal of the offender. Moreover, a defendant's access to resources also plays a part in whether alternative means of treatment or problem-solving are used to deal with their behavior. Perhaps, most important is the discretion of juvenile justice intake officers who ultimately decide whether young offenders are funneled toward formal probation or diverted from extensive contact with the system through informal probation services, which are often community-based and of short duration.

Impact of Disparate Contact

The impact of disparate contact with the justice system is far-reaching; affecting individuals, the community and law-enforcement at large. Quite simply, disparate contact naturally concentrates iatrogenic effects of the justice process in communities that experience the disparity. Moreover, we see iatrogenic effects across a broad spectrum of social living, from educational achievement to community health to political empowerment. For example, youth of varying levels of criminality are often mixed during interventions, creating deviant peer networks for first-time and minor offenders that may not have existed prior to contact with the system.

Thus, increasing the first-time and minor offenders propensity for continued offending and delinquency. Congress passed legislation in 1994 prohibiting prison inmates from receiving Pell grants in pursuing higher education, thus limiting prisoners' access to professional skill sets that ease re-entry to society (Fellner and Mauer, 1998). Thus, for groups such as that of the African American community, where males have a 29% chance of spending time in prison at one point in their lives, disparate contact with the justice system affects this group's very ability to gain upward social mobility through education.

Communities experiencing disparate contact with the criminal legal system have fewer informal mechanisms of crime control. Joblessness, poverty, and a highly transitory population are believed to be associated with poor neighborhood cohesion.

As a result, the ability of authority figures to transmit values in tune with the larger society expectations to children is highly threatened. These communities develop a somewhat antagonistic relationship with law enforcement, where police are perceived as equally as threatening as criminals. This leads to lower rates of participation in crime prevention programs or even basic reporting of crimes to the police.

The very basis of democracy is the presumption of equality; therefore it is generally agreed that it is wrong in principle to treat equals differently unless there is some reasonable circumstance warranting such treatment (May and Sharratt, 1994). In considering most crime theory, we see that crime reduction methods based on identifying differences saddles the line between violating our principles and addressing a social problem in the most practical way, despite iatrogenic effects.

A Comprehensive Theoretical Framework

Bronfenbrenner (1979) offered that the development of a child occurs within a larger relationship context between its biology and the various dimensions of its environment. Thus, as the child matures the interaction between the child's own biological make-up, his immediate family/communal environment and societal background collectively impact the child's development. When the child experiences a negative outcome or engages in undesirable social behavior like crime, the causal source lays not only in the realm of their environment or the individual (cognitive, genetic and physical attributes), but rather the cumulative interaction between the two, which are both multi-leveled. This ecological framework has implications for society's response to undesirable social behavior. At the macrosystem level our values and principles affect the basic determination of which undesirable behaviors are so egregious they warrant formal sanctions. They affect our attitudes, which in turn affect our implementation and consistency of application of these laws in the microsystems of youths' lives. These effects ripple into the exosystem of principle actors of the juvenile's life in many ways. For instance, attitudes in a community that reflect zero-tolerance for drug use exert considerable pressure on law enforcement officers to satisfy their expectation of having a drug-free community. This in turn affects the officer's relationship with the youth directly. It may even affect the youth indirectly through the parent or school via the mesosystem in a positive or negative manner depending on the internal environment of the child and their respective affinity for drug involvement.

When one traces these causal pathways from criminogenic factors to delinquent acts to justice response, the inordinate number of possible mediators and moderators becomes obvious. Moreover, one realizes that an interactive system such as this is primed for any number of differential outcomes and differential treatments of individuals. The system is then faced with a question of how to accommodate the complexity of the system yet manage the group with the single relevant outcome of offending. In juvenile justice, when powerful individuals and groups have sole discretion in deciding what those relationships are and in turn what those relationships mean with regards to differences between groups and individuals in behavior, the system becomes highly reflective of the beliefs and prejudices most prevalent in that population. Therein lie the cost of change models that are informal, of limited causal attribution scope and unchecked for inconsistencies in implementation.

From this premise one arrives at the notion of creating additive ecological models that account for each of these factors at the various levels. When certain thresholds are met the likelihood of offending becomes so great, specific action from the justice system addressing those needs is warranted. This is the theoretical framework behind risk assessment. The problem then arises when we consider that typical risk assessment goes no further than assessing the micro and mesosystem. Rarely does this expand to include the macrosystem. Nor does the common practice of simply adding the number of risks that exist in a youth's life account for the interaction between those risks and how particular combinations of criminogenic factors either mitigate or exacerbate delinquency. So in considering risk assessment as a solution to disparate contact, we must also recognize that this solvency may be limited by the comprehensiveness of risk measures and the lack of validation with diverse populations.

In so much as risk assessments are valid predictors of recidivism with diverse populations, risk assessments by their very nature could reduce the systems contribution to disparities in adjudication rates through squeezing out the biases found at the early stages of the justice process. Theoretically these instruments should do a better job than informal assessments at identifying youth likely to offend repeatedly, regardless of race or gender, thus members of marginal groups that are low risk would conceivably be eligible for the same programming as their counterparts, which in many cases includes being refracted from the system. For these groups, this in turn results in "narrowing of the net", the reduction of disproportionate marginal group contact with law enforcement.

Practice: A Case Example of System Maturation

The challenge in system reform of this nature is identifying a mutually beneficial end that reflects best practice and does not indict the system on charges of institutional racism. Such charges inevitably become inflammatory and require extensive substantiation of both the effect and intent of a cross-section of actors in the system. These actors then have to work together subsequent of contentious debates over responsibility for racial discrimination and its effects on members of marginalized groups. In that context, it is of little surprise that communities often find change in this regard slow going and laden with frustration.

The DMC component of the JJDP Act actually outlines four phases in addressing disproportionate contact: identification, assessment, intervention, and evaluation. In a 2010 survey of state respondents fewer than half of states reported entering the intervention phase since the policy's original creation in 1974. The system of interest to this commentary had in fact been subject to considerable research on the extent of disproportionate minority contact. Like many systems, disparities were present at every level of the system, despite seemingly race neutral policies and practices. An ideological concession was made early on by those that were interested in reducing disproportionate minority contact in the community that the focus of reforms could not be on institutional racism, but the mutual disadvantages of its effects in terms of resource allocation and community safety. Although this point on its surface appears to be merely an issue of pragmatics versus principals, this type of common sense thinking around issues of race can be of limited usefulness over the long haul when the premise upon which the cooperation for mutual benefit was based becomes less germane. In this case, there was certain anticipatory anxiety on the part of DMC change advocates about what would happen once the economic picture or perceptions of community safety shifted.

That said, in the early part of the last decade, the community established several commissions involving local community leaders and members of law enforcement to brainstorm on how best to address the disproportionate minority contact issue. Although no official strategic plan was agreed upon, the benefit of bringing these various parties to the table was that it shed light on the fact that the respective options offered by those attributing DMC to the behavior of minorities and those attributing DMC to the behavior of the juvenile justice system were not mutually exclusive. The system could focus on reducing disproportionate criminal activity of minority groups in addition to reducing disparate attention given to the behavior of specific minority groups.

The community like many others was in desperate need of resources and under considerable pressure to reduce what was perceived at the time as a growing problem with juvenile delinquency. An annual report to the Board of Commissioners from the juvenile court suggested that delinquency was becoming more violent and frequent. The county successfully passed a millage, funding system efforts at juvenile delinquency prevention. The money was initially ear-marked for expanding capacity at the local detention facility, but it was ultimately decided that bringing in external consultants would be a prudent first step before addressing the juvenile delinquency problem. That external consultant conducted a community-wide study of programs used by the local family court. The key recommendations that the consultant made was that 1) the system needed to begin systematically gathering information about their youth and programs, 2) the system needed to move toward best practice, 3) The system needed to begin tracking the effectiveness of what they were doing, and 4) the system needed to collaborate with a local independent researchers and evaluators.

A collaborative team of university researchers, court administrators, and practitioners was set up, and their first action per the recommendation of the researchers was the selection of a risk assessment tool, the Youth Level of Service/Case Management Inventory (YLS/CMI). The YLS/CMI was chosen because it reflected the aforementioned profile of a valid, comprehensive risk assessment tool. The YLS/CMI has seven dynamic risk factors [e.g., family circumstances, education, peer group association, free-time usage, drug involvement, attitudes and orientation, and personality and behavior] associated with delinquency and recidivism. The instrument has 42 items and can be divided into several levels of risk [i.e., low, moderate, high, very high] with each level statistically associated with a certain probability of recidivism.

In theory, a valid comprehensive measure would ultimately identify the youth responsible for the greatest amount of delinquency, while serving as a stop-gap for lower risk youth caught in the ever expanding law enforcement net. Remember, a small percentage of offenders commit the majority of offenses and these offenders share characteristics in common that can be identified by valid risk assessments. As such, the higher the probability of recidivism, the smaller the portion of the young offender population; conversely, the lower the risk, the larger the portion of the young offender population. The DMC reduction method through risk assessment hinges on the assumption that much of the disparity in contact between minorities and the juvenile justice system exists within the low risk offender population. It thus stood to the reason of the change advocates that if minority offenders were overly attended to by law enforcement, the low risk youth would be diverted from extensive contact with the justice system as a result of their low risk scores. The benefit of a diversion strategy based on risk thus would disproportionately benefit groups receiving inordinate attention from law enforcement and the juvenile court.

The risk assessment appealed to the court system because it offered a cost-friendly delinquency reduction strategy that could reduce case-load sizes and delinquency in a way that was "scientific" and reflective of best practice, using a race-neutral method of potentially reducing disproportionate contact. At that time, risk assessment was just regaining popularity in juvenile justice systems and the evidence for their predictive validity was relatively scant. What literature did exist, mainly produce by Andrews and Dowden (2006), and Bonta (1996)primarily based in Canada suggested that the YLS/CMI was in fact a valid measure, so the system incorporated the measure in its case management protocol. Given the relatively small body of research conducted on populations similar to that of their community, the researchers were very clear that the risk assessment had to be validated on the county's juvenile probation population. The applied research project that emerged focused on collecting risk assessment information, classifying youth, predicting their outcomes, and checking those outcomes for accuracy longitudinally.

In that time, court staff received nearly 3,600 hours of training on administering the YLS/CMI and the risk-need-responsivity model. By the time, the YLS/CMI was administered to probationers inter-rater reliabilities were well over 90% consistently in training exercises. In other words, practitioners consistently rated cases the same over 90% of the time, emboldening the system to rely on the indicator in case-management decision-making. The system was comprised of two probation divisions, informal and formal probation. Informal probationers had limited contact with the system, and were diverted to community based programs. Formal probation required weekly contact, and a minimum of 90 days on probation with a formal case plan, devised by a probation officer. Prior to the incorporation of the risk assessment protocol, the decision as to who be eligible for informal probation was based primarily on the discretion of the intake officer.

The intake officer used their professional judgment regarding the elements of the offense or characteristics of the offender to decide which cases to push forward and which cases to divert for informal programming. Although some level of review and accountability was specified in the guidelines through oversight and random case reviews by the court administrators, this left considerable discretion and subjectivity at the intake point of decision-making.

Informal discussions with court personnel did not reveal any overt bias against particular racial groups, but rather a sense of protectiveness for youth entering the system. Intake officers often noted that youth from single parent homes or those with dual status in the child welfare system had greater need for formal interventions by the court. Consequently, it was essential to provide a strong basis for reducing their discretionary power and institute a protocol connecting the formal versus informal probation decision to risk of recidivism. This was no easy task. The instrument would have to correctly classify youth as recidivist or non-recidivist substantially better than the officers themselves. Finally, the instrument itself had to be valid with both genders and minority populations.

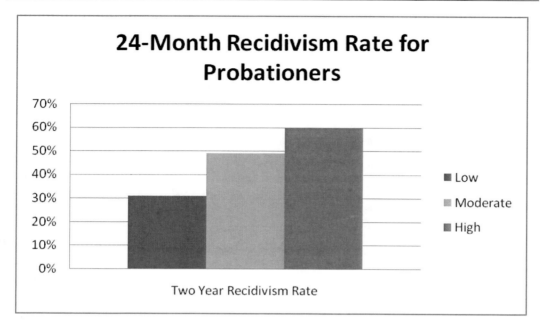

Figure 1. Validity of Risk Assessment.

Over a five-year period, over 5,000 assessments were administered in the county to all youth formally and informally probated by the juvenile court. The risk assessment itself after repeated validations over 12, 24, and 48 months was able to correctly class recidivist and non-recidivist nearly 70% of the time. The two-year recidivism rate for the probation population was 46%. Recidivists on average scored over twice as high on the risk assessment as non-recidivists. Thirty percent of low risk offenders received a new delinquency petition within a 24-month period. Forty-eight percent of moderate risk offenders received a new delinquency petition within that period, and over sixty percent of high risk probationers re-offended. Time to event (recidivism) analysis revealed significant differences in lag between low, moderate, and high risk offenders, with the majority of recidivism taking place within 90 days of probation termination for high risk offenders. Using ROC curve analysis we found that there was a 63% chance of selecting a recidivist with a higher score than a non-recidivist at random from the population, reinforcing the confidence of practitioners and researchers alike in the predictive validity of the risk assessment instrument.

These results were all discerned over a five year period in which significant turnover had occurred in the system, with the induction of a new court administrator, new lead personnel on the project, and new probation officers. The political climate had changed with less emphasis on the DMC problem and less concern with the juvenile delinquency rate. The project had annual meetings with the Board of Commissioners, Judges, and court administrators directly reporting risk assessment and delinquency data. Given the outsider status of the research component of project, the reported results seemed to have greater credibility with County Commissioners and the public.

This was another lesson learned from the project that collaboration with neutral third parties often makes system change easier. The researchers showed that the original numbers that had prompted so much concern about the delinquency rate in 2002 were based on the number of petitions rather than the number offenders, let alone the number of offenders per

10,000 youth as is the norm in reporting delinquency rates. The actual number of offenders was actually relatively low for a system of that size in an urban environment. The original consternation had been brought on by a simple misinterpretation of the increase in number of offenses committed by a small number of offenders. This reinforced the importance of correctly identifying that small group of youth with a high probability of repeatedly offending. The change over in probation personnel facilitated easier training in reliance on the formal risk assessment for this identification process rather than personal judgment.

Armed with the validation evidence, the case was made to court administrators and judges that the driving factor in the informal probation decision should be risk score rather than offense level or other factors. The researchers showed how family structure, race, gender, level of offense or even type of offense were less likely than simply flipping a coin at correctly predicting which offenders would return to the system within a 24 month period. After much consideration and debate, the court ultimately decided that low risk offenders would be placed on informal probation given no extenuating circumstances related to their offense. High-risk offenders would also be sent to formal probation. This was a huge policy and practice win for advocates of system reform, in particular those with interest in the DMC problem. The numbers suggested that this would lead to a considerable drop in the size of formal probation caseloads as was originally surmised during the conception of the project. Low risk offenders comprised nearly half of the probation caseload overall, and reshuffling offenders between the informal and formal probation division would free up considerable system resources that could be dedicated to the high-risk offenders.

As one can see in the second chart, there was a considerable drop-off in the offender rate over time for formal probationers. The decision to divert low risk offenders to informal probation and community programming was related to over a 50% decline over a six-year period in formal probation caseloads.

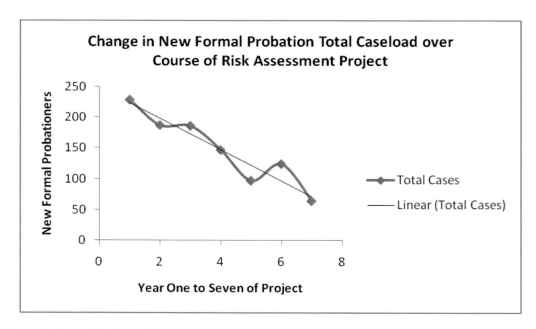

Figure 2. Formal Probation Caseload over Time.

It also resulted in a reduction of mixing offenders of different risk levels in the two probation divisions. However, as shown in figures 3 and 4, the majority of the reduction in mixing of different risk level probationers took place in the informal probation division with high risk and moderate risk offenders being placed on formal probation. There was a small drop off in the percentage of low risk kept on informal probation, but in a five-year period nearly 20% of low risk offenders were still being formally probated. If one recalls two of the four strategies recommended for reducing disproportionate minority representation were employed. One, subjectivity in decision-making had been reduced through the introduction of a risk assessment. Two, community programming outside of the court's purview had been ramped up through proper sorting of probationers based on risk level. With such dramatic changes in the system, concern was expressed by community members that the capacity of the community to hold down recidivism rates for informal probationers may by over-taxed. Follow-up studies of recidivism rates for informal probationers revealed no significant differences from formal probationers after controlling for relevant factors like initial risk level, race, gender, and offense type.

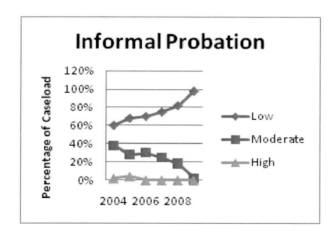

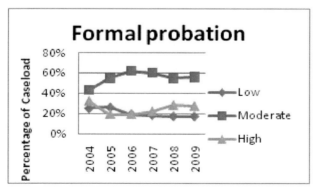

Figure 3 and 4. Informal and Formal Probation Caseloads over Time.

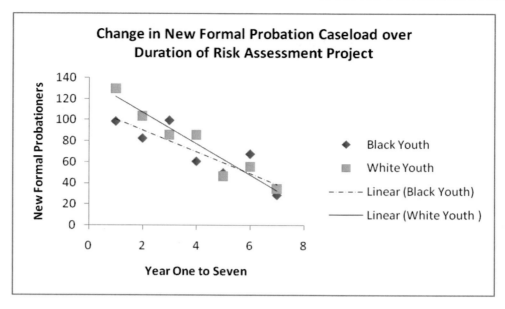

Figure 5. Black and White Formal Probation Caseloads over Duration of Project].

System reform advocates also began to question the necessity of formal probation for non-detention youth given the lower costs associated with informal probation and identical recidivism outcomes of youth. The system is currently struggling with properly evaluating and reviewing interventions employed by the two divisions given real world limitations precluding true experimental designs. System reform advocates that were particularly concerned with DMC also thought that reduction in formal probation caseload sizes would also mean a reduction in the African American formal probation population at the very least and could also mean a reduction in their over-representation in the system. Again, the theory was that over-representation was partly due to the existence of a wider net for low risk African American offenders than what exists for white offenders at the intake level. Thus, an objective decision-making tool could refract young offenders better suited for community interventions from the system, and this would naturally have greater impact on the African American population. As you can see in the chart below, this was not the case.

Although African American young offenders also experienced a substantial drop in their overall numbers over time in the formal probation division, that drop-off was shallower than that of whites. In fact, the general trend was for over-representation to increase as over-all case loads decreased. Over-representation varied from year to year, but never dropped below 200% over a six-year period. The immediate question was why. Despite the over-all validity of the risk assessment it could not be assumed that the risk assessment was equally valid with the various gender and racial groups of the youth offender population. The group simultaneously focused on exploring the dimensional identity of the risk assessment, that is to say they checked its validity with both girls and African Americans.

The results indicated that although the risk assessment performed better than chance and the discretion of practitioners at identifying recidivists and non-recidivists; the risk assessment performed better at predicting offense with whites and girls than African American boys. Where the risk assessment was regularly correctly classifying over 75% of white females, the risk assessment only correctly classified 62% of Black males. Black male offenders received new petitions at higher rates regardless of risk level. Moreover, the instrument appeared to have the greatest difficulty correctly predicting the outcomes of moderate risk offenders, especially those of African Americans.

The immediate question was again why, harking back to the original debate about whether over-representation was a result of differential offending behavior or discrimination within the system. System actors pointed out that the reform advocates had made a strong argument for reducing subjectivity in critical points of decision-making, pro-offering a purportedly objective risk assessment instrument as the solution to that problem. Now that the risk assessment had seemingly confirmed a disproportional risk of offense related to race and gender, the system reform advocates seemingly double backed to question the objectivity of the instrument. The counterargument rightly gave the system reform advocates pause in responding with little evidence to substantiate the claim that the instrument itself was biased. The researchers stepped back from the policy debate and redoubled their research efforts. Noting the conclusions from other community researchers that race effects are often proxies for other relations between relevant factors, the system reform advocates began systematically examine possible explanatory variables for differential predictive validity in the risk assessment instrument reflected in continued over-representation of African Americans in the formal probation caseload group. Those possible explanatory variables included: differential offending behavior as reflected in self report data, differential responsivity of offenders to intervention based on pattern of need, and differential validity of the instrument based on geographic location and socioeconomic status of neighborhood.

The community is currently launching several independent efforts at measuring offense behavior of youth separate of arrest and petition data. This is no small undertaking and requires leveraging of outside dollars to achieve that objective. It will be sometime before the results are collected, analyzed, and reported. On the second point, considerable research has been conducted identifying patterns of need within the population through cluster analysis. Cluster analysis of the offender population revealed two groups within the moderate risk level with different patterns of risk. One group of moderate risk level of offenders had criminogenic risks related to their environment; these probationers had exhibited lack of constructive use of their free time, were more likely to be involved with drugs, performed poorly in school and had extensive deviant peer groups. The other group appeared to have considerable needs related to personality, attitudes toward authority, and family circumstances.

Although their overall levels of risk were identical for the two groups, their recidivism outcomes were significantly different. Offenders with family risks appeared to be less responsive to formal probation interventions, recidivating at a higher rate over a two year period. The two groups also appeared to have significant differences in racial composition, with disproportionately high representation of African Americans in the family needs group. The researchers speculated that formal probation interventions typically had a better track record dealing with drug involvement, connecting youth with constructive things to do in their free time and breaking up deviant peer groups than they had improving attitudes toward authority or family circumstances of youth. This reflected an advantage within the system for youth with certain needs and risks, consequently it was quite possible that differential offending rates between racial groups could be related to that interaction between system response and youth responsivity to probation interventions.

The researchers were also interested in examining socioeconomic differences between neighborhood of origin for offenders and examining interaction effects with individual risks for recidivism. This was perhaps the most challenging issue to resolve research-wise, given the necessity of examining a cross-level interaction with a geographic component. The researchers again employed cluster analysis in their hiearachical linear modeling procedure. They found community was actually comprised of three distinct socioeconomic groups of neighborhoods. There was one high socioeconomic group of neighborhoods, and two low SES groups. The low SES groups were distinguishable by the level of education held by the residents. One low SES group had high levels of education despite low levels of income. Examinations of that group revealed that this group clustered around the university where there was high number of college students with low incomes but high levels of education compared to the rest of the neighborhood community. This mixing of residents of various education levels appeared to have an over-all suppression effect on the delinquency recidivism rate. This effect is currently being studied and confirmed as of the completion of this manuscript. The researchers also found that confounding nature of this possible effect appeared to destroy the risk-recidivism relationship upon which the risk assessment was based. For youth within this group of neighborhoods, the risk assessment had no predictive validity despite these youth comprising nearly a third of probationers. It was not possible to discern race effects related to this geographic factor due to sample size at the time so the researchers are still exploring the role this plays in the differential validity of the risk assessment with African Americans. The researchers are also interested in examining the role differential surveillance levels between the respective neighborhood groups has on the differential validity of the risk assessment. Unfortunately, this again investigation is easier said than done.

CONCLUSION

Reducing over-representation within the system of African Americans through risk assessment is no small undertaking and the suggestion that institutionalizing objective assessment will naturally reduce discrimination belies the complexity of institutional discrimination itself. Delinquency is very much a product of both social and psychological factors that interact in a multitude of ways. Even well intentioned systems face fluid policy environments making them amenable to change initially yet intractable when faced with the limitations of personnel, authority, and resources. DMC reduction efforts must certainly focus on system reform with watershed effects for all groups, but must be committed to discerning the interplay between multiple factors across levels related to race. Ssystems must tackle the issue of responsivity, improving the capacity of communities to respond to delinquency separate of formal juvenile justice system efforts, and differences in surveillance across communities.

Thus, there are multiple lines of inquiry that require additional interdisciplinary research and study. One, the etiology of undesirable behavior of youth is narrowly conceived, reflecting primarily the paradigmatic tradition of the researcher rather than causal pathways of the individual youth. Psychology, sociology, and other human science disciplines should accelerate their attempts to integrate their respective theories, as well as test these integrated theories of behavior in community settings. This certainly poses a challenge in cases where the benefits or harms could very well be concentrated into certain groups, given the nature of community science that utilizes true experimental designs (e.g. randomization). Moreover, it is rare that researchers are the primary stakeholders in deciding who receive particular community level interventions, especially in the realm juvenile justice. That said there are a number of techniques like matched pair sampling and experimental social intervention techniques innovated by ecological-community psychology that make such research possible.

Three, as this pertains to disproportionate minority contact, we know that both system and individual behavior contribute to delinquency rates and in turn disparities in offending. Risk assessment researchers must expand their domains to include mezzo- and macro- level factors, which requires greater utilization of sophisticated statistical analysis techniques that can ascertain interaction effects across multiple levels. Moreover, it will require greater use of tools outside the traditional repertoire on one's field; for example, psychologists and social workers should become abreast of recent developments in Geographical Information Systems. Doing so is absolutely necessary if we are to account for neighborhood and community process factors that both mediate and moderate the relationships between person level factors and undesirable behavioral outcomes.

Four, greater and more consistent evaluation of change efforts should be a priority. Researchers have a difficult time gaining access to juvenile justice data, and systems are understandably reluctant to subject themselves to rigorous review of their measures to protect the public in a just and equitable manner. The consequence of this has been a substantial degree of lag between identifications of problematic system behaviors, corrective responses, and sharing of experience with other practitioners. This is perhaps a common challenge of community-oriented translational research encountered by many disciplines.

Finally, this has broad implications for a number of fields investigating disparities affecting marginalized groups. Members of these groups rarely have adequate representation in constructing research plans, and have relatively little influence over how the results are interpreted and later implemented as change efforts. The system in this case deserves considerable credit for conferring on the community and researchers great latitude in analyzing and reflecting on the results before developing policies. Although this also allowed for conflict, it served as a model for cooperation for mutual benefit that was recognized by a cross-section of stakeholders in that community. This speaks to the necessity of participatory and empowering community practice techniques in implementing community level interventions pertaining marginalized groups. This also reflects on the necessity of increasing the research capacity of marginalized groups, not just as participants or subjects of inquiry but as powerful actors in the objective identification process.

REFERENCES

Albonetti, C. A. (1987). Prosecutorial discretion: The effects of uncertainty. *Law and Society Review*, 21, 291-313.

Andrews, D. A. and Dowden, C. (2006). Risk principle of case classification in correctional treatment. A meta-analytic investigation. *International Journal of Offender Therapy and Comparative Criminology, 50,* 88-100.

Bonta, J. (1996). Risk-needs: Assessment and treatment. In A. T. Harland (Ed.), *Choosing correctional options that work: Defining the demand and evaluating the supply (pp. 18-32)*. Thousand Oaks, CA: Sage.

Bronfenbrenner, U. (1979). *The Ecology of Human Development: Experiments by Nature and Design*. Cambridge, MA: Harvard University Press.

Bureau of Justice Statistics. Sourcebook Criminal Justice Statistics, 2002.30th Ed. (Pub NCJ 203301) Washington DC: BJS, 2004. Available at www.albany.edu/sourcebook.

Courtwright, D. T. (1996). The drug war's hidden toll. *Issues in Science and Technology*, 73.

Cullen, F. T., and Agnew, R. (2006). *Criminological theory past to present: essential readings. (Third edition)*. LA: Roxbury Publishing Company.

Eck, J. E., and Weisburd, D. (1996). *Crime in Place*. Monsey: Criminal Justice Press.

Fellner, J., and Mauer, M. (October 1998). "Losing the Vote: The Impact of Felony Disenfranchisement Laws in the United States," Human Rights Watch and The Sentencing Project.

Freudenberg, N. (2002). Adverse effects of US jail and prison policies on the health and well-being of women of color. *American Journal of Public Health, 92*, 1895-1899.

Hartley, R.D., Maddan, S., and Spohn, C. (2007). Prosecutorial Discretion: An Examination of Substantial Assistance Departures in Federal Crack-Cocaine and Powder-Cocaine Cases. Justice Quarterly : JQ, *24*(3), 382-407.

Harlow, C. W. *Profile of Jail Inmates—1996*. Washington, DC: US Dept of Justice; 1998:1–15. Bureau of Justice Statistics special report NCJ 164620.

Kent, S.L., and Jacobs, D. (2005). Minority threat and police strength from 1980 to 2000: A fixed-effects analysis of nonlinear and interactive effects in large cities. *Criminology, 43*, 731-760.

Kerstetter, W. (1990). Gateway to justice: Police and prosecutorial response to sexual assaults against women. *Criminology*, 81, 267-313.

Kraska, Peter B. (2006). Criminal Justice Theory: Toward Legitimacy and an Infrastructure. *Justice Quarterly*, 23 (2), 0741-8825. Retrieved September 13, 2007, from http://www.informaworld.com/10.1080/ 07418820600688735.

Loftin, C., and McDowall, D. (1982). The police, crime, and economic theory: An assessment. *American Sociological Review, 47*, 393-401.

Maguire, E. R. (2001). Research evidence on the factors influencing police strength in the United States. In Hiring and retention Issues in Police Agencies: Readings on the determinants of police strength, hiring and retention of officers and the federal cops program (pp. 7-25). A report to the National Institute of Justice by Christopher S. Koper, Edward R. Maguire, and Gretchen E. Moore. Retrieved from http://www.urban.org/pdfs/Hiring-and-Retention.pdf.

Mauer, M. (1999). *Race to incarcerate*. New York: New Press.

Maxfield, M.G., and C.S. Widom, "The Cycle of Violence: Revisited Six Years Later," *Archives of Pediatrics and Adolescent Medicine* 150 (1996): 390–395.

May, L. and Sharratt, S. (1994). *Applied Ethics: A Multicultural Approach,* Englewood Cliffs, NJ: Prentice-Hall.

Phillips S, and Bloom B. In whose best interests? The impact of changing public policy on relatives caring for children with incarcerated parents. *Child Welfare*. 1998;77:531–541.

Richie, B. E. Challenges incarcerated women face as they return to their communities: findings from life history interviews. *Crime Delinquency*. 2001;47:368–389.

Pope, C. and W. Feyerherm. (1992). *Minorities and the Juvenile Justice System*. Rockville, MD: U.S. Department of Justice, Office of Juvenile Justice and Delinquency Prevention, Juvenile Justice Clearinghouse.

Schrantz, D., and McElroy, J. (2000). *Reducing Racial Disparity in Criminal Justice: A Manual for Practitioners and Policmakers*. Sentencing Project. Washington, D.C.

Schwartz, I. M., Steketee, M. W. and Schneider, V. W. (1989). *The Incarceration of Girls: Paternalism or Crime Control?* Ann Arbor, MI: Center for the Study of Youth Policy

Steffensmeier, D. J., and Steffensmeier, R. (1980). Trends in female delinquency: An examination of arrest, juvenile court, self-report, and field Data." *Criminology* 18: 62-85.

Stucky, T.D. (2005). Local politics and police strength. *Justice Quarterly*, 22, 139-169.

Faye Taxman, James M Byrne, April Pattavina. (2005). Racial Disparity and the Legitimacy of the Criminal Justice System: Exploring Consequences for Deterrence. *Journal of Health Care for the Poor and Underserved*: Reducing HIV/AIDS and Criminal Justice Involvement in..., *16*(4), 57-77.

R.L. Weisman, J.S. Lamberti, N. Price. (2004). Integrating Criminal Justice, Community Healthcare, and Support Services for Adults with Severe Mental Disorders. *Psychiatric Quarterly*, *75*(1), 71-85.

Wilson, J. Q. (1968). Varieties of police behavior: The management of law and order in eight communities. Cambridge, MA: Harvard University Press.

In: Youth: Practices, Perspectives and Challenges
Editor: Elizabeth Trejos-Castillo

ISBN: 978-1-62618-067-3
© 2013 Nova Science Publishers, Inc.

Chapter 18

HUMAN CAPITAL DEVELOPMENT AMONG IMMIGRANT YOUTH

Elizabeth Trejos-Castillo[*], *Sherley Bedore and Nancy Treviño Schafer*
Human Development and Family Studies, College of Human Sciences,
Texas Tech University, Lubbock, TX, US

ABSTRACT

U.S. rapidly changing demographics raise important challenges for policy makers, practitioners and professionals when working with immigrant youth and families—1 in 5 children are born to immigrants (U.S. Census, 2004). It has been extensively documented that immigrant populations commonly experience limited opportunities in education, work and training, services, and housing that hinder the accumulation of human capital. However, the dynamics of how human capital is developed and transmitted across generations of immigrant populations, as well as the long-term socio-economic and political repercussions on American society, are phenomena that continue to puzzle scholars and policy makers alike. Furthermore, the assimilation and successful incorporation of immigrants' human capital into the country's labor market remains an urgent issue yet to be resolved but important because immigrants, particularly youth, represent a significant portion of the country's current and future workforce. Using a cultural lens, the authors aim to: first, review the main theoretical views on human capital (development and transmission), and second, conduct a critical review of extant empirical research on the development of human capital in immigrant families and youth. The proposed chapter will contribute to the scarce literature on the development of human capital among immigrants, particularly the most underserved minority groups such as refugees and illegal immigrants. Social and political implications will be also discussed.

---

[*] Address correspondence to: Elizabeth Trejos-Castillo, Human Development and Family Studies, Texas Tech University, MS 41230 Lubbock, TX 79409-1230 / Email: elizabeth.trejos@ttu.edu

INTRODUCTION

The United States experiences one of the most rapidly changing demographic trends among the world's industrialized nations. With a population estimated around 300 million people in 2011, the American society has become more diverse with approximately 1 in every 5 children being born to at least one immigrant parent as reported by the 2000 Census (U.S. Census Bureau, 2003). During the last two decades, the greatest concentration of immigrants has centered around a few states, namely California (3.3 million), New York (1.6 million), Texas (1.2 million) and Florida (1.2 million); these states together account for more than half (58%) of the legal permanent residents (LPR)[1] in the United Sates. Recent statistics show that immigrant groups come from all over the world with approximately 26% of legal residents migrating from Mexico, followed by the Philippines 5.3%, and 4.4% from People's Republic of China, 4% from India, 3.5% from Dominican Republic and 2.9% from Cuba (Rytina, 2011). In the case of illegal or unauthorized immigrants, the Pew Hispanic Center (2011) reports 11.2 million individuals were living in the U.S. as of March 2010, which suggests a slight decline from 12 million in 2007; illegal immigrants accounted for approximately 4% of the nation's population, 5.2% of the labor force and 8% of nationwide newborn babies in 2010 (Passel and Cohn, 2011). Beyond the changing demographics and growing immigration waves, a far more important issue continues to unfold: the well-being of immigrant families and their children.

Though it is well-documented that immigrants commonly experience limited opportunities as compared to the native population (e.g., education, work/ training, health services, housing), the dynamics of the development and generational transmission of human capital among immigrant families and their children have not been given much attention. Furthermore, the assimilation and successful incorporation of immigrants' human capital into the country's labor market remains an urgent issue yet to be resolved. Better understanding these issues is important because immigrants, particularly youth, represent a significant portion of the country's current and future task force. Using a cultural lens, the authors aim to: first, review the main theoretical views on human capital, both development and transmission, and second, to conduct a critical review of existing empirical research on the development of human capital in immigrant youth and families. This chapter will contribute to the scarce literature on the development of human capital among immigrants, particularly in the most underserved minority groups, such as refugees and illegal immigrants. Social and political implications will be also discussed.

WHAT IS HUMAN CAPITAL?

"Capital" can be defined as accumulated labor that is acquired by either single individuals or groups for their own benefit to further build their interest and increase their assets (Bourdieu,1986). The accumulation of capital is directly associated to the individual's availability to connect with other individuals and establish steady and supportive networks in which all individuals are benefited from their interactions. The first reference to human capital can be identified as early as 1776 when economist Adam Smith defined it as:

---

[1] Legal Permanent Residents (LPR) including relatives of U.S. residents, legally employed foreigners, refugees and asylees; and others who maintain a legal resident status due to special issues (Shrestha and Heisler, 2011).

"the acquired and useful abilities of all the inhabitants or members of the society. The acquisition of such talents, by the maintenance of the acquirer during his education, study, or apprenticeship, always costs a real expense, which is a capital fixed and realized, as it were, in his person. Those talents, as they make a part of his fortune, so do they likewise that of the society to which he belongs." (Smith, 1937).

Smith's economic approach was later revisited by Keynes (1920) and Lewis (1954) in an effort to justify the importance of labor inequality and its impact on savings and economic capital accumulation across different populations, specifically the less skilled to more skilled laborers, to support societal development at multiple levels.

A more contemporary definition of human capital states that it consists of the "inherent and acquired knowledge, skills, competencies, and other intrinsic attributes an individual commands to create personal, social, and economic well-being" (Grundy and Sloggett, 2003, pp. 207). From both the traditional and modern views, human capital is intrinsically embedded individual growth as it focuses on individual behaviors that facilitate the accumulation of knowledge and development of skills. Thus, enabling people to increase their economic productivity and accumulate capital over time. The accumulation of human capital directly affects the growth, wealth, and productivity of the society individuals live in (Schuller, 2000). Human capital is broadly described as a central predictor of individual's employment, socioeconomic status, and competitive advantage (Becker, 1964; Schultz, 1993). However, the dynamics of how human capital is developed, accumulated, and transmitted across individuals is directly affected by the context in which individuals live and thus, difficulties and opportunities could vary across populations (Schuller, 2000).

In the following sections, we describe the main theoretical views on human capital (development and transmission), and second, we provide a critical review of extant empirical research on the development of human capital in immigrant families and youth. The proposed chapter will contribute to the scarce literature on the development of human capital among immigrants particularly the most underserved minority groups such as refugees and illegal immigrants. Social and political implications will be also discussed.

DEVELOPMENT OF HUMAN CAPITAL IN IMMIGRANT YOUTH AND FAMILIES

Immigration and Assimilation into the Host Culture

Immigration represents a transitional process that places families and children in different and changing contexts. Often times, immigrant families and their children have a difficult multifaceted experience in the accumulation and transmission of human capital across generations due mostly to their particular needs and challenges as well as their unique societal interactions. One of the key factors affecting the development of human capital among immigrant youth and their families is the adaptation to the host culture.

The assimilation of oneself into a host country is a very complex process that has many dimensions. Assimilation includes taking on the "normal" traits of the host nation. These traits usually differentiate immigrants from those in the host nations and may include: income, human capital, occupational status, housing, education, health services, etc. Even though some immigrant families choose to embark on a journey in search of better opportunities, others are forced by multiple circumstances to leave their countries and their families behind. The latter is the case for refugees or asylees[2] who are removed from their countries and relocated without being able to chose where they are placed to live and, with limited or no contact with their families remaining in their countries of origin (Landale, Thomas, and Van Hook, 2011; Potocky-Tripodi, 2004). Children and youth seem to assimilate at a different rate than their parents, depending on the assimilating activity or dimension. It has been discovered that immigrants are more vulnerable in terms of accumulating a strong human capital because of assimilation complexities (Djajić, 2003).

As discussed by Portes and Rumbaut (2001) immigrants often experience what is called "segmented assimilation"—that is, physical "barrio" barriers where immigrants are physically isolated from the host culture by living within a "barrio" made up of other immigrants from their home culture; this might prevent immigrants from assimilating fully to the host country. This problem is very commonly a consequence of immigrants living choices where they tend to move where they "fit in" the most or can afford to live which are often lower class neighborhoods where interaction with the host country culture is minimal. Because the interactions with the host culture can be almost obsolete, especially in bigger cities like New York, Miami, and San Diego, the context can hinder the assimilation of human capital assets that are needed to fully assimilate into the host culture. The accumulation of human capital among immigrant youth and families is not only a topic of interest for the American society but for many other countries around the world with a great influx of immigrant populations. For instance, skill transference and educational opportunities were found to be stronger predictors of human capital accumulation among Suriname and Duth Antilles immigrant youth in the Netherlands (Van Tubergen and Van De Werfhorst, 2007). The acquisition and transmission of financial capital from a native country to the host country can also minimize the income gap that often occurs as a result of social policies in hiring immigrants, educated and not, in countries (i.e. Canada) where the immigrant population is similar to that of the American immigrant population influx (Finnie and Meng, 2002; Bartlett, 2007).

Living in an environment where immigrants have very little in common with others has the potential to positively and/or negatively affect the transaction trade-offs with the locals. To start with, immigrants already have very little in common with others in a host country and this dissimilarity only restricts or limits the transactions with others that would otherwise help the immigrant start to build human capital (McKenzie, 2008; Portes and Rumbaut, 2001). As a consequence, immigrants commonly have great difficulty in finding places to live, jobs, accessing health care services, and this can possibly even lead to experience associated problems such as discrimination, rejection, and segregation. On the other hand, in the presence of strong social ties and supportive networks in their living environments, immigrants with lower levels of human capital have a greater chance to access multiple resources and increase their capital accumulation over time compared to those lacking a supportive system (Portes and Rumbaut, 2001). In summary, greater networks facilitate assimilation into the host culture, promote job advancement, higher earnings, healthcare access, and better education for children; on the contrary, lack of a supportive network

---

[2] Refugee or asylum status is assigned to individuals who are unable to return to their country of origin due to potential persecution based on race, faith, nationality, membership in a particular social group, or political affiliations (Martin, and Yankay, 2011, Department of Homeland Security).

negatively affects assimilation, language proficiency, lost of cultural heritage, social support for the family and the children.

Generational Differences in the Accumulation of Human Capital

Depending on the family resources and the circumstances of the immigration, the adaptation process to the host culture might follow a different path and experience a different pace for acquiring human capital from one generation to the next in immigrant families (Djajić, 2003; Portes and Rumbaut, 2001).One generational cohort, for example, might have to enter the labor market in younger years with lower educational levels, would contract at some point personal household responsibilities, and might spend a great amount of their lives in the labor market. On the other hand, other cohorts might enter the labor market during middle age years after pursuing a career and would spend less time in the labor market. Large scale immigration across particular generations might create a "crowding effect" affecting the acquisition and accumulation of human capital across generations due to the competition for available resources (Connelly and Gottschalk, 1995; Fertig, Schmidt, and Sinning, 2009).

Intergenerational dependence in educational and employment attainment has been found to be highly correlated with generational differences in the accumulation of human capital. Empirical evidence shows that higher levels of education and professional careers are strongly associated with intergenerational dependence between parents and their children and the accumulation of human capital stock over a number of years (Fertig, Schmidt, and Sinning, 2009). Over time, the weakening of family ties and cultural values deteriorate parental influence across generations of immigrant children and this has been linked to the loss of human capital among immigrant families. On the other hand, there have been multiple family and cultural protective factors linked to intergenerational dependence such as the presence of extended family members in the household, cultural traditions, native language use, family responsibilities and chores. Similarly, other factors such as discrimination and segregation might affect generational cohorts differently. For instance, there is more tolerance among 3rd and later generations than among first and second generations which can negatively affect how the generational cohort values educational and employment attainment and in turn, impactings the accumulation of human capital for the following generation (Portes and Rumbaut, 2001).

Evidence has been provided that the second generation youth fare the same as the first generation in terms of participating in work; the local neighborhood job market has been suggested to have little to no effect on whether the youth will participate in the workforce (Bean and Bell-Rose, 2004). It has even been suggested that those immigrants who are living in neighborhoods that consist of predominantly one culture and are lower income, are less likely to participate in the work force. If this is the case, generations thereafter are more affected by the local labor market circumstances than anything else (Bean and Bell-Rose, 2004). This may be because the third and subsequent generations are considered more native, have the skills and traits (i.e. language use and education level) of the natives, and may rely on local sentiment to work whereas the first and second generation may have cultural skills that help them network within culture (Bean and Bell-Rose, 2004; Djajić, 2003). Also, taking family size into consideration within the second and third generations, those youth who had siblings were more likely to be working than youth who were an only-child (Perreira, Mullan, Harris and Lee, 2007).

For second generation immigrants, language exposure and use is stronger in terms of fluency. Since second generation immigrants have a longer exposure to the host language, they are better able to join the job market more easily and at faster rates than first generation immigrants (Djajić, 2003).

This makes second and subsequent generations thereafter important in terms of integrating into the host economy's higher-wage jobs. This is especially important for acquiring and sustaining the financial capital resource immigrants have (e.g. higher income jobs), how they are transferred from generation to generation, how the income of the family is affected, and what sort of policies can be established to minimize the income gap (Finnie and Meng, 2002).

TRANSMISSION OF HUMAN CAPITAL ACROSS GENERATIONS OF IMMIGRANT YOUTH

Different factors have been identified as key elements in the development and transmission of human capital among immigrants including personal networks (e.g., transnational families), group membership, social transaction of services, knowledge, labor market and skills, language proficiency, and education (Bean and Bell-Rose, 2004; De Flores, 2010; Perreira, Mullan, and Lee, 2007; Smith, 2012).

Labor Market

The accumulation and transmission of human capital across immigrant groups have been reported to follow different paths depending on the families' cultural background. Perreira and colleagues (2007) found that non-white immigrant youth worked more hours, on average, than Whites. Mexican, Cuban and African American immigrant youth work participation increased over time from generation to generation compared to whites in 1st to 3rd generations. On the other hand, Chinese and Filipino immigrant youth reported decreased work participation over time compared to Whites (Perreira, Mullan, and Lee, 2007). Bean and Bell-Rose (2004) argue that the primary influence of job market participation amongst immigrants is the submersion into the host society and its ethnic hierarchy. Speaking English and school networking skills with other students whose families had a higher socioeconomic status were important factors for first generation immigrant youth to participate in the labor force (Bean and Bell-Rose, 2004). This is taking into account the neighborhood and the job market they are entering into, which have been found to have no effect on the participation of youth in the work forces.

Immigrant youth in the workforce provide the host economy with another avenue in finding workers although this should not be a primary source, as immigrant youth should focus on higher educational attainment. In part, the phenomenon of different paths has been explained based on the premise that some groups have a "premigratory" advantage that supports a better adaptation to the host country and thus, a greater accumulation of human capital (Li, 2004; Suárez-Orozco, Gaytán, Bang, Pakes, O'Connor et al., 2010; Tseng, Chao, and Padmawidjaja, 2007). On the contrary, lacking a premigratory advantage, such as less educated parents, having a working mother in the household, increases the chances that first generation youth will participate in the workforce as well (Checchi, 2006; Perreira, Mullan, and Lee, 2007).

In addition to different trajectories in the development and accumulation of human capital in immigrant youth, empirical evidence also reports that individual trajectories might be related to cohort effects. As reported by Glick and White (2003) and supported by Portes and Rumbaut's (2001), "segmented assimilation" perspective, or birth cohort[3], might be a salient factor in the accumulation of human capital over time. A potential explanation for the lower accumulation of human capital in immigrant families is that skill acquisition concentrates at young ages, youth migrating at a younger age might have more or less schooling opportunities than second or subsequent generations which could affect their accumulation of human capital over time.

This explanation is consistent with the economic perspective of human capital accumulation which suggests that age-earnings vary according to learning ability and accumulated skills (Huggett, Ventura, and Yaron, 2006). School "orientation" or involvement in the school system, has not been reported as a predictor of work participation though it has been found to be strongly associated with greater job opportunities (Bean and Bell-Rose, 2004; Crosnoe andLopez Turley, 2011). Perhaps this lack of predictive association can be related to the idea that those who worked more were less school oriented. Furthermore, Smith (2012) suggests that there is a great overlap between jobs performed by youth and less educated adults and thus youth labor opportunities could be responsible for large waves of immigrant youth who would be paid similar to non-educated adults but with greater potential performance for longer periods of time.

Language Use

Language proficiency plays a significant role in the accumulation of human capital as well as support, learning ability, and skill acquisition among immigrant populations. For instance, if an available employment opportunity requires language use as part of maintaining efficiency, this may not be a realistic employment opportunity for an immigrant with low language skills, thus, forcing the immigrant to take on low skilled jobs that do not require language use. Language skills are also important in accessing other services that are available in the community but require some paperwork (Djajić, 2003; Portes and Rumbaut, 2001). Furthermore, a positive correlation between language ability in children and their academic and professional ambitions has been documented in previous studies so that aspirations will predict how hard the children are willing to work for the accomplishment of the dream (Crosnoe and Lopez Turley, 2011; Portes and Shauffler, 1994).

Different patterns of language acquisition are observed among children, youth, and adults and these patterns might affect their performance at school, at work, in interactions with

---

[3] According to Green and Worswick "differences between immigrants and the native born in the same cohort may move because of differences in ability and initial human capital stocks across native born cohorts" (2011, pg. 246).

others and so on. English speaking immigrant families are more likely to have youth who are more active in the job market than families who do not speak English at home. Indeed, English language use and proficiency among immigrant youth has been identified as a significant contributor to work participation (more, less, or at all) as well as a greater likelihood of having more educated parents (Perreira, Mullan, and Lee, 2007; Portes and Rumbaut, 2001). Immigrant children and youth who acquire language faster than their parents often become "language brokers"—translators or interpreters for their parents, relatives, and other adults. Thus, immigrant youth become responsible for supporting their parents' survival and completion of everyday tasks, their adaptation to the host culture, and they help bridge the family's cultural heritage with the host culture supporting the entire family well-being (Dorner, Orellana, and Grining, 2007; Hall and Sham, 2007; Trickett and Jones, 2007).

Education and the Immigrant Paradox

As described by Sam and colleagues (2006) the immigrant paradox is the "counterintuitive finding that immigrants have better adaptation outcomes than their national peers despite their poorer socioeconomic conditions" (Sam, Vedder, Ward, and Horenczyk, 2006, pp. 125). Empirical evidence has shown that the immigrant paradox extends to not only immigrant youth affecting their education attainment levels and socioeconomic opportunities but also their parents socio-cultural and psychological adaptation to the host culture (Fulgini, 1998; Sam et al., 2006).

Recent evidence has also found that immigrant youth, particularly 2nd and 3rd generation, are struggling more than the foreign-born youth in areas such as education, health, behavioral outcomes, and socioeconomic adaptation (Crosnoe and Lopez Turley, 2011; García Coll and Kerivan Marks, 2012). An example of the Immigrant Paradox is supported by Haskins and Tienda (2011) in which they provide evidence that Mexican immigrant families of the first generation tend to focus on strong work ethics and education, and family. On the other hand, in accordance with immigrant paradox assumptions, the second generation is less likely to attain the education human capital that is experienced by the first generation (Haskins and Tienda, 2011).

Educational differences based on the ethnicity of the immigrant youth have also been found. For instance, some findings suggest that Asian immigrant youth show a greater performance advantage across standardized tests in elementary and secondary schools than their Latin American, especially Mexican, and other immigrant peers (Crosnoe and Lopez Turley, 2011; Haskins and Tienda 2011).

Furthermore, other factors such as socio-economic resources, parental education, and language proficiency have been also related to increased academic performance among immigrant youth (Crosnoe and Lopez Turley, 2011; Kao and Tienda, 1995).

In addition, English-language background and ability are factors that are closely linked to both generational status and achievement in school (Grenier 1984; White 1997). Ideally, to be successful in society and for the sake of generations after them, incoming families must be able to join the job market.

In order to join the job market, immigrants have to have language and education capital and have to be received into an economy that is willing to incorporate these ideas (Bean and Bell-Rose, 2004).

SOCIAL AND PUBLIC POLICY AND THE ACCUMULATION OF HUMAN CAPITAL

The development of human capital is affected by social and public policy alike. Human capital accumulation is highly influenced by the amount of public and social policy resources legislated by governmental lawmakers. Not only is it important in national government public policy making but also in state policy, especially in states such as California, New York, Texas, and Florida where more than half of all immigrants in the United States reside (Rytina, 2001).

Public policy's effects on human capital accumulation among immigrants are especially important in determining the quality of capital obtained and sustained. According to the Department of Homeland Security's Office of Immigration Statistics, there are approximately 12,630,000 legal permanent residents in the United States as of January 1, 2010 (Martin and Yankay, 2011, Department of Homeland Security Office of Immigration Statistics).. This number of legal permanent residents does not include those immigrants who have been granted citizenship. Intuitively, most of these immigrants come from Mexico, which is approximately 26 percent of the immigrant population. (Rytina, 2011).

As immigrants come from all over the world, policy should take into consideration that there are cultural differences among various immigrant groups, immigration generations, and waves of immigrants, differences which lawmakers should at least be aware of when drafting and passing policies that are directly related to immigration, immigrants, and immigrant family units. The human capital components that are especially affected by public policy are: language use and acquisition, income, and education (Bean and Bell-Rose, 2004; Djajić, 2003; Haskins and Tienda, 2011; Portes and Raumbaut, 2001). In order to help support the large populations of incoming immigrants and their human capital accumulation, a strong, supportive public policy framework needs to be set in place.

A public policy framework that strengthens the accumulation of human capital and its consumption is imperative for integrating immigrants into a host society and minimizing the consequences of negative assimilation of capital (Djajić, 2003). A social policy structure that helps to support and promote the diversity of the host nation's current citizens as well as the diverse influx of the immigrant population is imperative in helping people gain the human capital they need.

This can provide incoming immigrants, as well as second and third generation immigrants, with better resources to maintain and accumulate human capital like language skills, better income and wages, and success in higher education levels. The success of a governmental public and social policy framework can benefit the host country in terms of maximizing labor market profit through the support of language and education programs and diversifying the job market.

The beginnings of this framework can be exemplified by recent national law debates for education, one of the major influences in the job market today. Haskins and Tienda (2011) discuss the Development, Relief, and Education for Alien Minors Act (DREAM Act)[4]. This

---

[4] A recent communication from the U.S. Library of Congress states that *"Development, Relief, and Education for Alien Minors Act of 2011 or DREAM Act of 2011 - Authorizes the Secretary of Homeland Security (DHS) to cancel the removal of, and adjust to the status of an alien lawfully admitted for permanent residence on a conditional basis, an alien who: (1) entered the United States on or before his or her 15th birthday and has*

Act aims to benefit both parties, undocumented immigrants as well as economy of the United States, in that it will allow undocumented immigrant workers to obtain a higher education degree in exchange for government service or out of pocket tuition for two years. For immigrants, undocumented and legal permanent residents alike, to have the opportunity for postsecondary education capital, would not hinder the U.S. economy but benefit it in the long run by stimulating competition in the job market and generating an educated society. This Act would help to curtail the subclass emergence from the lack of education capital consumption especially amongst Mexican immigrants and their children (Haskins and Tienda, 2011).

Education Policy

Part of the goal of education policy is for students to be successful and for teachers to encourage student's growth and success in a positive environment. Language acquisition plays a key role particularly in preschool education programs. Because preschool education is a choice in the U.S., many immigrant children or second generation children, children born to immigrant parents, are more likely to stay at home until it is necessary for them to go to school (Haskins and Tienda). This decision, in terms of "school readiness" sets immigrant children behind in learning even before they start kindergarten. There are some programs like Head Start and even state-wide school readiness programs that target low-income and immigrant groups and which emphasize learning and prepare children and parents for elementary school with very positive results (Haskins and Tienda, 2011).

Despite of the success of those programs, additional federal and state funds could help in participants gaining a more high quality transition from the home to school environment. One important question is how money should be allotted and what percent should be apportioned for teacher/educator training. This is especially important where there are large populations of immigrant students like California, Texas, New York, and Florida where it is important that educators know how to welcome the students and their families, how to teach English as a Second Language learners, and create a positive learning environment that would benefit current and future teachers and students (Rytina, 2001). Another salient goal of education policy is that students learn the host language before the third grade to minimize any achievement gaps that might begin at that grade level. Some states have bilingual education programs that promote the use of both the native language and the host language (e.g. Spanish-English dual language programs). In terms of readiness, the overlying idea is to linguistically prepare children to integrate into the host culture.

One innovative way to address the linguistic and cultural barriers faced by immigrant families with teenagers is combining English as a Second Language (ESL) instruction with social support, addressing topics such as dating norms, dangers of gang involvement, and postsecondary education opportunities. However, in contrast to programs for preschool children, few programs target immigrant families with adolescent children. One example is

---

been present in the United States for at least five years immediately preceding this Act's enactment, (2) is a person of good moral character, (3) is not inadmissible under specified grounds of the Immigration and Nationality Act, (4) has been admitted to an institution of higher education (IHE) in the United States or has earned a high school diploma or general education development certificate in the United States, and (5) was age 32 or younger on the date of this Act's enactment." See for further information: http://thomas.loc.gov/cgi-bin/bdquery/z?d112:HR01842:@@@Landsumm2=mand

Asian Community Teen's Youth Voice Radio, which broadcasts parenting advice from the youth perspective (Morse, 2005). Another successful program – AVANCE, based in Texas – serves predominantly low-income Latino families through parent education, early childhood development, literacy, and English language acquisition (AVANCE, 2012). Despite the fact that 91 percent of the parents in the program are high school dropouts, 94 percent of their children complete high school, 43 percent attend college, and half of the parents continue their education as adults. Avance started as a preschool and school readiness program but has also been successful in improving parent outcomes. AVANCE is funded by federal, state, county and city governments, United Way, foundations and corporations and serves more than 13,000 parents and children annually. Another approach is to help parents overcome language barriers, the lack of familiarity with the public school system, and cultural conceptions of the role of teachers.

For example, Montgomery County, Maryland created a parents' guide called "Navigating the System" in multiple languages (e.g., English, Spanish, French, Korean, Chinese; Morse, 2005). Topics include enrollment, graduation requirements, opportunities for parent involvement, instruction, specialized programs, school safety and security, and services for students and parents. This is the national conference of state legislature's website and is from the year 2005. Some of these programs and statistics might be beneficial in giving researchers an idea of the education of youth in the U.S. This provides us with an insight of what *is* being done and what still *needs* to be done. There are some government programs that are already in place in assisting immigrant students in achieving the educational capital they need to be successful.

The Emergency Immigrant Education Program (EIEP, Osorio-O'Dea, 2001) is a grant that helps education agencies who receive large numbers of immigrant students. It was created in 1984 and currently appropriates according to the number of Limited English Proficiency students the agencies have and recent immigrant students. More than $150 million has been dispersed and serves more than 800,000 students. Other programs and Acts in public policy are the No Child Left Behind Act of 2001 (NCLB, 2002), and Title III to enhance English Language acquisition for LEP (Limited English Proficiency) students. Of these funds, 95 percent of the NCLB and Title III funds are dispersed by states for their qualifying student population. These programs are intended for instruction, family literacy and parent outreach, personnel, tutorials, technology, and other educational related programs (ncsl.org). Although these millions of dollars seem staggering, it is not enough and there needs to be a larger allotment of money allocated for professional training and enhancements in order to properly serve those immigrant students. States get millions in government grants for the students who fall under these Titles, but teachers and educators still do not have the proper training to educate LEP students at the same level as native English speaking students.

Conclusion

Recent statistics show that approximately twenty five percent of all births in the United States are to foreign-born mothers and that the proportion of youth born to an immigrant parent compared to youth born to a native parent will increase in modest levels during the next decades ((Passel and Cohn, 2011; Passel and Taylor, 2010). In 2009, it was estimated that approximately 1.1 million unauthorized, or foreign-born, children were living in the U.S. and that approximately 4 million U.S. born children were born to unauthorized parents (Passel and Taylor, 2010). As noted by Shrestha and Heisler (2011): "The U.S. is getting bigger... and more diverse" (pp. 1). The influx and establishment of immigrant families and youth in the U.S. are impacting multiple domains of the American society, income, work, health care, and education, further than just the rapidly changing demographics and thus, it is important to understand the implications of human capital development and accumulation among immigrant populations.

The "*income gap is a result of education and experience returns*" (Finnie and Meng, 2002, pp. 19)—though immigrants might be well educated and have quality experience, it doesn't guarantee they will be getting paid as much as native born citizens or will be incorporated in the national workforce.

Thus, current public policy structure needs to address the immigrant population assimilation by developing education policies that support the success of future generations of citizens and also provide equal labor opportunities. This is important in preventing subclass citizens who do not have the human capital gains they need in order to provide for their family (Haskins and Tienda, 2011).

The discrepancy in the discrimination associated with hiring immigrants and also the social stigmas associated with their education and skills needs to be addressed. The education that is acquired by immigrants is not always acquired from the native country but can also include education received in the host country. What this means is that although an immigrant's education is obtained in the host country, they most likely will still receive a lower income than native born citizens (Finnie and Meng, 2002). In addition, family education, whether received in the host or native country, does not provide immigrants with any benefit in terms of income because of social policies that do not promote equality in hiring. Thus, skills acquisition, education achievement, and labor market warrant some attention in terms of policy making for expanding the stock of human capital among immigrants.

Appropriate policy changes could help narrow the income gap between immigrant and native-born citizens. This is especially important for those coming from countries that are a major contributor to the expatriate immigrant population in the United States. Mexico, for example, is the Organization for Economic Cooperation and Development's leading country in providing other countries with expatriates (Bartlett, 2007). In addition, because of its geographical location, higher rates of immigrant families and youth are reported coming from Mexico (Bartlett, 2007).

Although policies or changes can be made and would help immigrant youth and their families adapt to the host country, the ultimate goal is for them to accumulate human capital through education and skill acquisition over time. Substantial evidence shows that the lack of human capital among immigrant families and youth directly affects the host country's economy causing a greater income gap (Haskins and Tienda, 2011). Thus, if appropriate policies are not implemented, the problems associated with learning gaps as well as skill acquisition will only increase and will continue to impact the development and accumulation of human capital among immigrant youth and their families.

REFERENCES

AVANCE (2012). Early Childhood and Parenting Education at its Best. Retrieved from: http://www.avance.org/press-releases/.

Bartlett, D.L. (2007). U.S. Immigration Policy in Global Perspective: International Migration in OECD Countries, special report, Immigration Policy Center. Available at: http://www.immigrationpolicy.org/special-reports/us-immigration-policy-global-perspectiveinternational-migration-oecd-countries.

Bean, F. D., and Bell-Rose, S. (2004). *Immigration and opportunity: Race, ethnicity, and employment in the United States.* New York: Russell Sage Foundation Publications.

Becker, Gary S., (1964). *Human Capital: A Theoretical and Empirical Analysis with Special Reference to Education*, Chicago, Ill.: The University of Chicago Press.

Bourdieu, P. (1986) The forms of capital. In J. Richardson (Ed.) Handbook of Theory and Research for the Sociology of Education (New York, Greenwood), 241-258.

Checchi, D. (2006). *The economics of education: Human capital, family background and inequality.* Cambridge, UK: Cambridge University Press.

Connelly, R. and Gottschalk, P. (1995). The effect of cohort composition on human capital accumulation across generations. *Journal of Labor Economics*, 13, 155-176.

Crosnoe, R. and Lopez Turley, R. N., (2011). K-12 Educational outcomes of immigrant youth. *The Future of Children, 21,* 129-152.

De Flores, C. (2010). A conceptual framework for the study of social capital in new destination immigrant communities. *Journal of Transcultural Nursing, 21*(3), 205-211. doi:10.1177/1043659609358783.

Djajić, S. (2003). Assimilation of immigrants: implications for human capital accumulation of the second generation. *Journal of Population Economics*, *16*, 831-845. doi: 10.1007/s00148-003-0162-1.

Dorner, L. M., Orellana, M. F., and Li-Grining, C. P. (2007). I helped my mom and it helped me: Translating the skills of language brokers into improved standardized test scores. *American Journal of Education, 113*, 451-478.

Fertig, M., Schmidt, C.M., and Sinning, M. (2009). Human Capital Accumulation: Family Background, Cohort Effects and Unemployment. *Labour Economics,* 16, 659-668.

Finnie, R., and R. Meng (2002) "Are immigrants' human capital skills discounted in Canada?" School of Policy Studies, Queen's University, Working Paper JEL codes: J61, J31.

Fulgini, A. 1998. "The Adjustment of Children from Immigrant Families." *Current Directions in Psychological Science* 7:99–103.

García Coll, C., and Kerivan Marks, A. (Eds) (2012) The Immigrant Paradox in Children and Adolescents: Is Becoming American a Developmental Risk? Washington, DC: American Psychological Association.

Glick, J. E., and White, M.J. (2003). The academic trajectories of immigrant youths: Analysis within and across cohorts. *Demography*, 40,759- 83.

Grenier, G. 1984. "The Effects of Language Characteristics on the Wages of Hispanic American Males." *Journal of Human Resources* 19:35–52.

Grundy, E., and Sloggett, A. (2003). Health inequalities in the older population: The role of personal capital, social resources and socio-economic circumstances. *Social Science and Medicine, 56*, 935-947.

Hall, N., and Sham, S. (2007). Language Brokering as Young People's Work: Evidence from Chinese Adolescents in England. *Language and Education,* 21,16-30.

Haskins, R. and Tienda, M. (Spring 2011). The future of immigrant children. *The Future of Children, 21*, 1-7.

Huggett, M., Ventura, V., and Yaron, A. (2006). *Human Capital and Earnings Distribution Dynamics.* Journal of Monetary Economics, 53, 265-290.

Kao, G., and Tienda, M. (1995). Optimism and Achievement: The Educational Performance of Immigrant Youth, *Social Science Quarterly* 76, 1–19.

Keynes, J. M. (1920), The Economic Consequences of the Peace", Macmillan and Co. Limited.

Landale, N. S., Thomas, K. A., and Van Hook, J. (2011). The living arrangements of children of immigrants. *Future of Children*, 21, 43-70. doi:10.1162/jeea.2007.5.5.927.

Lewis, W.A. (1954), Economic Development with Unlimited supply of Labor", *The Manchester School*, 22, 139-91.

Li, J. (2004). "I learn and I grow big": Chinese preschoolers' purposes for learning. *International Journal of Behavioral Development, 28*(2), 116–128.

Martin, D.C., and Yankay, J.E. (2011). Refugees and Asylees: 2011Asylum Division, U.S. Citizenship and Immigration Services (USCIS), of the Department of Homeland Security. Retrieved from: http://www.dhs.gov/xlibrary/assets/ statistics/publications/ois_rfa_fr_2011.pdf

McKenzie, D. J. (2008). A profile of the world's young developing country international migrants. *Population and Development Review, 34,* 115-135. doi:10.1111/j.1728-4457.2008.00208.x.

Morse, A. (2005). *A Look at Immigrant Youth: Promising Prospects and Promising Practices.* National Conference of State Legislatures, Children's Policy Initiative. Washington, D.C. Retrieved from :http://www.ncsl.org

NCLB (2002). No Child Left Behind Act of 2001. Retrieved from: http://www2.ed.gov/policy/elsec/leg/esea02/107-110.pdf.

Osorio-O'Dea, P. (2001). The Federal Emergency Immigrant Education Program. The Library of Congress Retrieved from:http://www.policyarchive.org/handle/10207/bitstreams/3254.pdf.

Passel, J.S., and Cohn, D. (2011) *Unauthorized Immigrant Population: National and State Trends, 2010.* Pew Hispanic Center. Retrieved from http://www.pewhispanic.org/2011/02/01/unauthorized-immigrant-population-brnational-and-state-trends-2010/

Passel, J.S., and Taylor, P. (2010). *Unauthorized Immigrants and Their U.S.-Born Children* Retrieved from: http://pewhispanic.org/files/reports/ 125.pdf.

Perreira, K. M., Mullan Harris, K., and Lee, D. (2007). Immigrant youth in the labor market. *Work and Occupations*, 34, 5-34. doi: 10.1177/0730888406295394.

Portes, A., and Rumbaut, R. G., (2001). *Legacies: The store of the immigrant second generation.* Berkeley: University of California Press.

Portes, A., and Schauffler, R. (1994). Language and the second generation: Bilingualism yesterday and today. International Migration Review, 28(4), 640-661.

Potocky-Tripodi, M. (2004). The Role of Social Capital in Immigrant and Refugee Economic Adaptation. *Journal of Social Service Research, 31*(1), 59-91. doi:10.1300/J079v31n01_04.

Rytina, N. (2011). *Estimates of the Legal Permanent Resident Population in 2010.* Office of Immigration Statistics, Policy Directorate, U.S. Department of Homeland Security. Retrieved from http://www.dhs.gov/xlibrary/assets/ statistics/publications/ois_lpr_pe_2010.pdf.

Sam, D.L, Vedder, P., Ward, C., and Horenczyk, G. (2006). Immigrant Youth:"Psychological and Socio-cultural Adaptation of Immigrant Youth." Pp. 117–42 in *Immigrant Youth in Cultural Transition: Acculturation, Identity, and Adaptation across National Contexts*, edited by JohnW. Berry, Jean S. Phinney, David L. Sam, and Paul Vedder. New York: Lawrence Erlbaum.

Schuller, T. (2000). Social and Human Capital: The Search for Appropriate Technomethodology', *Policy Studies*, 21, 25-35.

Schultz, T.W. (1993). The economic importance of human capital in modernization. *Education Economics, 1*(1), 13-19.

Shrestha, L. and Heisler, E. (2011). *The changing demographic profile of the US*. Congressional Research Service. Retrieved from http://www.fas.org/sgp/crs/misc/RL32701.pdf.

Smith, A. (1937). *An Inquiry into the Nature and Causes of the Wealth of Nations Book 2 – Of the Nature, Accumulation, and Employment of Stock* (First Published 1776). The Modern Library, Random House, Inc.

Smith, C.L. (2012). The Impact of Low-Skilled Immigration on the Youth Labor Market. *Journal of Labor Economics*, 30, 55-89.

Suárez-Orozco, C., Gaytán, F.X., Bang, H.J., Pakes, J., O'Connor, E., and Rhodes, J. (2010). Academic trajectories of newcomer immigrant youth. Developmental Psychology, 46, 602-618.

Trickett, E., and Jones, C. (2007). Adolescent Culture Brokering and Family Functioning: A Study of Families from Vietnam. *Cultural Diversity and Ethnic Minority Psychology*, 13, 143-50.

Tseng, V., Chao, R. K., and Padmawidjaja, I. A. (2007). Asian Americans' educational experiences. In F. T. L. Leong, A. Ebreo, L. Kinoshita, A. G.Inman, L. Yang, and M. Fu (Eds.), *Handbook of Asian American psychology*(2nd ed., pp. 102–123). Thousand Oaks, CA: Sage. U.S. Census Bureau. *Statistical abstract of the United States: 2003.* Washington, DC: 2004, table no. 7; and U.S. Census Bureau. *Statistical abstract of the United States: 2002.* Washington, DC: 2003, table no. 43.

Van Tubergen, F., and Van De Werfhorst, H. (2007). Postimmigration investments in education: A study of immigrants in the Netherlands. *Demography, 44*, 883-898. doi:10.1353/dem.2007.0046.

White, M. 1997. "Language Proficiency, Schooling, and the Achievement of Immigrants." Washington, DC: U.S. Department of Labor.

INDEX

#

20th century, 68
21st century, 15, 21, 25, 34, 94, 170

A

A Bullying Prevention Program, 114
Aberrant Information Processing, 79
Abraham, 38, 49
abstraction, 146, 149, 209, 219
abuse, 81, 89, 90, 91, 92, 94, 104, 132, 209, 314, 322, 328
academic motivation, 161, 165
academic performance, 279, 296, 356
academic problems, 238
academic progress, 101
academic success, 160, 166, 170, 268, 270, 272, 273, 283
accelerometers, 27
access, ix, 89, 91, 104, 116, 118, 119, 127, 164, 172, 173, 211, 267, 282, 292, 298, 301, 312, 324, 333, 334, 345, 352
accessibility, 301, 302, 303
accountability, 100, 102, 165, 168, 169, 312, 323, 338
accounting, 264
acculturation, 263, 269
accumulation of human capital, 349, 351, 352, 353, 355, 357, 360
achievement test, xii, 167, 263, 267
acid, 47
acquisition of knowledge, 225
activity level, 18, 19, 23, 27, 28, 29, 36
acute schizophrenia, 57
AD, 44

adaptability, 247
adaptation, 4, 97, 211, 239, 253, 266, 281, 351, 353, 354, 356
ADHD, 216, 247, 254, 255, 258
adiponectin, 20
adipose tissue, 33
adiposity, 19, 22, 23, 24, 27, 28, 33
adjustment, 38, 41, 43, 49, 51, 53, 55, 68, 96, 184, 235, 296
administrators, 115, 167, 197, 200, 337, 338, 339, 340
adolescent adjustment, 284
Adolescent and Family Anger Management (AFAM), 193
adolescent behavior, 99, 127
adolescent boys, 183, 185
adolescent development, xi, 96, 99, 100, 102, 159, 257, 284, 331
adolescent female, 136, 202
adult learning, 202
adult obesity, 22, 51
adulthood, ix, xi, 14, 18, 19, 20, 22, 24, 29, 30, 31, 68, 95, 99, 113, 127, 131, 132, 135, 136, 139, 141, 149, 151, 173, 209, 219, 246, 259, 285, 307
adults, 17, 19, 20, 21, 22, 23, 24, 25, 27, 28, 29, 33, 34, 37, 38, 39, 50, 51, 52, 62, 67, 71, 79, 84, 89, 115, 131, 140, 161, 173, 186, 187, 191, 219, 247, 248, 249, 251, 252, 258, 259, 261, 290, 291, 292, 293, 294, 304, 305, 306, 313, 355, 359
advancement, 352
adverse conditions, 266
adverse effects, 38, 40, 43, 45, 47, 49, 60, 64, 249
adverse event, x, 37, 46, 53, 64
advertisements, 133
advocacy, 309

affective disorder, 55, 68, 261
affective reactions, 251
affirming, 298
Afghanistan, 220
African Americans, 46, 161, 332, 333, 342, 343, 344
African-American, 14, 132, 134, 136, 167, 168, 244
agencies, ix, 102, 109, 113, 137, 138, 148, 172, 200, 322, 359
aggression, 89, 91, 99, 101, 111, 112, 113, 114, 115, 126, 127, 181, 182, 185, 187, 191, 194, 197, 200, 202, 203, 204, 205, 218, 254, 318
Aggression replacement training, 181, 202
aggressive behavior, 95, 97, 101, 112, 182, 187, 190, 200, 202, 204, 218
agility, 25
agonist, 40
agranulocytosis, 46
akathisia, 44, 45, 60
Alcohol, 97, 135, 136
alcohol abuse, 97
alcohol consumption, 17, 18, 19, 29
alcohol use, 95, 97, 109
alienation, 97
allele, 62
altruism, 152
American Academy of Child and Adolescent Psychiatry, 249, 260, 261, 262, 283
American College of Sports Medicine, 26, 34
American culture, 271
American Heart Association, 30, 31, 34
American paediatrics, 38, 49
American Psychiatric Association, 68, 74, 81
American Psychological Association, 361
amino, 47
amino acid, 47
Amisulpride, 40, 43, 58
amplitude, 302
anger, xi, 97, 150, 170, 181, 182, 184, 185, 187, 188, 190, 191, 192, 193, 194, 195, 197, 200, 202, 204, 205
Anger control training, 182, 204
Anhedonia, 67, 72, 73, 74, 75, 76, 77, 78, 79
ANOVA, 120
antagonism, 41, 42, 43
anthropology, 153, 176
anticholinergic, 38, 42, 45, 65
antidepressant, 42, 44, 46, 58, 62
antidepressants, 42, 62

antipsychotic, 37, 38, 39, 40, 45, 46, 48, 49, 50, 51, 54, 55, 56, 58, 59, 60, 61, 62, 63, 64 , 494
antipsychotic drugs, 37, 39, 40, 46, 48, 49, 54, 55, 56, 59, 63
Antipsychotic drugs, 59
antisocial acts, 182
antisocial adolescents, xi, 184
antisocial behavior, 95, 100, 104, 181, 182, 187, 203, 204, 327
antisocial children, 104
antisocial personality, 93
anxiety, 42, 44, 57, 127, 255, 258, 279, 285, 337
anxiety disorder, 44, 258
Appearance of environment, 143
appointments, 301, 302
appraisals, 279
aptitude, 151
aripiprazole, 38, 39, 40, 43, 44, 45, 48, 58, 59, 249
arousal, 183
arrest, 187, 316, 320, 321, 334, 343, 347
artery, 30
articulation, 301, 302
Asia, 325
Asian Americans, 363
assault, 91, 94, 97, 183, 184, 196
Assertivity, 152
assessment tools, 4
assets, 30, 32, 280, 307, 350, 352, 362, 363
assimilation, 349, 350, 351, 352, 355, 357, 360
asthma, 18
asylees, 350, 352
asylum, 352
asymmetry, 75
atherosclerosis, 32
atmosphere, 213
attachment, 170, 210, 211
Attention Deficit Disorder (ADD), 216
Attention Deficit Hyperactive Disorder (ADHD), 216
Attenuated Psychotic Symptoms Risk Syndrome, 80
attitudes, xii, 5, 9, 93, 101, 115, 196, 197, 205, 247, 259, 263, 271, 275, 276, 277, 305, 335, 337, 343
attribution, 217
Austria, xi, 54, 207, 214, 220
authenticity, 276
Authoritarian parenting, 122

Index

authority, 97, 98, 104, 143, 153, 154, 155, 168, 169, 317, 320, 322, 335, 343, 344
autism, 44, 64
autonomy, 93, 141, 142, 153, 211, 251, 271, 272, 273, 291, 292, 296, 297
Autonomy Development and Integration Project, 295
Auxiliary Ego, 212, 216
avoidance, 43, 45, 136, 211
awareness, x, 50, 51, 90, 98, 101, 108, 114, 115, 153, 210, 215, 222, 253, 255, 271, 272, 303, 305

B

barriers, 172, 258, 304, 305, 352, 358
base, 27, 52, 107, 127
basic needs, 213, 273
Batshaw Youth and Family Centres, 193
BD, xi, 31, 245, 246, 247, 248, 249, 250, 251, 252, 253, 254, 255, 257, 258, 259
behavioral change, 184
behavioral disorders, 202, 205
behavioral problems, 191, 296
behaviors, 5, 6, 9, 14, 29, 68, 89, 94, 101, 104, 105, 114, 116, 117, 118, 122, 124, 126, 127, 136, 167, 182, 193, 198, 215, 218, 219, 222, 247, 250, 255, 259, 266, 275, 332, 333, 335, 345, 351
belief systems, 175
beneficial effect, 49
beneficiaries, 294, 299
benefits, 26, 27, 28, 35, 59, 162, 191, 193, 194, 199, 201, 220, 226, 257, 290, 291, 292, 294, 303, 304, 305, 306, 345
beverages, 12
bias, 4, 14, 45, 133, 167, 338
bile, 52
bilingual, 164, 263, 265, 272, 274, 275, 276, 277, 279, 280, 281, 358
biomarkers, 20, 39
bipolar disorder, xi, 61, 245, 246, 257, 259, 260, 261, 262
bipolar illness, 245, 246, 249, 250, 253, 257, 258, 259, 262
birth cohort, 83, 85, 355
births, 283, 359
BJS, 346
blame, 90, 95, 247

blood, 4, 18, 22, 24, 34, 35, 37, 39, 48, 49, 50, 52, 53, 54, 55, 58
blood flow, 52
blood pressure, 4, 22, 24, 34, 35
blood vessels, 18
blueprint, 167
BMI, 21, 22, 23, 24, 27, 28, 34
Board of Commissioners, 337, 339
body composition, 22, 24, 25, 52
body fat, 22, 24, 27, 34, 35, 52
body mass index, 4, 21, 32, 33
body weight, 4, 13, 28, 51, 57
Bogalusa Heart Study, 18, 20, 24, 30, 32
bonding, 92, 93, 97, 169, 211
bonds, 92, 171, 172, 215
bone, 26, 27
borderline personality disorder, 63
boredom, 165
bottom-up, 149
brain, 39, 175, 212
Brazil, 21
breast cancer, 27
breathing, 183
breeding, 96
Brittany, 241
Bronfenbrenner, 335, 346
brutality, 96
budget cuts, 319
budgetary resources, 323, 324
bullying, x, 90, 94, 111, 112, 113, 114, 115, 116, 117, 120, 121, 122, 123, 124, 125, 126, 127, 128, 129
Bureau of Justice Assistance, 327
Bureau of Justice Statistics, 128, 346
bureaucracy, 301
businesses, 146

C

cabbage, 10
caffeine, 132
caliber, 237
California Institute for Mental Health, 188
campaigns, 98, 294, 306
candidates, 11, 53, 276, 277, 278
cannabis, 71, 80, 131, 132, 134, 136
capacity building, 293, 306
capital accumulation, 351, 352, 357
capital consumption, 358
carbamazepine, 48, 55, 62

cardiomyopathy, 46, 61
cardiovascular disease, x, 14, 17, 31, 33, 35, 46
cardiovascular morbidity, 29, 30, 51
cardiovascular risk, 20, 29, 30, 31, 32, 34, 35
Cardiovascular Risk in Young Finns Study, 18, 30
cardiovascular system, 18
caregivers, xi, 181, 184, 192, 193, 194, 196, 197, 200, 201, 251, 262
caregiving, 247, 259
cartoon, 103
case studies, 98
Caucasians, 23, 46, 47, 62
causal attribution, 336
causal relationship, 29, 183, 245, 246
causality, 191
cell membranes, 52
cell phones, 112
Census, 160, 161, 163, 178, 265, 283, 284, 328, 349, 350, 363
Center for Education and Drug Abuse Research (CEDAR), 131
central nervous system, 51, 52
central obesity, 23, 24
certificate, 145, 358
certification, 275, 281
CFI, 230, 231
challenges, xii, 4, 13, 21, 31, 49, 104, 110, 146, 154, 159, 160, 162, 163, 171, 254, 282, 289, 296, 303, 307, 308, 331, 349, 351
chaos, 260
character traits, 194
chemical, 38, 48, 81
Chicago, 85, 117, 240, 241, 361
chicken pox, 272
child abuse, 94, 104
child benefit, 147
child development, 100, 103, 176, 245, 246
child labor, 94, 95
child protection, 307, 308
childcare, 106, 139
childhood, 4, 14, 17, 18, 20, 22, 24, 29, 30, 92, 95, 96, 127, 132, 139, 140, 207, 208, 209, 245, 246, 256, 258, 262, 271, 281, 359
childhood disorders, 258
ChildLine India, 95
China, xi, 21, 220, 223, 224, 350
Chlamydia, 136
cholesterol, 31
chronic diseases, 22
cigarette smoking, 31, 55

circadian rhythm, 253, 256
CIS, 289, 295, 299, 307
cities, 89, 91, 94, 95, 284, 312, 324, 346, 352
citizens, 93, 145, 147, 151, 152, 165, 264, 306, 309, 357, 360
citizenship, 265, 291, 292, 307, 357
City, 170, 223
Civil Rights Project at UCLA, 166
clarity, 267
classes, 50, 97, 139, 166, 173, 216, 228, 230
classification, xii, 20, 51, 114, 263, 345
classroom, 6, 7, 9, 14, 73, 115, 128, 143, 161, 164, 167, 168, 175, 177, 194, 215, 216, 225, 228, 268, 272, 278, 279, 284, 285
classroom management, 284
classroom teacher, 6, 14
clients, 213, 214, 217, 219, 220
climate, 115, 161, 297, 339
clinical application, 42
clinical judgment, 53
clinical symptoms, 19
clinical trials, 50, 259
close relationships, 269
clothing, 97, 213
clozapine, 38, 39, 40, 41, 45, 46, 48, 49, 55, 56, 61, 63
Clozapine, 40, 41, 56, 61
cluster analysis, 343, 344
cluster sampling, 73
clustering, 14, 18, 31, 226, 230, 231, 234, 235
clusters, 218
CNS, 52, 53, 58, 62
coaches, 148
cocaine, 131, 132, 134
coding, 38, 47
cognition, 42, 43, 45, 61, 203, 205
cognitive ability, 3, 4, 5
cognitive development, 224
cognitive function, 46, 59
cognitive impairment, 57
cognitive perspective, 211
cognitive skills, 182, 202, 272, 305
cognitive testing, 4, 10
cognitive-behavioral therapy, 252, 262
coherence, 168
collaboration, 27, 226, 339
collectivism, 168, 169
College Entrance Examination, 279
college students, 94, 111, 124, 125, 269, 281, 344
colleges, 99, 139, 173, 174

Index 369

color, 166, 170, 171, 177, 346
combination therapy, 59, 249
combined effect, 57
Commitment Reduction Program (CRP), 320
common sense, 214, 337
communication, 94, 95, 96, 100, 101, 103, 104, 112, 113, 117, 124, 125, 126, 138, 140, 145, 147, 150, 151, 155, 203, 213, 220, 251, 252, 253, 254, 258, 271, 291, 357
communication patterns, 103
communication skills, 140, 253, 271
Community Assessment of Psychic Experiences-42 (CAPE-42), 72
Community Juvenile Accountability Act, 187
community psychology, 345
community service, 303, 318
community support, 104, 289, 299, 300
Community Youth Investment Project (CYIP), 319
community-based services, 316, 321
comorbidity, 53, 258, 259, 260
comparative analysis, 33
compassion, 272, 273
compensation, 152, 239
competition, 96, 238, 353, 358
competitive advantage, 351
competitiveness, 238
complexity, 211, 236, 238, 246, 335, 344
compliance, 41, 45, 49, 53, 55, 249
complications, 29, 97, 100
composites, 230, 235
composition, 25, 52, 164, 232, 277, 343, 361
comprehension, 73, 292, 299
computer, 115, 141
computing, 11
conception, 340
conceptual model, xi, 290
conceptualization, 291
concordance, 110
conduct disorder, 100, 101, 110, 203, 204, 216, 258
conductor, 215
conference, 133, 177, 271, 359
confidentiality, 75, 293, 302, 303, 305
confinement, 108, 312, 313, 314, 315, 316, 317, 318, 319, 320, 321, 322, 323, 324, 325, 328
conflict, 96, 100, 105, 107, 111, 121, 122, 125, 126, 150, 183, 209, 211, 212, 213, 215, 216, 217, 218, 247, 248, 252, 257, 262, 298, 299, 345

conflict resolution, 216, 298, 299
conformity, 72, 73
confrontation, 212
Congress, 334, 357, 362
consciousness, 168, 170, 210, 272
consensus, 33, 50, 93, 133, 169, 190
Consensus, 63
consent, 4, 9, 117, 121, 127, 197, 296, 298
constipation, 43
Constitution, 265
construct validity, 83
construction, 69, 70, 73, 74, 214
consulting, 305, 306
consumers, 256
consumption, 9, 15, 141, 155, 357
content analysis, 296, 300
contingency, 197, 198
control condition, 183, 184, 185, 186, 188, 191
control group, 115, 116, 183, 184, 185, 186, 188, 190, 191
control measures, 108
controlled studies, 58
controlled trials, 35, 58, 59, 249
controversial, 245, 257
convention, 290, 309
convergence, 274
conversations, 169
conviction, 94, 108, 211, 217
cooking, 214
cooperation, 106, 142, 152, 154, 155, 337, 345
coping, 80, 170, 171, 200, 221, 249, 251, 253, 254, 255, 258, 266, 279, 280, 292
coping strategies, 80, 200, 251, 253
coronary heart disease, 25, 27, 30
correlation, 7, 12, 75, 78, 81, 82, 114, 118, 122, 165, 170, 196, 217, 234, 236
correlation coefficient, 7
cost, 13, 21, 53, 151, 165, 200, 220, 301, 311, 312, 314, 315, 316, 317, 318, 319, 320, 321, 323, 328, 336, 338
cost effectiveness, 53
cost saving, 319
Council of Europe, 156
counseling, 90, 98, 103, 105, 195, 200, 315, 321
country of origin, 264, 352
course work, 229
covering, 109, 213, 216, 296
cracks, 165
C-reactive protein (CRP), 20
Creative Circle, 208

creativity, 213
crimes, 98, 108, 183, 217, 314, 332, 333, 335
criminal activity, 337
criminal behavior, x
criminal justice system, 196, 328, 333
criminality, 334
criminals, 91, 109, 334, 335
crises, 107, 323
crisis management, 253
critical thinking, 273
criticism, 248, 250, 257
cross-sectional study, 30, 64, 128, 132, 134
CRP, 20, 320
crystallization, 208
CT, 14, 31, 85, 243
Cuba, 350
cues, 183, 194
cultural beliefs, 168
cultural differences, 168, 357
cultural diversity, 263
cultural heritage, 277, 353, 356
cultural influence, 239
cultural norms, 269
cultural tradition, 353
cultural values, 104, 150, 353
culture, 95, 100, 108, 146, 149, 152, 155, 159, 160, 161, 167, 168, 169, 171, 172, 174, 176, 178, 185, 239, 265, 269, 271, 273, 274, 277, 293, 304, 305, 308, 334, 351, 352, 353, 356, 358
Curfews, 334
curricula, 9
curriculum, 15, 29, 103, 114, 166, 167, 168, 170, 173, 273, 278, 281
CVD, x, 17, 18, 19, 20, 22, 23, 24, 25, 27, 28, 29
CVD risk profiles, 19, 22
cyberbullying, 111, 112, 113, 114, 116, 117, 118, 119, 120, 121, 122, 123, 124, 125, 126, 127, 128
Cyberbullying Survey, 117, 118, 120, 121, 124
Cybervictimization, 117, 121, 123
cycles, 253
cycling, 249
cytochrome, 38, 47, 50, 56, 60, 61, 62
Cytochrome P450 (CYP450), 48

D

daily living, 291
dance, 139, 143, 216
danger, 91
data analysis, 188
data collection, 4
data set, 162
database, 220
deaths, 18, 25, 97
decision makers, 306, 325
decision-making process, 291, 292, 304, 305
decomposition, 147
deduction, 141
defensiveness, 276
deficiency, 51
deficit, 72, 93, 160, 161, 162, 170, 171, 174, 216, 247, 316
delinquency, 89, 181, 196, 200, 202, 273, 331, 333, 334, 336, 337, 338, 339, 344, 345, 347
delinquent acts, 104, 335
delinquent adolescents, 193
delinquent behavior, 101, 107, 115, 196
delinquent friends, 91, 97
delinquent group, 271
delusions, 71
democracy, 152, 293, 305, 335
Democracy, 152, 241
demographic characteristics, 111
demographic factors, 133, 300
Demographic Information and Access to Technology Survey, 117, 121
demographics, 167, 197, 276, 349, 350, 360
Denmark, 20, 27, 31, 32
dentist, 148
Department of Education, 75, 128, 167, 191, 274, 279, 280, 284
Department of Education of the Principality of Asturias, 75
Department of Health and Human Services, 26, 27
Department of Homeland Security, 352, 357, 362, 363
Department of Justice, 114, 128, 347
Department of Youth Services (DYS), 317
dependent variable, 120, 198
depression, 19, 27, 42, 44, 46, 58, 69, 80, 94, 98, 101, 105, 113, 129, 217, 246, 247, 251, 252, 254, 255, 269
Depression, 64, 65, 216
depressive symptomatology, 252
depressive symptoms, 81, 247, 248, 252, 254
deprivation, 64
depth, x, 4, 5, 13, 18, 19, 67, 83, 115, 142, 145, 214, 291, 294, 306

Index

desensitization, 92
detachment, 272
detection, 29, 33, 57, 69, 70, 73, 75, 78, 80, 238
detention, 90, 108, 136, 139, 207, 318, 321, 337, 342
deterrence, 332
developed countries, 18
developmental change, 38, 49, 52
developmental factors, 38
developmental psychology, 280
developmental psychopathology, 261, 280
DHS, 357
diabetes, 17, 18, 19, 22, 29, 31, 33, 38, 45, 54, 68, 82
Diagnostic and Statistical Manual of Mental Disorders, 81
diagnostic criteria, 74, 134
dialogues, 155, 294
dichotomy, 84
diet, 4, 15, 17, 19, 29, 32, 298
dietary habits, 18
dietary intake, 4, 13, 14
differential treatment, 335
diffusion, 52
digital cameras, 12
digital communication, 111, 127
Digital Image Food Records (DIFR), x, 3
dignity, 166
direct observation, 4
directionality, 259
disability, 80, 246, 261
disadvantaged youth, 215, 221
discrimination, 96, 173, 224, 227, 230, 232, 271, 305, 336, 343, 344, 352, 353, 360
diseases, 19
disorder, 18, 45, 57, 58, 60, 68, 69, 71, 80, 81, 84, 85, 134, 136, 203, 204, 214, 216, 246, 247, 251, 253, 254, 255, 256, 257, 258, 259, 260, 261
displacement, 24
disposition, 55, 65, 315
dissatisfaction, 297
dissociation, 60
Distortion of Reality, 73
distortions, 183
distress, 80, 81, 113, 247
distribution, 20, 38, 47, 52, 72, 74, 97, 121
divergence, 69
diversity, 62, 100, 151, 168, 172, 173, 174, 177, 263, 264, 276, 281, 293, 357

division of labor, 226
DNA, 46
doctors, 98, 148
DOI, 56, 63
domestic tasks, 298
domestic violence, 196
Dominican Republic, 350
dopamine, 39, 40, 42, 43, 44, 45, 46, 59, 60
dorsolateral prefrontal cortex, 43
dosage, 39, 46, 48, 50, 51, 52, 53, 55, 56
dose-response relationship, 43
dosing, 39, 41, 42, 44, 50, 52, 53, 57
Doubling, 213, 214, 215, 216, 219
draft, 6
drawing, 216
dream, 62, 212, 282, 283, 355
drug abuse, 94, 102, 273
drug action, 51
drug addict, 97
drug interaction, 43, 45, 50, 53, 57, 62
drug metabolism, 48, 49, 51, 60
drug offense, 316, 334
drug reactions, 48
drug safety, 39
drug targets, 51, 65
drug therapy, 49, 53, 60
drug treatment, 45, 249
drugs, 37, 38, 40, 41, 42, 45, 46, 47, 48, 50, 51, 52, 53, 59, 62, 89, 91, 95, 96, 97, 132, 134, 249, 343
DSM, 132, 133
DSM-IV-TR, 74
dynamic risk factors, 337
dyslipidemia, 17, 18, 19, 22, 29
dysphoria, 45
dysthymic disorder, 255
dystonia, 45

E

earnings, 352, 355
East Asia, 23
economic development, 89, 170
economic resources, 356
economic status, 104, 160, 304
economic theory, 346
economic well-being, 351
economics, 361
editors, 34, 55
Education Commission of the States, 172

Education Development Center, Inc., 171
education policy, 358
educational attainment, ix, 270
educational experience, 277, 363
educational institutions, 139
educational opportunities, ix, xi, 159, 168, 352
educational policy, 112
educational psychologists, 160
educational research, 175
educational services, 186
educational settings, 70, 80
educational system, 146, 270
educators, 13, 161, 165, 167, 168, 169, 171, 172, 173, 175, 258, 265, 270, 271, 274, 277, 297, 298, 299, 303, 358, 359
Eductive reasoning, 227
EEG, 40
Effective programs, 190
Efficacious programs, 190
elaboration, 223, 284
elders, 168, 169
elementary school, 5, 6, 9, 11, 91, 103, 218, 272, 282, 285, 358
elementary students, 115
eligible youth, 322
elucidation, 39
e-mail, 67, 289
emergency, 145, 147, 301
emotion, 138, 181, 182, 192, 194, 201, 221, 247, 259
emotion regulation, 182, 194
emotional distress, 113
emotional problems, 188
emotional responses, 247
emotional state, 214
empathy, 101, 146, 186, 271, 297
empirical studies, 160, 306
employees, 212
employment, 99, 100, 102, 110, 139, 145, 149, 152, 156, 162, 243, 269, 270, 284, 296, 297, 298, 333, 351, 353, 355, 361, 363
employment attainment, 353
employment opportunities, 333
empowerment, 102, 170, 293, 334
encouragement, 106, 109
endocrine, 51
endophenotypes, 84
end-users, 295
energy, 14, 19, 24, 25, 26, 28, 33, 34, 42, 212
energy expenditure, 25, 26

enforcement, 108, 166, 334, 338
England, 21, 27, 30, 32, 84, 187, 308, 325, 362
English dominant, 263
English Language, 163, 164, 165, 265, 274, 278, 280, 282, 359
English learners, 263, 279, 280
enrollment, 178, 359
environmental factors, 89, 162, 165, 171, 204
environmental stress, 249, 250
environments, xi, 4, 137, 138, 139, 140, 141, 142, 143, 144, 145, 147, 155, 159, 160, 161, 162, 163, 167, 168, 172, 173, 247, 248, 263, 270, 344
enzyme, 38, 41, 42, 43, 44, 46, 47, 48, 51, 52, 62
epidemic, 22, 89, 90, 93
epidemiologic, 84, 246
epidemiologic studies, 246
epidemiology, 261
epigenetics, 47
EPS, 38, 39, 41, 42, 43, 44, 45, 46
Equal Educational Opportunities Act, 266
equality, 142, 335, 360
equity, 163, 168, 174, 177
Estonia, 20, 27, 28, 31
ethics, 275
ethnic groups, 4, 47, 52, 168
ethnic minority, 164, 173
ethnicity, 117, 120, 121, 160, 161, 162, 163, 174, 195, 293, 356, 361
etiology, x, 17, 32, 132, 252, 344
Etiology, 204
Europe, 20, 21, 28, 32, 33, 35, 114, 186, 326
European Medicines Agency (EMEA), 46, 61
European Youth Heart Study, 18, 27, 30, 31, 33, 35
everyday life, 105, 182, 208, 213
evidence-based policy, 31
evidence-based program, 125
Evidence-Based Program Directory, 114, 115, 128
evil, 90
evolution, 174, 306
examinations, 276
Excessive Social Anxiety, 73, 74, 75, 76, 77, 78
exclusion, 160, 161, 177, 278, 305
excretion, 38, 52
executive function, 43
executive functioning, 43
exercise, 4, 25, 26, 28, 34, 35, 214, 216, 226, 255, 256, 308
expenditures, 311, 312, 313, 315, 321, 323

experimental design, 114, 342, 345
expertise, 53, 220, 301, 302
exploitation, 151
exposure, 11, 15, 20, 45, 46, 60, 89, 92, 93, 96, 97, 110, 177, 230, 256, 266, 267, 354
Expressed emotion, 247, 259
expulsion, 167
Extensive metabolizers (EM), 47
external validity, 201
extrapyramidal effects, 45
extreme poverty, 163

F

face validity, 15
facial expression, 216
facilitators, 183, 192, 194, 290, 293
factor analysis, 74, 85, 196, 230
factories, 166, 173
Factors for physical health, 298
Factors for psychological health, 297
fairness, 275
faith, ix, 352
false belief, 150
Family Assessment System, 121, 122, 123
family characteristics, 89
family conflict, 121, 122, 124, 125, 126, 187, 247, 250, 252, 258, 267
family environment, 111, 116, 126, 245, 246, 247, 248, 249, 250, 251, 252, 257
family factors, 246, 283
family functioning, xi, 245, 246, 247, 248, 251, 259
family income, 171
family interactions, 256
family life, 99, 121
family literacy, 359
family meals, 13
family members, 91, 92, 93, 94, 95, 98, 103, 111, 122, 126, 182, 184, 192, 195, 203, 247, 251, 259, 353
family planning, 147, 301
family relationships, 297
family studies, 50
family support, 102, 267, 301, 302
family system, 211, 245, 251, 254, 261
family therapy, 201, 250, 318
Family Tree, 214
family units, 357
fantasy, 210, 216

fat, 10, 19, 21, 22, 23, 24, 33
FDA, 42, 44, 58, 61
fear, 89, 93, 103, 213, 220, 269, 272
federal law, 265
feelings, 97, 165, 182, 183, 192, 194, 209, 210, 214, 215, 216, 218, 255, 297
female rat, 64
FFT, 200, 251, 252, 253, 254, 258
fibrinogen, 20
fidelity, 114, 190
fifth grade teachers, 268
fights, 99, 103, 182, 196
Filipino, 354
financial, ix, xii, 18, 146, 154, 162, 163, 171, 173, 282, 296, 298, 299, 302, 305, 311, 312, 313, 314, 315, 316, 318, 319, 320, 322, 352, 354
financial capital, 352, 354
financial incentives, xii, 311, 313, 314, 315, 319
financial resources, 305, 312, 319, 322
financial stability, ix
financial system, 154
Finland, 21
firearms, 89, 91, 97
first degree relative, 69
first generation, 45, 353, 354, 355, 356
First Universe, 210
fish, 5
fitness, 23, 25, 26, 27, 28, 31, 33, 34, 35
FITNESSGRAM test assessment programme, 24
flexibility, 169, 220, 271, 299
fluctuations, 311, 320
fluid, 344
focus groups, 4, 296, 300, 301, 308
food, 4, 5, 6, 7, 9, 10, 11, 12, 13, 15, 97, 106, 218, 297
food intake, 13
food safety, 6, 10
Food Taste Test Tool (TTT), x, 3
force, 90, 176, 225, 350, 353
Ford, 226, 241
formal education, 140, 155, 164
formation, 137, 138, 208, 209, 238, 246, 256, 270
formula, 316, 322
foster youth, 308
foundations, 138, 156, 157, 168, 279, 359
framing, 13
France, 21, 324, 326
Free time, 141
freedom, 209, 264, 298
Freud, 159, 175

friendship, 97, 104
fruits, 7, 9, 11, 13
Functional family therapy, 201
funding, 5, 163, 228, 312, 313, 315, 316, 317, 319, 322, 323, 325, 326, 327, 332, 337
funds, 108, 311, 315, 316, 317, 319, 323, 358, 359
fusion, 208

G

gambling, 91
gangs, 95, 96, 97, 139, 271, 334
gastrointestinal tract, 52
gender differences, 116, 125, 128
gender role, 270
gene regulation, 51
general education, 358
General Education Diploma (GED), 165
generalizability, 201
generalized anxiety disorder, 44, 57, 59
generational differences, 353
generational factors, 263
generational status, 356
genes, 38, 45, 46, 47
genetic background, 80
genetic factors, 48, 80
genetic predisposition, 74
genetics, 60
genital warts, 134
genomics, 65
genotype, 43, 45, 47, 53, 60, 62
genotyping, 41, 47, 48, 50, 53, 54, 62
Geographical Information Systems, 345
Georgia, 202, 220, 274
Germany, 21, 54, 220, 282, 324, 326
gifted, 236, 268, 272
glasses, 220
global scale, 292
globalization, 173
glucose, 4, 51
goal setting, 202
God, 272
gonorrhea, 134
Goodness-of-Fit Index, 230, 231
governance, 299
government funds, 108
governments, xii, 108, 152, 311, 312, 313, 323, 324, 359
governor, 319, 323, 326

grades, xi, 112, 120, 162, 223, 224, 225, 226, 227, 228, 229, 230, 231, 232, 234, 235, 236, 237, 238, 263, 267, 278, 279
grading, 225, 226, 236, 238
Graduation Really Achieves Dreams, 172
grants, 135, 169, 314, 334, 359
gravitation, 239
Great Britain, 186, 190
Greece, x, 37
group activities, 182, 214
group membership, 333, 354
group size, 51
group therapy, 192, 222
group treatment, 204, 205, 254
group work, 212, 214
Group-Centered Psychodrama, 218
grouping, 137, 225
growth, ix, 22, 23, 25, 102, 160, 248, 255, 264, 283, 317, 351, 358
guardian, 103, 121, 193
guidance, 33, 96, 100, 109
Guided Affective Imagery, 217
guidelines, 10, 26, 27, 50, 51, 74, 84, 121, 248, 260, 281, 300, 303, 323, 334, 338
gun control, 108

H

hallucinations, 82, 84
harassment, 93, 94, 113, 127, 129
harmony, 138
Hart, 291, 292, 306, 307
Harvard Growth Study, 32
Hawaii, 282
HE, 358
healing, 301, 302
health care, 49, 68, 80, 258, 262, 289, 290, 295, 298, 300, 301, 302, 303, 333, 352, 360
health care costs, 68
health care professionals, 258, 302
health care services, 295, 298, 300, 302, 303, 352
health care system, 302
health education, 303
health insurance, 175
health practitioners, 23, 200
health services, xii, 289, 308, 350, 351
health status, 19, 26, 27
healthier meal, 6
health-promoting behaviors, 30
heart attack, 34

heart disease, 30, 45
height, 13, 33, 94
helplessness, 270, 279
heritability, 133, 250
heroin, 132, 134
herpes, 134
heterogeneity, 39, 68, 191, 296
high blood cholesterol, 33
high blood pressure, 25
high school, 111, 112, 116, 117, 120, 124, 125, 126, 128, 162, 164, 165, 167, 170, 171, 172, 177, 215, 266, 267, 268, 271, 273, 280, 283, 358, 359
high school diploma, 358
high school dropouts, 359
higher education, 170, 175, 177, 225, 279, 280, 334, 354, 357, 358
hiring, 274, 346, 352, 360
Hispanic, viii, xi, 35, 120, 159, 160, 161, 162, 163, 164, 165, 166, 167, 168, 169, 170, 171, 172, 173, 174, 175, 176, 177, 178, 263, 264, 268, 270, 273, 274, 277, 279, 280, 281, 282, 283, 284, 285, 350, 361, 362
Hispanic adolescents, 159, 160, 162, 163, 165, 169
Hispanic population, 160, 161, 164, 165, 172, 264, 265
Hispanic/Latino student population, 263
histamine, 40, 43
historical data, 265
history, 49, 97, 104, 132, 133, 134, 173, 196, 215, 260, 265, 271, 278, 279, 325, 346
HIV, 134, 347
HIV/AIDS, 347
home culture, 352
homelessness, 90
homes, 90, 92, 94, 95, 126, 207, 213, 218, 219, 270, 271, 307, 311, 315, 319, 324, 338
homework, 192, 225, 267, 268, 270
homicide, 91, 97, 108
homicide rates, 108
homogeneity, 201
honesty, 194, 275
Hong Kong, xi, 223, 224, 227, 228, 230, 239, 240, 241, 242, 243, 244
hopelessness, 113, 170, 270
host, 214, 220, 351, 352, 353, 354, 356, 357, 358, 360
host country, 220, 351, 352, 354, 357, 360
host economy, 354

hostility, 91, 168, 193, 247, 257
House, 188, 213, 217, 220, 222, 363
housing, 105, 164, 213, 269, 278, 296, 298, 349, 350, 351
human, xii, 25, 48, 52, 55, 61, 62, 65, 91, 95, 109, 127, 151, 152, 154, 169, 175, 196, 208, 215, 222, 273, 293, 305, 344, 349, 350, 351, 352, 353, 354, 355, 356, 357, 360, 361, 363
human behavior, 127
human capital, xii, 349, 350, 351, 352, 353, 354, 355, 356, 357, 360, 361, 363
Human capital, 351, 357, 361
human development, 175
human health, 25
human resources, 109, 293, 305
human right, 152
human rights, 152
Hungary, xi, 137, 146, 155
Huskins, 291, 292, 308
hygiene, 256
hyperactivity, 247
hyperglycemia, 46
hyperlipidemia, 20, 38, 45, 46
Hyperlipidemia, 54
hyperprolactinemia, 38, 45
hypersensitivity, 46
hypertension, 17, 18, 19, 20, 27, 29, 31, 51
Hypertension, 31
hypothesis, 48, 60, 68

I

iatrogenic, 191, 202, 334, 335
Iatrogenic, 204, 205
ideal, 29, 30, 48, 101, 150, 209, 217, 218, 295, 299, 300, 301, 302, 303
ideals, 215
identification, xii, 20, 23, 24, 33, 37, 39, 53, 83, 100, 104, 175, 223, 227, 230, 232, 237, 263, 272, 290, 293, 297, 300, 302, 333, 336, 340, 345
identity, 104, 140, 145, 152, 159, 164, 171, 172, 173, 176, 208, 211, 213, 217, 220, 246, 251, 269, 270, 272, 278, 342
illicit substances, 132
Illinois Department of Juvenile Justice (IDJJ), 318
Illinois General Assembly, 318
image, 11, 12, 13, 15, 116, 117, 118, 119, 120, 121, 124, 127, 209, 214, 217, 218, 270, 294, 303

imagination, 216
imitation, 211
immigrant groups, 350, 354, 357, 358
Immigrant Paradox, 356, 361
immigrant youth, 349, 350, 351, 352, 354, 355, 356, 360, 361, 363
immigrants, xii, 264, 279, 282, 283, 285, 349, 350, 351, 352, 353, 354, 355, 356, 357, 358, 360, 361, 362, 363
immigration, 269, 279, 283, 350, 353, 357, 361
Immigration and Nationality Act, 358
impairments, 247
improvements, 18, 28, 42, 45, 101, 115, 181, 183, 186, 187, 188, 190, 191, 193, 199, 254, 256, 257
impulses, 152
impulsive, 93, 184
impulsiveness, 72, 184
In the relationship between residents, 298
in vivo, 127
inadmissible, 358
incarceration, 90, 166, 311, 312, 314, 315, 317, 320, 323, 324, 325, 326
incidence, 19, 38, 39, 45, 49, 84, 113, 132, 162
income, 4, 15, 91, 104, 164, 271, 333, 344, 351, 352, 353, 354, 357, 358, 359, 360
independence, 96, 103, 168, 169, 176, 209, 246, 291, 298, 307
independent living, 289, 295, 296, 298, 299, 303, 307, 308
independent variable, 197, 198
India, x, 89, 93, 94, 95, 98, 99, 103, 109, 240, 350
Indian Child Welfare Association (ICWA), 95
indirect effect, 136
individual character, 160
individual development, 281
Individual Family Psychoeducation (IFP), 251, 256
individual students, 9
individualism, 168, 169
individualization, 39, 48
individuation, 217
induction, 339
industrialization, ix
industry, 4
inequality, 271, 351, 361
INF, 74
infants, 51, 55, 91
infection, 40, 134
Inference, 71, 98

inflammation, 40, 55
Informal learning, 149
informed consent, 5, 9, 10, 75, 117, 133, 293, 296
ingredients, 4
inhibition, 212
inhibitor, 20, 42
initiation, 97, 107, 133, 151
injuries, 91, 133, 261
inmates, 334
insecurity, 297
insomnia, 57
Institutional overcrowding, 314, 324
Institutional Review Board, 5, 9, 117, 120, 133
institutionalisation, 143
institutions, 102, 108, 139, 140, 142, 143, 152, 154, 155, 162, 171, 203, 216, 276, 289, 294, 295, 296, 300, 304, 305, 333
instructional time, 166
insulin, 4, 18, 20
insulin resistance, 18
integration, 81, 151, 209, 266, 289, 296, 297
intelligence, xi, 160, 168, 223, 224, 225, 226, 227, 228, 229, 230, 231, 232, 234, 235, 236, 237, 238, 239, 283
Intelligence, viii, xi, 223, 224, 225, 229, 234, 235, 236, 240, 241, 242, 243, 244
interaction effect, 344, 345
interaction process, 157
Inter-analyst reliability, 12
intercourse, 134
Intercultural learning, 151
interdependence, 154, 168, 169, 176
interface, 141
intergenerational dependence, 353
internal consistency, 5, 67, 70, 75, 78, 79, 121, 196, 230
internal controls, 92, 250
internal environment, 335
internal processes, 212
Internal structure, 82
internal validity, 187
internalization, 228
International Diabetes Foundation (IDF), 23
interpersonal conflict, 255
Interpersonal Disorganization, 67, 73, 74, 76, 78, 79
interpersonal relations, 96, 126, 150, 159, 303
interpersonal skills, 184, 193
interrelations, 149, 222

Intervention, viii, ix, xi, 100, 102, 105, 106, 107, 115, 179, 295, 299
intervention strategies, 4, 14, 19, 73, 256
intima, 30
intimacy, 96, 211
intoxication, 41, 46, 53
Intra-Psychic Psychodrama, 214
investment, 30, 161, 303, 363
Involvement, vii, x, 96, 97, 99, 111, 116, 152, 242, 347
iron, 60
irritability, 44, 58
isolation, 94, 96, 104, 105, 220, 269, 297
Israel, 113
issues, ix, x, xi, 90, 93, 98, 103, 104, 105, 107, 109, 115, 116, 128, 147, 153, 163, 165, 169, 176, 214, 217, 249, 251, 263, 276, 279, 294, 302, 308, 314, 316, 322, 337, 350

J

Jews, 168
Jordan, 242, 278, 281
jumping, 220
junior high school, 112, 117, 128
Junior Schizotypy Scales (JSS), 70
jurisdiction, 324
Jurisdictions, 324
Juvenile Assessment Center/Care Management Organization (JAC/CMO), 321
juvenile crime, 95, 311, 316
Juvenile Crime Prevention Council (JCPC), 319
juvenile delinquency, 324, 337, 339
juvenile delinquents, 204, 205, 221, 312
juvenile justice, xii, 174, 181, 188, 195, 196, 199, 200, 201, 311, 312, 314, 315, 316, 319, 320, 321, 322, 323, 324, 325, 326, 327, 328, 331, 332, 333, 334, 336, 337, 338, 344, 345
Juvenile Justice and Delinquency Prevention Act, 332
Juvenile Justice Reform Act (JJRA), 319
juveniles, 64, 311, 312, 313, 314, 315, 316, 317, 318, 319, 320, 321, 325, 328

K

Keynes, 351, 362
kidnapping, 217
kindergarten, 139, 140, 143, 144, 358
kinetics, 50

knowledge acquisition, 292
Kohlbergian stages of moral development, 183

L

labor force, 350, 354
labor market, 96, 349, 350, 353, 354, 357, 360, 362
labour market, 147, 149
Lack of Close Friends, 73, 74, 75, 76, 77, 78
lack of confidence, 304
landscape, 274
language acquisition, 263, 355, 359
language barrier, 159, 169, 278, 359
llanguage development, 165
language diversity, 279
language proficiency, 269, 353, 354, 356
language skills, 271, 355, 357
language use, 353, 355, 356, 357
languages, 95, 172, 238, 266, 271, 359
Latent Trait of Intelligence, 227
Latin America, 356
Latinos, 162, 164, 167, 168, 174, 176, 177, 270, 271, 281, 283, 284
law enforcement, 166, 331, 333, 335, 336, 337
laws, 94, 108, 153, 265, 278, 312, 333, 335
lead, 18, 46, 48, 51, 71, 93, 161, 172, 181, 208, 211, 216, 250, 251, 257, 271, 339, 340, 352
leadership, xii, 104, 174, 294
leaks, 162, 165
learners, 165, 170, 263, 265, 266, 273, 279, 280, 281, 282, 358
learning difficulties, 147
learning environment, 139, 161, 164, 168, 267, 268, 275, 285, 358
learning outcomes, 160, 161, 164, 173
learning process, 139, 149, 202, 225
legal protection, 153
legislation, 108, 112, 153, 312, 314, 315, 316, 319, 322, 324, 328, 334
leisure, 137, 143, 149, 156, 224, 298, 301, 303
leisure time, 143
lending, 239
lens, 349, 350
level of education, 104, 344
LIFE, 84
life changes, 269
Life context, 297
life expectancy, 46
lifestyle behaviors, 18

lifetime, 19, 52, 68, 132, 134, 300
light, 44, 81, 97, 116, 126, 127, 214, 215, 258, 337
Likert scale, 77, 117, 121, 196
linear model, 344
lipids, 24
liquid chromatography, 57
literacy, 5, 175, 359
lithium, 249
Lithuania, 113
liver, 41, 44, 48, 52
living arrangements, 362
living environment, 352
lobbying, 155
local community, 168, 337
local government, ix, 141, 148, 155, 312, 313, 315, 320, 324, 333
local youth, 152, 316
locus, 272
loneliness, 113, 269
longevity, 27, 34
longitudinal study, 70, 84, 114, 131, 132, 134, 135, 136, 163, 284, 285
Louisiana, 274
love, 98, 138, 142, 273
low risk, 20, 266, 331, 336, 337, 339, 340, 341, 342
low-level youth offenders, 317, 319, 322
loyalty, 218

M

Mackintosh, 225, 226, 227, 242
magazines, 139
Magic Shop, 213, 214, 216
magical thinking, 69, 72, 76
magnitude, 44, 93, 99, 199
major depression, 58, 136
major depressive disorder, 42, 44
major issues, 90
majority, 17, 38, 45, 100, 124, 125, 151, 161, 164, 171, 191, 277, 315, 322, 337, 339, 341
man, 273
management, xi, xii, 19, 33, 54, 141, 150, 151, 154, 181, 184, 191, 192, 193, 194, 195, 200, 203, 251, 252, 254, 256, 294, 297, 298, 299, 301, 303, 305, 311, 320, 329, 338, 347
mania, 41, 42, 44, 58, 246, 249, 251, 252, 254, 255, 256, 260
manic, 58, 247, 248, 252, 254

manic symptoms, 247, 252, 254
manipulation, 150
manufacturing, 212
mapping, 332
marginalization, 155, 166, 171, 173, 271
marijuana, 97, 132, 215
marital conflict, 94, 105
marketing, 49
marriage, 93, 94, 99
Maryland, 359
mass, 14, 21, 32, 33, 95, 138, 140, 145
mass communication, 138, 140, 145
mass media, 95
material resources, 109
materials, 104, 116, 125, 229
maternal mood, 259
mathematical achievement, 225
mathematics, 230, 231, 234, 235, 237, 238, 267
matter, 94, 98, 99, 150, 212
Maturation, viii, xii, 331, 336
MB, 14, 15, 33
measurement, 21, 22, 23, 24, 29, 33, 34, 38, 48, 49, 54, 60, 67, 69, 70, 71, 72, 74, 79, 81, 82, 190, 192. 239
meat, 12
media, 30, 90, 93, 95, 99, 103, 138, 139, 140, 142, 147, 155, 173, 177, 221, 305, 314
media messages, 173
median, 68, 161
mediation, xi, 215, 223, 235, 298
medical, 22, 108, 133, 145, 150, 204, 246, 301, 303
medical care, 303
medical history, 22
medication, 39, 41, 42, 48, 51, 54, 69, 248, 249, 250, 251, 252, 258
medication compliance, 252
medicine, 49
mellitus, 22
membership, 97, 167, 196, 352
memory, 43, 46, 84
mental disorder, 50, 68, 69, 78, 132, 133, 255, 261
mental health, x, 80, 110, 113, 115, 188, 195, 199, 200, 217, 221, 257, 258, 259, 262, 279, 296, 318, 321
mental health professionals, 115
mental illness, 83, 250
mental image, 210
mental retardation, 133

messages, x, 15, 111, 117, 121, 124, 126, 127, 272, 295, 307
meta-analysis, 28, 35, 45, 55, 59, 85, 204, 205, 248, 259
Metabolic, 33, 47
metabolic disorder, 19, 42, 43, 46
metabolic disorders, 19, 46
metabolic disturbances, 46
metabolic syndrome, 23, 30, 31, 33, 51, 54
metabolism, 38, 40, 41, 47, 48, 49, 50, 52
Metabolism, 31, 32
metabolites, 40, 61
metabolized, 48, 50
methodology, 146, 150, 153, 296
methylation, 47
metropolitan areas, 165, 177
Mexican American, xi, 4, 31, 170, 263, 264, 265, 266, 267, 269, 273, 274, 275, 276, 277, 278, 279, 280, 282, 283
Mexico, 264, 274, 350, 357, 360
Miami, 204, 352
Michigan Department of Human Services, 321
Middle East, 21, 47
migrant population, 283
migrants, 362
migration, 52, 220, 269, 361
military, 217
milligrams, 41
miniature, 38, 49
Ministry of Women and Child Development, 93
minority, xii, 91, 104, 140, 151, 160, 163, 164, 167, 168, 173, 176, 177, 216, 271, 277, 304, 331, 332, 336, 337, 338, 341, 345, 349, 350, 351
minority groups, xii, 163, 164, 168, 337, 349, 350, 351
minority students, 164, 167, 168, 277
minors, 333
misconceptions, 150, 276
mission, 91, 138, 145, 156, 173, 318, 322
mixing, 341, 344
mobile phone, 95
Model programs, 190
Modeling, 241, 242
models, xii, 51, 72, 81, 90, 95, 96, 103, 136, 137, 138, 150, 171, 173, 200, 230, 231, 254, 265, 266, 289, 291, 306, 311, 331, 333, 336
moderate activity, 28
moderates, 262
moderators, 296, 335

modernisation, 139, 146
modernization, 363
modifications, 312
mold, 169, 170
molecules, 51
monopoly, 150
Monotherapy, 249
mood disorder, 57, 248, 250, 255, 256, 260, 261
mood states, 255
Moon, 317, 327
moral development, 183, 204
moral reasoning, xi, 181, 182, 183, 184, 185, 188, 190, 191, 192, 193, 201
moral training, 194
morbidity, 22, 32, 246
mortality, 18, 19, 20, 22, 23, 24, 25, 26, 29, 30, 31, 32, 33, 34, 45, 68, 84, 91, 136, 246, 261
mortality rate, 18, 29
motivation, 168, 175, 177, 183, 253, 267, 272, 273, 275, 279, 297
movement disorders, 38, 45, 60
Mplus, 230, 243
MR, 35
mucosa, 48
multicultural education, 276, 277
multiculturalism, 171
multidimensional, 72, 84
Multifamily Psychoeducation Groups (MFPG), 251
multiple factors, 128, 344
multiple regression, 118, 119, 120, 122, 123, 124
multiple regression analyses, 119, 123
multiple school system, 263
multiple-choice questions, 229
Multi-Systemic Therapy, 319
murder, 99, 184, 217, 317
muscarinic receptor, 40, 43
Muscatine Study, 18
music, 141, 301
mutations, 47
mutuality, 138, 143
myocardial infarction, 24, 31
myocarditis, 46, 61
MyPyramid food, 12

N

NAACP Legal Defense and Education Fund School to Prison Pipeline report, 166
narratives, 170, 215, 253

national borders, 154
National Center for Education Statistics, 128, 164, 174, 175, 265, 274, 279, 280, 282, 284
National Cholesterol Education Program (NCEP), 24
National Council for La Raza (NCLR), 166
national identity, 155
National Opinion Research Center, 168
nationality, 352
native population, 350
NCS, 261
negative attitudes, 274, 277
negative consequences, 159
negative effects, 164, 266, 269
negative influences, 103
negative mood, 255
negative outcomes, 126
negative relation, 27, 124
negativity, 91, 95, 257
neglect, 92, 94, 212, 214, 279, 328
negotiating, 194, 217, 269, 270
Nelson Mandela, 93
Nepal, 220
nervous system, 51, 52
Netherlands, 113, 240, 244, 352, 363
network members, 239
networking, 151, 354
neuroleptics, 56
neurons, 52
neuropsychology, 203
neurotransmission, 44
neurotransmitter, 39, 52
neutral, 230, 336, 338, 339
New England, 32, 33, 34
New Zealand, 70, 85
nicotine, 132
nightmares, 272
No Child Left Behind, 165, 172, 275, 359, 362
non-smokers, 42
norepinephrine, 40, 42, 43, 44, 57
normal development, 82
North Africa, 21
North America, 20, 32, 128, 260
Northern Ireland, 27
Norway, 27, 114, 115, 203
NRT, 47
nucleotides, 47
null, 223
nurses, 107
nursing, 301

nutrition, x, 3, 4, 5, 6, 9, 10, 12, 13, 14, 15

O

obedience, 142
obesity, x, 3, 4, 14, 15, 17, 18, 19, 21, 22, 23, 25, 29, 30, 31, 32, 33, 46, 51, 68, 217
Obesity, vii, x, 14, 17, 21, 31, 32, 33, 34
obesity prevalence, 19, 21, 25
obesity prevention, 4
objective tests, 191
objectivity, 343
observed behavior, 190, 191
obstacles, xi, 107, 159, 160, 161, 164, 176, 265, 278, 303, 304, 306
Oceania, 21
ODD, 216, 247, 255, 258
Odd Behavior, 73, 74, 75, 78
Odd Thinking and Language, 73, 74, 75, 76, 77, 78
OECD, 361
offenders, xii, 91, 93, 97, 126, 128, 186, 187, 190, 191, 201, 202, 203, 204, 205, 217, 311, 312, 313, 314, 315, 316, 317, 318, 319, 320, 322, 323, 324, 325, 327, 334, 337, 339, 340, 341, 342, 343, 344
Office of Justice Programs, 128
officials, 166, 312, 314, 321, 323, 324, 334
OH, 44, 181, 204, 327, 328
Ohio Department of Youth Services, 317, 328
Oklahoma, 274
olanzapine, 38, 39, 41, 42, 57, 58, 64, 249
Olanzapine, 40, 42, 43, 57, 58
Olweus Bullying Prevention Program, 114, 115
openness, 151
operations, 311, 312
opportunities, ix, 47, 93, 96, 99, 105, 106, 127, 139, 150, 152, 154, 160, 161, 163, 166, 168, 172, 173, 184, 192, 195, 238, 254, 273, 304, 309, 349, 350, 351, 352, 355, 356, 358, 359, 360
Oppositional-Defiant Disorder (ODD), 216
oppression, 175, 272
optimism, 272, 273
organ, 49, 290
organism, 53
Organization for Economic Cooperation and Development, 360
organs, 94, 95
outpatient, 54, 55, 72, 187, 245, 246, 261

outreach, 169, 359
overlap, 139, 189, 230, 355
oversight, 315, 320, 324, 338
overweight, x, 4, 14, 17, 18, 19, 20, 21, 22, 25, 29, 30, 32, 33, 35, 217
overweight adults, 4
Oviedo Questionnaire for Schizotypy Assessment (ESQUIZO-Q), 67, 70, 74, 76, 79
ownership, 104, 169, 292, 293, 306
Oxford-Liverpool Inventory of Feelings and Experiences, 84
oxidation, 65

P

Pacific, 110
pacing, 267, 268
paediatric patients, 38, 49, 52
pain, 93
pairing, 11
panic disorder, 44, 59
paradigm shift, 109
parallel, 107
Paranoid Ideation, 73, 74, 76, 77, 78
paranoid personality disorder, 68
parental consent, 4, 12
parental influence, 353
parental involvement, 192, 258, 268
parental support, 169, 170, 256
parenting, x, 94, 96, 99, 100, 101, 102, 104, 105, 111, 116, 121, 122, 124, 125, 126, 194, 251, 319, 359
parenting styles, x, 111
parkinsonism, 45
parole, 185, 318, 323
Participation, viii, xii, 102, 152, 177, 193, 280, 289, 290, 291, 292, 293, 295, 303, 304, 308, 309, 319
Participatory research, 294
path analysis, 134
pathology, 208, 218
pathophysiology, 31, 46
pathways, 43, 52, 110, 126, 170, 259, 335, 344
peace, 109
Pearson correlations, 75, 77
pedagogy, 154, 168
Pediatric bipolar disorder (PBD), xi, 245
peer group, 95, 97, 112, 138, 140, 141, 142, 143, 219, 293, 297, 299, 337, 343
Peer groups, 142

peer rejection, 97
peer relationship, 254
peer review, 187
peer support, 267
pelvic inflammatory disease, 134
penalties, 313
percentile, xii, 4, 263, 267, 268
perfusion, 52
permission, 117
permit, 9, 194, 221
perpetration, 97, 128
perpetrators, 96, 109, 121, 126
perseverance, 225
person environment fit theory, xi, 159
personal choice, 169
personal control, 217, 284
personal development, 146, 297
personal qualities, 214
personal relations, 72
personal relationship, 72
personality, xi, 68, 75, 79, 81, 82, 83, 84, 85, 133, 138, 146, 150, 207, 208, 209, 211, 218, 219, 221, 247, 337, 343
personality characteristics, 68, 75
Personality Disorder, 69, 81, 82, 83, 213, 214
personality test, 218
personality traits, 68, 81
PET, 57, 59
Pew Research Center, 161, 264, 283
pharmaceutical, 47, 50
pharmaceutics, 39, 48
Pharmacodynamics, 40
Pharmacogenetic, 37, 47, 48, 52, 53, 61, 62, 63
pharmacogenomics, 53, 63
Pharmacokinetic, 58, 64, 65
pharmacokinetics, 38, 39, 48, 52, 53, 58, 65
pharmacological treatment, 50, 51, 248, 249
pharmacology, 49, 55, 58
pharmacotherapy, x, 37, 38, 39, 49, 51, 52, 53, 248, 249, 250, 251, 252, 255, 258
phenomenology, 260
phenotype, 38, 45, 47, 48, 62, 71, 73, 80, 85, 136, 250, 260
Philadelphia, 203
Philippines, 350
phrenology, 333
physical abuse, 91, 92, 94
physical activity, x, 6, 17, 18, 19, 20, 23, 25, 26, 27, 28, 29, 30, 31, 32, 33, 34, 35, 68
Physical activity, 25, 26, 30, 31, 33, 34, 35, 36

physical education, 29
physical environment, 164
physical fitness, 25, 27, 31
physical health, 213, 262, 298
physical inactivity, 17, 19, 25, 29
Physical space, 298, 302
physicians, 49, 80
physiology, 38, 52, 176
pilot study, 9, 10, 195, 255, 257
pipeline, xi, 47, 159, 160, 162, 163, 167, 172, 174, 175, 178
placebo, 46, 54, 57, 58
plasma levels, 40, 41, 42, 43, 44, 46, 54, 55, 56, 57, 58, 61, 63
plasma proteins, 52
plasminogen, 20
platform, 100, 142, 173
plausibility, 236
playing, 103, 104, 143, 221, 222, 278
pleasure, 72
plethysmography, 24
pluralism, 151
PM, 15, 47
police, 90, 94, 167, 177, 195, 201, 334, 335, 346, 347
policy, xi, 14, 28, 30, 110, 159, 171, 173, 220, 238, 246, 258, 280, 282, 304, 306, 308, 312, 313, 336, 340, 343, 344, 349, 357, 358, 360, 361, 362
policy makers, xi, 28, 30, 159, 171, 173, 220, 258, 349
policy making, 220, 357, 360
policymakers, 93, 109, 190, 312, 318, 323, 324
political affiliations, 352
political participation, 305
political party, 265
politics, 140, 155, 347
polymorphism, 38, 45, 46, 47, 51, 56, 59, 60, 61, 62
population group, 162
population growth, 173, 264
Portugal, xii, 20, 27, 31, 289, 295, 299
positive attitudes, 196
positive correlation, 75, 124, 355
positive feedback, 252
positive mood, 255
positive reinforcement, 103
positive relationship, 122, 171
posttraumatic stress, 57
postural hypotension, 38, 45

poverty, 90, 96, 155, 160, 161, 162, 163, 164, 166, 169, 174, 175, 176, 177, 263, 269, 271, 278, 335
poverty line, 163
poverty trends, 163, 164
predictability, 225, 235
predictive validity, 68, 69, 81, 338, 339, 343, 344
Predispose, viii, 131
pregnancy, 96, 101, 273
prejudice, 271
premigratory advantage, 355
preparation, 109, 170, 171, 172, 269, 270, 274, 275, 276, 281
pre-pubertal adolescents, 22
preschool, 6, 11, 14, 15, 18, 127, 128, 283, 358
preschool children, 128, 358
preschoolers, 15, 91, 362
Presence of authority, 143
president, 109, 170
pressure on students, 224
prevalence rate, 71
prevention, 3, 4, 25, 29, 31, 33, 43, 69, 85, 89, 90, 100, 104, 108, 111, 115, 125, 126, 127, 128, 135, 136, 172, 248, 252, 253, 258, 282, 300, 301, 302, 319, 328, 335, 337
Prevention program, 114
primary school, 164, 228
Principal Components Analysis, 75, 76, 78
Principality of Asturias, 73
principles, 53, 105, 143, 145, 171, 207, 253, 289, 294, 298, 335
prisoners, 203, 334
prisons, 183, 320, 323, 324, 325, 334
private information, 117
private schools, 228
probability, 44, 108, 133, 337, 340
Probation, 313, 314, 315, 328, 340, 341, 342
probation officers, 187, 193, 313, 339
Probation Subsidy Act of 1965, 313
problem behavior, 198
problem-solving, 104, 107, 182, 186, 192, 194, 200, 201, 248, 251, 252, 253, 254, 255, 258, 271, 333, 334
problem-solving skills, 201, 252, 253, 255, 271
problem-solving strategies, 194, 253
professional careers, 353
professional development, 161
professional growth, 275
professionals, 80, 148, 152, 200, 217, 220, 349
profit, 145, 154, 155, 321, 357

program outcomes, 9, 14
programming, 162, 314, 315, 316, 318, 332, 336, 338, 340, 341
project, 106, 151, 293, 295, 296, 299, 300, 302, 306, 308, 338, 339, 340
Project for the Assessment of Risk/Protection Factors and Institutional Social Support in Health Care, 295, 299
proliferation, 275, 334
Promising programs, 190
promoter, 47, 60
prophylactic, 80
prophylaxis, 65
proposition, 141, 276
prosocial behavior, 102, 188, 195, 204
prosperity, ix
protection, xii, 29, 78, 93, 97, 138, 289, 290
protective factors, 169, 170, 252, 269, 271, 272, 276, 353
protective role, 280
prototype, 9
psychiatric disorders, 46, 49, 50, 51, 248, 259, 261
psychiatric illness, 246
psychiatric morbidity, 81
psychiatric patients, 51, 53, 55, 56, 58, 59, 203
psychiatrist, 133
psychiatry, 50, 51, 54, 63
psychoactive drug, 52, 97
psychoanalytic tradition, 159
Psychodrama technique, xi, 207, 212, 213, 214, 216, 217, 219, 220
Psychodramatic role-level, 210
Psychodynamic and Family Therapy, 213
Psychoeducation, 252, 254, 256
Psychoeducational Drama, 215
psychoeducational intervention, 250
psychological assessments, 318
psychological distress, 208, 220
psychological health, 296, 297
psychological well-being, 68
psychologist, 133, 150
psychology, 117, 137, 174, 176, 202, 302, 363
psychometric properties, x, 67, 70, 81
Psychometric properties, 83
psychopathology, 84, 133, 245, 246, 250, 257, 261
Psychopathology, 239, 260, 261, 281, 285, 327
psychopharmacological treatments, 80
psychopharmacology, 48, 57, 58, 61, 64

psychoses, 222
psychosis, 41, 42, 44, 63, 68, 69, 70, 71, 73, 74, 78, 80, 82, 83, 84, 85, 133, 214, 248, 249, 254
psychosocial development, 162
psychosocial factors, 69, 245, 246, 253
psychosocial functioning, 110, 133, 196, 254
psychosocial interventions, 200, 249, 250, 257, 258, 259, 260
psychosocial stress, 17, 19, 29, 282
psychosomatic, 208, 210, 211
Psychosomatic role-level, 210
psychotherapy, 186, 195, 197, 201, 221, 222, 248, 258
psychotic symptoms, 68, 71, 80, 83, 84
psychotropic drugs, x, 37, 38, 39, 48, 51, 52, 54, 61
psychotropic medications, 49, 63, 64
public education, 155, 160, 165, 177
public health, x, 21, 25, 32, 34, 90, 100, 113, 246, 334
Public health, 17
public investment, 93
public life, 152
public opinion, 334
public policy, 279, 293, 346, 357, 359, 360
public safety, 327
public schools, 159, 160, 162, 164, 165, 167, 170, 171, 173, 177, 265
public service, 133, 149, 294
public welfare, 220
punishment, 102, 121, 125, 138, 324, 332

Q

qualifications, 148
quality of life, 68, 89
quality of service, 256
questioning, 159
questionnaire, 14, 84, 85, 115, 205, 215, 300
quetiapine, 38, 39, 40, 41, 42, 46, 56, 57, 58, 61, 63, 249

R

Rab, 158
race, 91, 133, 134, 160, 162, 163, 168, 170, 173, 174, 177, 178, 331, 333, 336, 338, 340, 341, 343, 344, 352
racial/ethnic minority, 164
racism, 96, 215, 336

radio, 77, 139
RAINBOW, 253, 254
random assignment, 188, 189, 190, 191
rape, 94, 184, 217, 317
rating scale, 45, 74
RE, 32
reactions, 105, 216
reactivity, 253
reading, 141, 148, 215, 272
reality, 62, 139, 162, 202, 208, 212, 215, 217
Reasoned and Equitable Community and Local Alternatives to the Incarceration of Minors (RECLAIM Ohio), 317
reasoning, 181, 183, 184, 190, 191, 224, 225, 226, 227, 228, 236, 237, 238, 320
reasoning skills, 181
rebelliousness, 72
recall, 12, 216, 220, 273
reception, 142, 152
receptors, 39, 40, 43, 44, 46, 52
recession, 139, 176
recidivism, 181, 184, 185, 186, 187, 188, 190, 191, 193, 195, 196, 197, 198, 199, 312, 318, 321, 328, 331, 336, 337, 338, 339, 341, 342, 343, 344
recidivism rate, 185, 312, 318, 321, 339, 341, 344
recognition, 38, 49, 114, 256
recommendations, x, 18, 23, 26, 27, 28, 39, 48, 50, 53, 90, 159, 246, 255, 262, 304, 337
recovery, 215, 246, 252, 258, 260
recreational, 255, 256
Redeploy Illinois, 318, 319, 326, 327, 328
reform, xii, 165, 212, 241, 282, 283, 311, 312, 313, 315, 318, 319, 320, 321, 322, 324, 325, 326, 327, 328, 336, 340, 342, 343, 344
refugees, xii, 213, 349, 350, 351, 352
regression, 55, 118, 122, 131, 133, 134, 208, 230
regression analysis, 55, 134, 230
regression equation, 118
regulations, 153, 312
rehabilitation, 90, 186, 311, 315, 318, 319, 320, 322, 332
rehabilitation program, 315, 319, 320
reinforcement, 100, 182, 192, 257
Reinforcement, 97
Reinvestment strategies, 313, 324
rejection, 97, 168, 352
relapses, 250
relatives, 80, 93, 139, 140, 144, 152, 247, 259, 269, 346, 350, 356

relaxation, 255
relevance, xi, 51, 96, 208, 224, 225, 239, 294
reliability, x, 4, 5, 9, 10, 12, 15, 67, 70, 73, 75, 79, 82, 140, 230, 296
religion, 140, 176, 293
remediation, 239
replication, 85, 115, 261
requirements, 38, 39, 52, 95, 97, 139, 146, 149, 165, 359
Research and Ethics Committee, 75
researchers, 4, 5, 10, 12, 23, 25, 29, 91, 93, 112, 127, 166, 184, 185, 186, 187, 188, 190, 192, 218, 246, 249, 264, 265, 268, 296, 337, 338, 339, 340, 343, 344, 345, 359
Residential, 205, 212, 214, 221, 297
resilience, 109, 170, 209, 266, 267, 269, 277, 280, 281, 282, 283, 284, 285, 291, 297
Resiliency, 266, 271, 280
resilient students, xii, 263, 266, 267, 268, 278
resistance, 49, 96, 107, 212, 214, 219, 257, 272, 300, 304
resolution, 107, 209, 211, 212
resource allocation, 336
response format, 74
responsiveness, 115, 271
restructuring, 212, 253
retaliation, 128
rewards, 7, 96, 311, 313
RH, 31
rhythm, 260
rights, 153, 177, 183, 289, 291, 295, 308, 309
risk assessment, xii, 20, 196, 331, 332, 333, 336, 337, 338, 339, 340, 341, 342, 343, 344
risk factors, 4, 17, 18, 19, 20, 22, 23, 27, 29, 30, 31, 32, 33, 34, 35, 45, 54, 68, 71, 80, 89, 91, 94, 107, 109, 111, 126, 197, 200, 249, 252, 261, 283, 337
risk management, 151
risk profile, 18, 19, 20, 22, 27
risks, 38, 45, 46, 59, 96, 160, 266, 269, 336, 343, 344
risperidone, 38, 39, 40, 41, 43, 44, 45, 48, 59, 63, 64, 249
RMSEA, 135, 230, 231
Role Play Tests, 212
Role Theory, 207, 208
role-playing, 104, 221, 222, 252, 294
romantic relationship, 246
root, 95, 108, 230, 312, 318
root-mean-square, 230

roots, 176
Roses, 48, 62
routes, 126, 165
routines, 250, 298, 303
rowing, 147
Royal Society, 204
rules, 98, 102, 103, 115, 121, 137, 139, 140, 143, 145, 155, 213, 227, 293, 296, 297, 298, 299
Rules and functioning, 298
rural areas, 94
Russia, 113

S

sadness, 218
safety, x, 37, 39, 48, 51, 54, 57, 62, 63, 64, 128, 253, 311, 336, 359
sanctions, 108, 325, 335
sarcasm, 170
saturation, 41
Saudi Arabia, 21
savings, 315, 319, 321, 351
Schedule for Affective Disorders, 133
schizophrenia, 38, 39, 40, 41, 42, 44, 50, 54, 55, 56, 57, 58, 59, 60, 61, 62, 63, 68, 69, 70, 71, 72, 74, 79, 80, 82, 84, 85, 133, 248
Schizophrenia for School-Age Children-Epidemiologic Version (K-SADS-E), 133
schizophrenic patients, 56, 57, 60, 61
Schizotypal, vii, 67, 69, 70, 71, 76, 81, 82, 83, 84
Schizotypal Personality Disorder, 83
Schizotypal Personality Questionnaire (SPQ), 70
schizotypy, 68, 69, 70, 72, 73, 74, 79, 81, 82, 83, 84, 85
Schizotypy, 68, 70, 72, 77, 78, 82, 83, 84
Schizotypy Traits Questionnaire (STA), 70, 82
scholarship, 306
school achievement, 170, 226, 227, 238
school activities, 267, 319
school adjustment, 177
school climate, 126
school community, 167
school culture, 168
school enrollment, 164
school environment, xi, 6, 29, 30, 114, 115, 159, 160, 161, 165, 167, 171, 263, 272, 358
school failure, 97, 170, 171
School grades, 224
school performance, 238
school success, 165, 169

school support, 267
schooling, 161, 163, 166, 167, 168, 170, 174, 228, 239, 269, 270, 273, 355
science, 25, 146, 162, 175, 344
scientific knowledge, 295
scope, 109, 133, 142, 165, 336
SCORE, 172
scripts, 176
second generation, 41, 45, 46, 283, 353, 354, 356, 358, 361, 362
secondary education, 162, 165, 167, 171, 265, 280
secondary schools, 74, 174, 176, 228, 230, 284, 356
Secondary socialisation, 140
Secretary of Homeland Security, 357
secretion, 52
security, 93, 162, 167, 185, 298, 359
security guard, 167
segmented assimilation, 352, 355
segregation, 155, 164, 177, 352, 353
seizure, 46, 61
selective serotonin reuptake inhibitor, 42
selectivity, 225
self-awareness, 101, 209
self-concept, 161, 267, 268, 280, 285
self-confidence, 218
self-control, 101
self-discipline, 99
self-efficacy, 96, 99, 101, 217, 224, 272, 273, 279
Self-efficacy, 244
self-esteem, 101, 127, 209, 216, 217, 268, 273, 276, 278, 292
self-expression, 151, 152, 169, 214
self-identity, 264
self-image, 146, 209, 210, 217, 219
Self-improvement, 152
self-knowledge, 146, 150
self-monitoring, 253
Self-realization, 152
self-reflection, 209, 225
self-regulation, 126, 250
self-reports, 14, 67, 69, 70, 74, 79, 81, 116, 188, 191
self-sufficiency, 296
self-worth, 113, 277
Senate, 314, 322, 323
Senate Bill 103, 322
Senate Bill 681, 314
Senate Bill 81, 322, 323
sensation, 210

sensitivity, 15, 51, 52, 81, 98
sentencing, 317, 334
Sequelae, 113
serotonin, 40, 42, 44, 46, 64
sertraline, 65
serum, 34, 56, 58
service provider, 126, 139, 315, 321
services, 102, 146, 149, 154, 187, 188, 217, 256, 258, 262, 289, 292, 293, 294, 295, 297, 298, 299, 300, 301, 302, 303, 304, 306, 307, 312, 313, 315, 316, 317, 320, 321, 322, 324, 328, 329, 333, 334, 349, 352, 354, 355, 359
SES, 133, 267, 344
settlements, 152
sex, 21, 24, 55, 85, 91, 117, 125, 127, 176, 178, 303
sexual abuse, 93, 94, 214
sexual assaults, 346
sexual behavior, 132, 134, 136
sexual harassment, 93, 114
sexual intercourse, 136
sexual violence, 114, 128
sexuality, 103, 301
sexually transmitted diseases, 131, 132
shame, 174, 176, 270
shape, 99, 155, 159, 170, 320
shelter, 185, 204
Shier, 291, 292, 309
short supply, 109
shortage, 93, 273, 274, 280, 283
showing, 9, 42, 44, 99, 103, 140, 166, 186, 190, 193, 196, 223, 274, 296, 302
sibling, 250, 253, 257, 270, 271, 354
side effects, x, 37, 38, 39, 41, 42, 43, 45, 46, 47, 49, 51, 52, 54, 55, 56, 59, 65, 249, 256
signal transduction, 51, 52
signals, 210
signs, 80, 146, 194, 320
skeletal muscle, 25
skill acquisition, 190, 193, 355, 360
skills training, 200, 203, 251, 318
Skillstreaming, 182, 202
skinfolds, 24, 28, 34
sleep disturbance, 254
sleeping problems, 272
smoking, 17, 18, 19, 29, 40, 56, 57
Smoking, 83
snack choices, 6
snacking, 5
sociability, 302

social activities, 98, 224
social adjustment, 96
Social and family relationships, 297
Social Anxiety, 73
Social Atom, 213, 218
social behavior, 332, 335
social capital, 361
social care, 290
social class, 90, 91, 168
social competence, 182, 190, 196, 197, 198, 203, 219, 271
social consequences, 96
social construct, 331
social context, 138, 168, 170, 250
social control, 96, 104, 332
social development, 137
Social Disorganization, 73, 79
social environment, 138, 151, 152, 161, 177, 262
social exchange, 212
social group, ix, 154, 305, 352
social image, 297
social injustices, 171
social integration, 295
social interactions, 115, 165, 255
social justice, 168, 171, 275
social learning, 192
Social Maladjustment, 214
social network, 102, 124, 143, 152, 294
social organization, 96
social perception, 174
social policy, xii, 220, 357
social problems, 183, 298, 333
social psychology, 153
social relations, 125, 170, 296
social relationships, 125, 170, 296
social resources, 105, 267, 269, 282, 362
social services, ix, 212, 326
social situations, 138, 184
social skills, xi, 99, 181, 182, 184, 185, 186, 187, 188, 190, 191, 192, 193, 194, 195, 199, 200, 216, 254, 291, 308
social skills training, 194, 200
social status, 90
social structure, 98, 104, 170, 305
social support, 104, 126, 170, 185, 192, 193, 256, 298, 299, 333, 353, 358
social workers, 80, 200, 220, 297, 324, 345
socialization, x, 109, 137, 138, 142, 156, 157, 237
society, 21, 62, 68, 89, 90, 92, 93, 94, 95, 96, 98, 99, 104, 108, 137, 140, 143, 145, 150, 151,

152, 154, 168, 211, 224, 272, 278, 290, 292, 293, 295, 308, 331, 332, 333, 335, 349, 350, 351, 352, 354, 356, 357, 358, 360
Sociodramatic role-level, 210
socioeconomic background, 168
socioeconomic status, 104, 263, 267, 343, 351, 354
Sociogram, 214
sociology, 137, 146, 153, 176, 344
Sociometric Tests, 212
Sociometry, 208, 214, 221, 222
sodium, 249
solidarity, 146, 152
solution, 67, 89, 90, 147, 236, 252, 254, 336, 343
somnolence, 42
Southern Poverty Law Center, 166
SP, 14, 15
Spain, x, 67, 74, 324, 325
spatial ability, 225
specialists, 323
speech, 68, 72, 208, 209, 210, 216, 219
spending, 118, 126, 165, 220, 319, 320, 335
spontaneity, 213
Spring, 14, 362
SS, 31
stability, 100, 196, 213, 250, 251, 297, 303
stabilizers, 249, 252, 256
staff members, 106, 115, 184, 185, 215
staffing, 280, 284
stakeholders, 14, 294, 325, 345
standard deviation, 75, 117, 118, 120, 122, 133, 197, 198, 199, 229
standardization, 197, 198, 199
standardized testing, 80, 165
State Correctional Institution at Camp Hill, 315
state laws, 278
state legislatures, 278
state oversight, 323
state schools, 278
states, 42, 58, 93, 160, 164, 246, 255, 264, 265, 270, 272, 273, 278, 282, 290, 311, 312, 313, 315, 319, 324, 327, 332, 336, 350, 351, 357, 358, 359
Statistical Package for the Social Sciences, 75, 85
statistics, 30, 75, 76, 162, 187, 188, 270, 274, 316, 328, 350, 359, 362, 363
steel, 98
stereotypes, 159, 160, 161, 164, 166, 167, 168, 173, 174, 270
stereotyping, 163

stigma, 81, 249
stimulus, 19
stock, 353, 360
stomach, 272
Stop-Think-Plan-Do-Check, 255
storms, 159
storytelling, 294
strategy use, 44
stratification, 53, 153, 224, 228
stress, 64, 94, 96, 98, 104, 105, 159, 177, 182, 194, 200, 249, 266, 269, 279, 280, 282, 291
stressful life events, 253, 267
stressors, 247, 269, 270
stroke, 27, 30
structural equation modeling, 231
structure, 47, 67, 72, 73, 75, 79, 81, 82, 83, 84, 85, 90, 102, 138, 139, 146, 154, 170, 208, 212, 213, 223, 227, 228, 230, 232, 236, 250, 255, 298, 302, 315, 316, 340, 357, 360
structuring, 212
student achievement, 165, 267
student development, 164
student motivation, 268
student populations, 162, 167
style, 105, 111, 116, 121, 122, 124, 126, 139
Styles, 241, 243, 244
subjectivity, 332, 338, 341, 343
subsidy, 314, 328
substance abuse, 45, 136, 196, 216, 258, 296, 301, 318, 321
substance use, xi, 96, 97, 131, 132, 133, 134, 136, 196, 204
substance use XE "substance use" disorders, xi, 131, 132, 134
substrate, 44
subtraction, 227
success, 96, 106, 115, 143, 159, 160, 161, 162, 165, 166, 168, 169, 170, 172, 176, 224, 226, 266, 268, 270, 272, 273, 276, 280, 281, 283, 285, 312, 318, 321, 327, 357, 358, 360
Success in Stages, 114, 115, 125
SUD, x, 131, 132, 133, 135, 136
suicidal ideation, 113
suicide, 68, 95, 98, 112, 113, 128, 246, 314
Suicide, 91, 115, 128
Suicide Prevention Resource Center, 115
supervision, 75, 89, 91, 92, 94, 96, 106, 196, 267, 298, 299, 311, 312, 313, 314, 320, 322, 323, 324, 325
supervisor, 106

supervisors, 314
support services, 296, 301
support staff, 314
suppression, 344
Supreme Court, 323, 325, 334
surplus, 275
surveillance, 18, 334, 344
survival, 356
survivors, 285
susceptibility, 51, 160, 162, 172
suspensions, 166, 169
Suspiciousness, 73
sustainability, 295
Sweden, 28, 113
Switzerland, 30, 54
Symbol-Drama, 214
symptoms, 27, 38, 39, 41, 45, 46, 54, 58, 68, 69, 71, 72, 76, 80, 82, 84, 109, 128, 246, 248, 250, 252, 254, 255, 256, 257, 258, 260, 302
synapse, 52
synaptogenesis, 52
synthesis, 209, 238
syphilis, 134
systemic risk, 200

T

tachycardia, 42
tactics, 101, 103, 192
Taiwan, 128, 241
takeover, 321
tandem repeats, 47
tangible benefits, 185
tardive dyskinesia, 38, 39, 45, 60, 61
target, 5, 10, 13, 40, 41, 42, 44, 45, 49, 52, 58, 90, 94, 104, 105, 125, 126, 127, 148, 162, 191, 200, 220, 256, 258, 269, 303, 318, 332, 333, 358
target number, 318
Taste Test Tool, 5, 9, 10
teacher expectations, xii, 168, 263, 271
teacher identification, xii, 263
Teacher Observation Tool (TOT), x, 3, 5, 7
teacher preparation, 263, 275, 276, 283
teacher support, 267
teacher thinking, 285
teachers, 3, 5, 6, 9, 11, 13, 14, 80, 81, 107, 115, 138, 143, 148, 163, 164, 165, 167, 168, 172, 177, 186, 205, 215, 224, 225, 236, 238, 263, 267, 268, 269, 271, 273, 274, 275, 276, 277, 278, 280, 281, 282, 283, 284, 358, 359
teacher-student relationship, 161
teaching effectiveness, 276
teams, 80, 195, 270
technician, 301, 302, 303
techniques, xi, 15, 24, 37, 48, 69, 72, 101, 104, 155, 183, 192, 194, 195, 200, 207, 211, 212, 213, 214, 215, 216, 217, 218, 219, 220, 252, 253, 276, 345
technological advances, ix
technology, 3, 14, 15, 116, 118, 119, 127, 202, 309, 346, 359
teens, 94, 103, 177, 247, 248
telephone, 15, 133, 192, 193
temperament, 93
tension, 183, 209, 210, 217
territory, 165
test scores, 162, 163, 166, 265, 268, 361
testing, 4, 15, 47, 53, 62, 165, 174, 204, 225, 228, 242
Tests of Spontaneity, 212
Texas Juvenile Justice Department (JDD), 322
Texas Juvenile Probation Commission, 322, 328
Texas Youth Commission, 320, 322, 328
text messaging, 111, 118, 124, 125
textbook, 175
The Empty Chair, 214
The family, 124, 138, 247
theatre, 139, 141, 221, 301
theft, 98, 183, 196, 297
theoretical approaches, 307
theoretical support, 122
therapeutic approaches, 220
Therapeutic Bond, 219
Therapeutic Drug Monitoring (TDM), x, 37
therapeutic effects, 49, 53
therapeutic use, 42
therapeutics, 65
therapist, 185, 214, 215, 219, 252, 254
therapy, 45, 49, 51, 54, 55, 58, 59, 192, 193, 197, 199, 203, 205, 211, 213, 214, 217, 219, 221, 249, 254, 256, 258, 260
think critically, 272
Thinking and Perceptual Style Questionnaire (TPSQ), 70
third dimension, 73
thoughts, 77, 80, 113, 165, 192, 210, 214, 253, 255
threats, 187

threshold level, 42
time frame, 91
tissue, 38, 47
Title I, 359
Title II, 359
tobacco, 25, 68
toddlers, 51
tokenism, 307
torture, 98, 213
total cholesterol, 34
toxicity, 42, 45, 53, 56
toxicology, 49
tracks, 22
trade, 155, 352
trade union, 155
trade-off, 352
Traditional Bully and Cyber-bully Questionnaire, 117
traditions, 94, 332
trainees, 212
training, xi, 26, 100, 104, 106, 111, 133, 139, 148, 151, 154, 160, 165, 171, 181, 182, 183, 184, 185, 192, 194, 195, 200, 202, 203, 204, 205, 220, 251, 274, 293, 303, 308, 318, 319, 332, 338, 340, 349, 350, 358, 359
training programs, 104
traits, 68, 69, 70, 74, 82, 84, 85, 95, 194, 228, 230, 231, 234, 236, 266, 273, 351, 353
trajectories, 84, 266, 279, 355, 361, 363
trajectory, 257
transactions, 352
transduction, 52
transference, 352
transformation, 103, 266, 294
translation, 224, 307
Transmissible Liability Index (TLI), xi
transmission, xii, 44, 349, 350, 351, 352, 354
transmission of human capital, 350, 351, 354
transport, 203
transportation, 106, 304
trauma, 80, 98, 213, 219, 221
traumatic experiences, 217, 266
Treseder, 291, 292, 309
trial, 57, 59, 60, 108, 115, 141, 205, 252, 254, 256, 257, 261, 321
triceps, 24
triggers, 183, 193, 194
triglycerides, 4
Trinidad, 174
Tucker-Lewis Fit Index (TLI), 230

tuition, 358
turnover, 297, 309, 339
tutoring, 169, 319
type 2 diabetes, 18, 27

U

U.S. Department of Education Office for Civil Rights (OCR), 167
U.S. Department of Health and Human Services, 26, 27
U.S. Department of Labor, 363
U.S. economy, 358
UK, x, 17, 21, 23, 26, 27, 242, 308, 361
UN, 289, 290, 307
UN Convention on the Rights of the Child, 289, 290
unauthorized immigrants, 350
underserved students, 167, 175
unemployment rate, 96
uniform, 223
United Nations, 309, 325
United States, 14, 20, 35, 85, 113, 114, 115, 135, 159, 161, 162, 163, 175, 176, 185, 187, 190, 191, 214, 263, 264, 265, 271, 279, 280, 282, 311, 312, 324, 331, 346, 350, 357, 358, 359, 360, 361, 363
United States Department of Education, 191
United States Office of Juvenile Justice and Delinquency Prevention, 191
United Way, 359
universities, 139, 173
University of Oviedo, 67, 75
unusual perceptual experiences, 72
updating, 227
Upward Bound, 172, 214
upward mobility, 169
urban, 69, 71, 80, 90, 94, 98, 164, 165, 214, 221, 267, 268, 272, 282, 308, 340, 346
Urban Institute, 177
urban life, 282
urban youth, 165
urbanicity, 69, 71, 80
US Department of Health and Human Services, 34

V

valence, 296
Valencia, 171, 172, 174

validation, 4, 5, 14, 15, 69, 70, 83, 151, 203, 253, 263, 307, 336, 340
variables, 19, 21, 30, 53, 56, 116, 118, 119, 120, 122, 123, 124, 125, 127, 200, 221, 230, 231, 267, 343
variations, 38, 41, 46, 47, 49, 50, 62
vegetables, 6, 7, 9, 11, 12, 13, 15
venlafaxine, 42
Verhofstadt-Deneve's Phenomenological-Dialectical personality model, xi, 207
victimization, x, 80, 93, 97, 111, 113, 115, 116, 117, 118, 122, 124, 125, 126, 127
victims, 91, 92, 94, 96, 98, 109, 112, 113, 124, 125, 128, 167, 213
video games, 89, 98
videos, 116
Vietnam, 264, 363
vigorous physical activity, 23, 27, 28, 35
violence, x, 89, 90, 91, 92, 93, 94, 95, 96, 97, 98, 99, 100, 101, 102, 103, 104, 107, 108, 109, 110, 114, 202, 204, 205, 213, 267, 271, 307, 308
violent behavior, 92, 94, 96, 97, 98, 99, 100, 104, 107
violent crime, 97
violent offenders, 91, 92, 97, 320
Virtual youth work, 152
vision, 43, 95, 176, 275
vocabulary, 176
vocational tracks, 173
vocational training, 74
voicing, 212
Voluntariness, 151, 152
vote, 305
voters, 265
voting, 304
vulnerability, 51, 68, 71, 116, 156, 308

W

wages, 278, 357
Wales, x, 17, 27, 30, 325
war, 109, 213, 220, 322, 346
Washington, 14, 34, 61, 81, 128, 131, 136, 175, 176, 177, 187, 201, 202, 245, 279, 280, 281, 283, 284, 325, 327, 328, 346, 347, 361, 362, 363

water, 12, 24, 52, 218
watershed, 344
wealth, 162, 172, 173, 174, 178, 211, 351
weapons, 91, 99, 108
web, 6, 17
websites, 113, 294
weight gain, 38, 42, 43, 44, 45, 46, 51, 60, 61, 256
weight loss, 22
weight management, 33
weight status, 19, 20, 21, 22, 24, 29
welfare, 95, 102, 216, 309, 326, 338
welfare system, 338
well-being, 19, 22, 26, 27, 28, 126, 139, 224, 295, 297, 300, 346, 350, 356
wellness, 11, 309
WHO, 19, 21, 26, 32
windows, 48, 50
Wisconsin, 70, 79, 83, 315, 316, 326
Wisconsin Schizotypy Scales, 70, 79
withdrawal, 97
work ethic, 356
workers, 106, 138, 148, 151, 153, 156, 184, 265, 270, 308, 354, 358
workforce, 173, 309, 349, 353, 354, 360
workplace, 138, 139, 140, 141, 145, 148
World Bank, 262
World Health Organization, 18, 26, 27, 30, 32, 34, 262
worldwide, 23, 32, 246, 265
Worldwide Health Survey, 71

Y

yes/no, 196
yield, 3, 132, 190, 191, 193, 194, 200, 235
young adults, 29, 32, 79, 81, 85, 183
young people, 26, 32, 51, 91, 93, 138, 140, 147, 149, 151, 152, 156, 217, 219, 222, 223, 289, 290, 291, 292, 293, 294, 295, 296, 297, 298, 299, 300, 302, 303, 304, 305, 306, 308, 309
young women, 212
Youth community development, 151
youth populations, 17, 18, 19, 21, 22, 23, 24, 25, 27, 29
youth transition, 131
youth unemployment, 110
Youth work, 146, 147, 150